*Evaluating Health
Promotion Programs*

Evaluating Health Promotion Programs

THOMAS W. VALENTE, Ph.D.

Keck School of Medicine
University of Southern California

Bloomberg School of Public Health
Johns Hopkins University

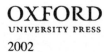

2002

OXFORD
UNIVERSITY PRESS

Oxford   New York
Athens   Auckland   Bangkok   Bogotá   Buenos Aires   Cape Town
Chennai   Dar es Salaam   Delhi   Florence   Hong Kong   Istanbul   Karachi
Kolkata   Kuala Lumpur   Madrid   Melbourne   Mexico City   Mumbai   Nairobi
Paris   São Paulo   Shanghai   Singapore   Taipei   Tokyo   Toronto   Warsaw

and associated companies in
Berlin   Ibadan

Copyright © 2002 by Oxford University Press, Inc.

Published by Oxford University Press, Inc.,
198 Madison Avenue, New York, New York 10016
http://www.oup-usa.org
1-800-334-4249

Oxford is a registered trademark of Oxford University Press.

Library of Congress Cataloging-in-Publication Data
Valente, Thomas W.
Evaluating health promotion programs/
Thomas W. Valente
p. cm.   Includes bibliographical references and index.

ISBN 978-0-19-514176-4

1. Health promotion—Evaluation
2. Communication in medicine—Evaluation.
I. Title.
RA427.8.V35 2002   613—dc21   2001036417

To 'Becca:

Your quick laugh and pretty smile
    that precious twinkle of an eye
Makes this journey ever more joyous
    as the milestones glide on by

Preface

Traditional and modern communication channels (from storytelling to satellites) are used to entertain, promote values, share ideas, and influence behavior. In the past few decades, there have been deliberate attempts to use communication to promote health-related values and behaviors by disseminating information on topics such as the following:

1. The dangers of alcohol abuse, drug abuse, and cigarette smoking
2. Behaviors that elevate the risk of cardiovascular disease (CVD)
3. The advantages of seat belt use
4. The importance of early screening for cancer and other diseases
5. The availability of family planning services and the importance of preventive behaviors designed to protect individuals from sexually transmitted diseases (STDs).

Many of these health promotion programs have been accompanied by evaluation strategies designed to measure their effectiveness. This book was written with the intent of facilitating such assessments.

The evaluation of health promotion programs is an exciting but challenging field of research. It is exciting because researchers work directly with projects that affect people's lives everywhere. Many of these projects include messages created with unique and fascinating methods to convey ideas to a public often using mass media. For example, radio and television soap operas have been produced to promote literacy, entrepreneurship, safe sex, and a host of other goals. Health promotion program evaluation is challenging because it requires skill and training to determine the effects of these programs in naturalistic settings.

Although health promotion projects are exciting to create, their true worth is measured not in how much people like them, but rather in their impact on the community. The impact of these interventions on health, well-being, and quality of life will be the ultimate verdict passed on these activities. Some people may gain satisfaction from the quality and appeal of an intervention, but the crucial element is whether it improved the quality of life for those it reached.

Novel and creative media used to disseminate information and persuade people to adopt new practices add to the excitement of evaluation efforts. As the number and variety of health promotion programs expand, there is a pressing need to determine which ones worked, how they worked (or did not), and what their relative effectiveness was in relation to other programs. For example, street theater and drama productions are commonly used at the community level to get messages across to the general public and "hard-to-reach" populations. Evaluating their effectiveness is critical for future planning to determine if they should be continued.

Health promotion program evaluation is exciting also because evaluators often improve the interventions they evaluate. The presence of an evaluation plan results in more focused objectives and better message creation and dissemination, thus increasing its impact. Evaluation, then, should be integrated into the design, management, and dissemination of a health promotion program.

Health promotion program evaluation is challenging because it requires skill, talent, and sometimes luck. Evaluation skills enter into study design, data collection, data management, and the statistical analysis needed to understand the effects. Talent, however, is often required to work with disparate groups who often have competing interests. Since many things can go wrong during an evaluation, an evaluator is indeed lucky if every component of the evaluation gets implemented as planned. This book provides information that will help evaluators improve their skills, exercise their talents, and increase their chances of conducting a successful evaluation.

Finally, health promotion program evaluation is challenging because it combines theory and applied research to achieve meaningful objectives. The potential of health promotion programs to improve society is increased dramatically by well-conducted and precise evaluation. Evaluation is a rewarding endeavor at the nexus of theory, research, and application.

ABOUT THE BOOK

This book provides an introduction to the logic, theories, and steps used to evaluate health promotion programs, an area where few sources currently exist. It is an introductory text designed to be accessible to students and researchers both within and outside the fields of public health, medicine, health promotion, health education, health communication, social work, the behavioral sciences, and related disciplines.

The book is written to take readers from the first steps in understanding behavior theory and the nature of interventions to more advanced steps such as statistical techniques in meta-analysis and power calculations. Many readers will choose to skip these more advanced topics and be satisfied with the step-by-step guides to successful evaluation, returning to the advanced topics at a later date. Others may find that topics such as power analysis are what make the book interesting.

A dataset from an evaluation of a reproductive health campaign in Bolivia that is available on the Internet can be used with this book. Examples in the text may be replicated using the dataset and readers may experiment with further statistical tests. The datasets are in SPSS and STATA formats and the language in the statistical chapters will in part follow SPSS and STATA conventions. Funding for the Bolivia project was provided by the U.S. Agency for International Development (USAID).

This book does not assume prior familiarity with behavioral theory, statistics, or statistical packages. In general, I have tried to include examples from real-world situations based on my own and others' research and evaluation experience. The text is designed to provide both a review of existing theory useful in designing evaluations and a guide to conducting them. Whenever possible, I have included checklists and step-by-step instructions. The book primarily covers the logistical and computational steps needed to conduct an evaluation. Hence, it is written as a guide to help students and researchers learn how to do evaluation research. It is also intended for experienced researchers to use as a checklist for steps in the evaluation process.

The organization of the book attempts to follow the chronological order of the occurrence of each of these activities during an evaluation project. To be sure, however, an evaluation does not happen so neatly, and anticipated as well as unanticipated events that occur at various stages can influence one another. For example, anticipated dissemination vehicles might determine the choice of study design. Thus, being familiar with the full volume will help readers refer to specific sections or chapters when needed.

It is also the case that many evaluations involve a team of researchers with different people being responsible for different activities. For example, one person may be responsible for specifying program objectives and outcome measures, while another may be responsible for statistical analysis. While readers will probably focus their attention on those sections most relevant to their interests and responsibilities, the team will benefit if every person is familiar with the different aspects of the evaluation process.

The book is divided into three sections. The first, Chapters 1 through 5, addresses pre-program topics such as strategic planning, specification of goals and objectives, and frameworks and theories that guide the process. Part I also covers formative and process research needed to develop messages and monitor the program. These interrelated topics frame the evaluation study and are generally conducted before quantitative data are collected to measure and determine effects. Part II, Chapters 6 through 10, addresses topics such as data collection techniques, sample selection, sample size calculations, data management, data cleaning, scale creation, and data analysis. Part III, Chapters 11 through 14, deals with the calculation of program effects and their interpretation and dissemination. This final section provides examples of statistical analysis used to assess program outcomes. One barrier to more widespread evaluation is the perceived difficulty of conducting statistical analysis—which I try to simplify in this section. The final chapter discusses ethical issues and dissemination of findings.

Chapter 1 provides a history of program interventions from a communication perspective. It covers the motivation and rationales for conducting evaluation as well as the barriers to such a project. Finally, it provides an evaluation framework used to understand the steps in the evaluation process. These frameworks guide many of the activities covered in the book.

Chapter 2 describes the different types of intervention and offers some guidance as to how and when they should be used. Examples include entertainment–education programs in the mass media, such as soap operas; posters and billboards; radio and television spots; newspaper ads; distribution of brochures and flyers; training of service providers in interpersonal communication and counseling; community mobilization events; and community participation. This chapter also has a section on the conditions necessary for a program to be effective.

Chapter 3 describes behavior change theory from a variety of disciplines. Most health promotion programs—perhaps all—are designed to disseminate information and/or change certain behaviors. Over the years, many theories, models, and frameworks have been developed to explain processes of behavior change. These theories are used to aid in choosing specific instruments for program evaluation and help explain behavior change. They enable the development of theory-based intervention and evaluation (Chen and Rossi, 1983; Weiss, 1997).

Chapter 4 explains formative research using qualitative methods such as in-depth interviews, focus group discussions, and observational studies. It also covers methods for pilot-testing program materials and the use of simulations and ratings data in program evaluation. Formative research is an extremely important component of program evaluation, often making the difference between success and failure.

Chapter 5 discusses process research, which is used to document program implementation and dissemination. Process research can be conducted at six points during the implementation process from creation to product supply. The longer or more complex the program, the more critical process research becomes.

Chapter 6 describes study designs and the language of evaluation research. The logic of control and treatment groups, the importance of pre- and posttest measurements, and the distinction between experimental and quasi-experimental designs are discussed here. Evaluation logic and study design provide the key to understanding the scientific process and the means by which to determine program effects. This chapter shows how various study designs control for threats to validity so that the researcher can minimize these threats and make proper inferences from the data.

Chapter 7 covers sampling designs, sample size calculation, and sample selection. Discussed here are the language that researchers use to describe sample selection strategy and the advantages and disadvantages of various sampling strategies. Techniques for computing the sample size needed to conduct the evaluation are also provided. The emphasis here is on power analysis, a set of procedures that can be used to specify the sample size needed or the power of a statistical test, given a predetermined sample size.

Chapter 8 is an overview of data collection and data management procedures such as the construction of questionnaires and data encoding and entry. The many computer commands needed to collect and manipulate data successfully are covered here. When survey and other types of empirical data are collected for an evaluation, it often takes the researcher months to get the dataset ready for analysis. This chapter is designed to accelerate that process so researchers can know how to process data efficiently.

Chapter 9 deals with univariate statistical procedures used to describe the distribution for each variable in the data. Use of univariate statistics helps the researcher determine whether variables are normally distributed, which is important for later statistical tests. Also presented here are methods of constructing scales and indices, such as factor analysis, and means of understanding the validity and measuring the reliability of scales and indices.

Chapter 10 describes the procedures and computer steps needed to conduct statistical tests. Through a step-by-step approach, readers can learn how to test hypotheses and interpret the results of statistical tests. This chapter covers levels of measurement and the statistical tests that can be used to determine whether two variables are associated with one another. The tests are explained by running them on the same two variables and interpreting their respective results. Multivariate statistical procedures are also described.

Chapter 11 discusses in detail the measurement of program exposure—the degree to which the audience recognizes and recalls the program. Program exposure is the single most important measurement needed by designers to decide whether a program has reached its intended audience. Measurement of program exposure is used for future planning purposes as well as for outcome evaluation.

Chapter 12 presents a detailed example of an outcome evaluation from a health promotion campaign created to promote reproductive health and family planning in Bolivia. The evaluation of this program consisted of cross-sectional and panel studies of a diverse population of randomly selected lower-socioeconomic status (SES) Bolivians. The evaluation also entailed a comparison with a separately collected national dataset. The Bolivian project evolved over a 10-year period and is an example of a strategically planned, nationwide communication campaign effort that was linked to major policy and social changes.

Chapter 13 covers eight advanced topics in research design and statistical analysis: *(1)* stepwise regression, *(2)* three- and multi-wave data analysis, *(3)* structural equation modeling, *(4)* event history analysis, *(5)* time series analysis, *(6)* meta-analysis, *(7)* weighting data, and *(8)* cost–benefit and cost-effectiveness analysis. These eight advanced issues in statistical and logistical designs are relevant to health promotion program evaluation.

Chapter 14 discusses three ancillary topics that are critical to evaluation research but are under debate in the field: the ethical issues that evaluators face when collecting data, and techniques and issues in the dissemination of evaluation results. Perspectives on these topics depend largely on the purposes of the evaluation and the goals of the evaluator. Program evaluators need to be aware of these issues, as they often influence the evaluation itself.

This text will not answer all the questions that arise during a program evaluation, but it will help answer many of them. There is nothing like doing an evaluation to learn how it is done. My aim has been to provide a guide to the evaluation process that will enable evaluators to make a better contribution to the projects they evaluate, to our quality of life, and to academic scholarship.

Acknowledgments

I would like to thank my colleagues at Johns Hopkins University in the Center for Communication Programs (JHU/CCP), in the Department of Population and Family Health Sciences, and in other departments who have helped me learn from the evaluation experiences reported in this text. In particular I would like to thank Phyllis Piotrow for her guidance, leadership, and advice; Walter Saba for his insights from the designer perspective and for creating some really great interventions to evaluate; and my colleagues in the JHU/CCP Research and Evaluation Division.

The JHU/CCP receives most of its funding from the Agency for International Development and has been working for over 15 years in developing countries creating mass media and other communication interventions to promote reproductive health (Piotrow et al., 1997). The JHU/CCP has implemented communication interventions in over 60 different countries throughout the world and has made extensive use of communication theory and strategy in its efforts to promote health. The staff at JHU/CCP has, whenever possible, included research and evaluation in its communication programs. The JHU/CCP staff's attention to research and to understanding the processes and impacts of their programs has helped us draw many lessons from the programs. Phyllis Piotrow is often quoted as saying, "If you can't document it, it didn't happen." Her emphasis on research and evaluation has helped make possible the experiences relayed in this book.

I would also like to thank the students who took my Program Evaluation class at Johns Hopkins University's School of Public Health; they have supported and helped shape this book. I would also like to thank the following individuals for helpful comments on earlier drafts and/or discussions about evaluation: Eileen Cardenas, Martha Ann Carey, John Finnegan, Robert Foreman, Deborah Glick, Ronald Rice, Everett Rogers, Darleen Schuster, Anne Baber Wallis, and an anonymous reviewer recruited by Oxford University Press. Jeffrey House and Leslie Anglin provided patient and guiding editorial assistance throughout.

I also thank the National Institute on Drug Abuse for supporting my work through grant number DA-10172, and my new colleagues at USC for providing a stimulating environment to continue my work.

Most importantly, I thank Rebecca Davis, who has inspired this work and whose ongoing conversations about statistics, evaluation, teaching, learning, and life have made it worthwhile.

Contents

Part One

Theory

The first section of this book, Chapters 1 through 5, covers topics important to evaluators new to the field. It presents the reasons for conducting evaluations and provides background on the evaluation field. The first chapter provides a general introduction to evaluation frameworks, language, and logic. This section also describes interventions (Chapter 2) and behavior change theory (Chapter 3) used to set program goals and objectives. These chapters are particularly helpful in aiding study design and understanding how a program is expected to work. For evaluators of mature programs, these chapters may provide new insights and perspectives. Formative research (Chapter 4) describes qualitative methods used to develop messages and a rich understanding of the behavior of study. Process research (Chapter 5) describes techniques for measuring how a program is implemented. Scholars interested in the purely quantitative aspects of evaluation or who involved in secondary analysis may decide to skim this first section.

Chapter One

Frameworks, Models, and Rationales

This chapter offers an introduction to the motivation for evaluating health promotion programs. It begins by defining health promotion programs and evaluation, then discusses rationales for conducting evaluations as well as the barriers one may encounter. To plan health promotion programs, researchers and practioners have created many frameworks for organizing evaluation activities in specific settings. In the second part of this chapter, a general framework for evaluating health promotion programs is presented that is similar to frameworks discussed (Green and Kreuter, 1991) elsewhere. The different phases and components within this framework are explained, as is the distinction between frameworks, models, and theories.

HEALTH PROMOTION PROGRAMS

Health promotion programs are created to generate specific outcomes or effects in a relatively well-defined group, within a relatively short time period, often through a concentrated set of communication activities (Cartwright, 1949; Mendelsohn, 1973; McQuail, 1987; Rogers and Storey, 1987). Health promotion programs are usually designed to bring about changes in people's knowledge, attitudes, and/or behaviors by using multiple channels of communication operating at several levels: mass media, such as TV and radio; meso media, such as street theater, drama, and posters; and micro media, such as discussion groups or interpersonal persuasion. Today, many programs recognize that community norms influence behavior, and the current trend is to explicitly account for these community influences.

Promotional programs are one component of social change, which is constant and occurs through purposive efforts, unanticipated consequences, and random events. Social change can be radical or gradual and can occur evenly throughout society or in a highly segmented fashion. Many agencies use health promotion programs in an effort to direct social change. Their objectives may be related to health, safety, environmental protection, politics, or many other as yet unrealized aims.

EVALUATION

In this context, *evaluation* refers to the systematic application of research procedures to assess the conceptualization, design, implementation, and utility of social intervention programs (Shadish et al., 1991; Rossi et al., 1999). It is used to determine which programs have been effective and how they achieved that effectiveness thus enabling researchers to plan and implement more effective programs in the future (Suchman, 1967).

Evaluation techniques originated with the scientific method and first started to become a discipline when federal agencies began to address social problems. Evaluation research was refined partly because of political, ideological, and demographic changes that occurred during this century and partly because of the emergence of social science disciplines in universities. Commitment to evaluation first became commonplace in the fields of education and public health. Educators evaluated programs concerned with literacy and occupational training; public health practitioners evaluated initiatives to reduce mortality and morbidity from infectious diseases (Rossi and Freeman, 1993).

After World War II, many programs were created to address the need for improvement in urban development, housing, technological change, and occupational training. In public health there were domestic and international programs for family planning, health and nutrition, and community development, among others. By the 1960s and 1970s, evaluation had become a growth industry and many books and articles appeared throughout the social and medical disciplines. The journal *Evaluation Review* was first published in 1976, and now, 25 years later, there are a dozen journals devoted primarily to evaluation research (Rossi and Freeman, 1993).

Shadish and colleagues (1991) argue that evaluation has evolved through three stages. First, it emerged as a distinct endeavor aimed at applying rigorous scientific criteria to evaluate the effectiveness of programs designed to ameliorate society's ills. This first stage provided the language and concepts needed by practitioners to conduct evaluation research. Shadish and others (1991) note that Campbell and Stanley's 1963 book as well as the work of Scriven (1967, 1972) and Suchman (1967) are characteristic of this stage.

The second stage concentrated on the practicalities of doing evaluation research. Researchers encountered difficulties in defining objectives and producing socially and politically relevant results. Evaluation researchers such as Weiss (1972), Wholey (1979), and Stake (1980) developed numerous alternative methodologies and studied many programs in a wide variety of settings.

The third and current stage of evaluation (represented by researchers such as Cronbach and associates [1980] and Rossi and colleagues [1999]) is characterized by attempts to integrate lessons learned from the first two stages. Two major themes in contemporary evaluation research are that many different theories and techniques are used in program evaluation and that the results are usually best understood within the context of the program. The integration of evaluation techniques along with an appreciation for the context of implementation presents many challenges to researchers but also emphasizes a commitment to conducting evaluations that are fair, comprehensive, and useful.

Dividing the evolution of evaluation into three stages oversimplifies its complex development but provides an outline of the way evaluation research has changed as a field. The field has matured, and its theory and practice have acquired their own special character resulting from the interplay of the problems addressed, the programs evaluated, the perspectives of the evaluators themselves, and the interaction of these elements. There has been tremendous growth and development in evaluation research during its short history, and it has been characterized by vigorous debate over theoretical and methodological issues.

One noticeable trend in evaluation research is the use of more participatory and narrative approaches to understanding the impact of programs. Early evaluation research throughout the 1950s and 1960s relied almost extensively on experimental designs and rigorous outcome measures. Although these techniques are still greatly valued, there has been an increasing recognition of the importance of program implementation research (Chapter 5). Implementation research is useful to the people who run programs and is important when attempts are made to expand or replicate a program.

Evaluation as a field of study will continue to grow for a number of reasons. First, it is an integral component of the health promotion process and so should be included in all programs. Evaluation should not be seen as a separate activity but rather as one that helps define and measure objectives and provide guidance for future program activities. Second, constraints on resources make it imperative for policy-makers to know which programs work so that they can decide which programs to support, which to modify, and which to close down. Evaluation is often the only way to decide whether to continue an existing program or fund a new one. Third, resource constraints make it necessary to measure the impact of programs so that appropriate fund allocations can be determined. Finally, statistical and computing technology continue to improve and hence make evaluation research easier and more feasible in many situations.

Evaluation is often seen as threatening to those programs being evaluated. It often evokes the feeling that something is wrong with the way things are done, and that changes, particularly personnel changes, are likely to follow. Consequently, many evaluators use terms such as *assessment* or *quality control* to alleviate fears on the part of those being evaluated. While it is reasonable that employees in particular fear evaluation, it is in fact rarely used to find ways to fire personnel. Evaluation, if done properly, provides the means to improve the quality of work for everyone involved, since it provides the opportunity for those being evaluated to voice their opinions about how to improve the functioning of the organization or agency being evaluated.

Why Evaluate Health Promotion Programs?

Evaluation is important because it both improves the probability of creating a successful program and enables researchers to understand the effect (if any) of a program. Thus, it is integral to program planning and development and to the generation of useful knowledge. There are many compelling reasons for evaluating programs. First, evaluation of a health promotion program measures the degree of the program's impact (if any). For example, if a program was designed to raise awareness of the dangers of substance abuse, the program's evaluation would measure whether this goal was reached.

Second, the existence of an evaluation plan often prompts project planners to establish goals and objectives for a program. In the absence of an evaluation plan, many project planners fail to set measurable objectives for their program and hence have no objective criteria for decision-making. When the goals and objectives for a program are set, they become the criteria used to determine other elements of the program and evaluation. For example, setting the goals may help researchers decide when to broadcast a campaign and what kinds of messages to emphasize.

The lack of clear goals and objectives for a program can seriously undermine its effectiveness. For example, in the 1980s, the Advertising Council sponsored a series of drug abuse prevention commercials, the best-known being "this is your brain—this is your brain on drugs." The impact of these commercials on adolescents or other audiences has not been evaluated (Backer and Marston, 1993). Studies conducted to evaluate these commercials were either cross-sectional (Reiss et al., 1994) or incorrectly used secondary data to show changes in adolescents' attitudes toward and use of illicit substances. Thus, it is unclear whether the commercials had clearly defined objectives and whether these objectives were met. In fact, the campaign may have been counterproductive. We do not know how the audience reacted to these commercials, but adolescents at risk for abusing drugs might have decided that adults do not understand this behavior, judging by the way the drugs were portrayed in the media, and hence their alienation from adult society might have been reinforced. Moreover, the commercials may have stimulated further drug abuse by providing material for adolescents to satirize and thus may have worked to attract more users.

In an experimental study, Feingold and Knapp (1977) found that television commercials led to less negative attitudes toward substance abuse. Their research indicated that television ads about methamphetamine and barbiturate use may have demystified these substances. The point here is not that TV commercials are inappropriate or ineffective means to reduce substance abuse, but rather that media campaigns need to be carefully planned and evaluated to ensure that objectives are specified and measured.

A third reason to conduct health promotion program evaluation is that it helps planners and researchers understand why or how a particular program worked. Through study of qualitative and quantitative data, those aspects of a program that were effective in bringing about the desired behavior change can be specified. Thus, while it is important to know whether a campaign met its objectives, it is also important to know which aspects of the intervention worked and why.

Fourth, program evaluation provides information that is useful for planning future activities since the data can be used to specify who was and was not influenced by the program. Did it reach all members of the target audience, or did it reach women but not men? Determining who was reached and influenced by the program enables planners to decide whether a different audience should be targeted or a different message strategy used in the future. Suppose, for example, that in a campaign to promote seat belt use, investigators discover that it increased seat belt use from 55% to 65%. The evaluation might show that many people did not wear seat belts because they were "only going for a short drive." The next campaign could focus its message on telling people that most accidents occur "on short drives" within a short distance from home.

A fifth reason for conducting this evaluation is that it provides an opportunity for basic research on human behavior. Evaluation studies offer an applied setting for testing theories of behavior change. In addition, although evaluation is usually considered applied research, it also provides the opportunity to conduct basic research on the behavior of human populations. Research on program evaluation may yield new theoretical hypotheses or prompt new research questions.

Evaluations are often conducted also simply because they are required by granting agencies. In 1993, for example, the federal government passed the Government Performance Results Act (GPRA), which required federal agencies to develop measurable performance goals and indicators and then to use them to evaluate themselves. Most grants and other funded projects mandate an evaluation of their programs.

Finally, program evaluation can be interesting to do. There is real joy in specifying a theoretical model of behavior change and testing it in the field. This is particularly true when evaluating programs designed to improve the human condition, where success can be translated as improvements in the quality of people's lives.

One challenge facing program evaluators is the array of media and the proliferation of health education programs in contemporary industrialized societies. The Internet has spawned a new industry for disseminating health information and most hospitals and health-care facilities have health education programs on many topics. Deciding which programs warrant evaluation and how these activities influence existing or planned activities is not easy.

Barriers to Evaluation

Even when there are compelling reasons for conducting an evaluation, it is often difficult to do. The most often cited barrier to evaluation is cost. Program staff often believe that evaluation is expensive and argue that the money should be spent on the intervention, not the research. The cost of program evaluation will be considered in this book, along with guidelines on how to budget evaluation expenses. The perspective taken here is that evaluation, if done properly, is an extremely cost-effective enterprise that contributes more to the campaign than it takes away from it.

A second barrier is the specification of control groups. Evaluation designs often call for the comparison of treatment and control groups as a means of showing what happened in the absence of the program. The control group consists of people not exposed to the program and usually hypothesized to remain unchanged on the outcome relative to the intervention group. In communication campaigns it can be difficult to create a control group not exposed to the campaign because the message is often relayed via mass media, making it difficult to restrict dissemination of the campaign. For example, in a national reproductive health campaign in Bolivia (see Chapter 11), the campaign was broadcast over the national network, so no segment of the population could be prevented from seeing or hearing the campaign. Hence establishing a control or comparison group was not possible.

If a control or comparison community can be established, often it is not similar to the treatment communities, thus hampering inferences about the program's effect. It can be hard to find communities that are similar enough for one to act as a treatment group and the other as control, and still have those communities sufficiently removed from one another. Contamination of control groups occurs because people move between communities and hence are exposed to the program when they should be in the control group. Contamination also occurs because human beings tend to spread information by word of mouth so that information received as part of a program is often disseminated to people in the control group (Freedman and Takeshita, 1969). Thus, control and comparison groups may be difficult to create. There are many valid study designs that do not require control groups.

A third difficulty in evaluating health promotion programs is that they are often culturally specific. When a communication campaign is created to promote a specific behavior in a specific community, it is rarely possible to simply rebroadcast this campaign in another community and reevaluate its effectiveness. For example, the Bolivian communication campaign designed to promote family planning used the Bolivian Minister of Health as a spokesperson. This message would have little meaning in another country where this minister is not known. Rebroadcasting such an intervention can seriously harm an agency's credibility.

A fourth difficulty is that the effects of health promotion programs are often hard to detect because the behavior under study may be heavily influenced by background characteristics such as socioeconomic status, previous knowledge of the behavior, and prior behavioral dispositions. Controlling for the effects of background and moderating variables can be difficult. Statistical procedures, however, covered later in this book, can be used to control for these confounding factors.

A fifth barrier to evaluation is that many stakeholders or policy-makers who support a program fear evaluation because it may show that it was not effective. The evaluation would then undermine their support and attempts to advocate social change. In a related vein, many program staff members resist evaluation because they feel that it will not be able to measure the intended effects. For example, a program may be created to shift political or public opinion in a way that facilitates later widespread behavior change. Program staff may argue that the shift will not be adequately detected in the evaluation. Any expected outcome of a program can be measured and incorporated into the evaluation design.

These barriers to program evaluation, however, should not deter investigators from conducting an evaluation. This book provides the tools and guidelines needed to address and overcome these barriers, and it discusses the frameworks, models, and practical background needed to guide the researcher through a step-by-step approach to evaluate health promotion programs.

FRAMEWORKS

In this context, *frameworks* refer to schemes that specify the steps in a process. They are useful guides to carrying out studies and activities. Numerous frameworks have been designed to guide health promotion programs and this chapter will review two of them, the P-Process and PRECEDE/PROCEED. Most health promotion frameworks include evaluation as a specific or ongoing component of the process.

P-Process

The P-Process was developed in 1983 by the first Population Communication Services project team, which included staff from Johns Hopkins University, the Academy for Educational Development; Porter, Novelli and Associates; and the Program for Appropriate Technology in Health. The P-Process provides a communication campaign framework for strategy development, project implementation, technical assistance, institution building, and training. Similar frameworks have been developed by other individuals and organizations to guide the health promotion process (e.g., Green and Kreuter, 1991). Over the past 15 years, many family planning and reproductive health communication programs around the globe have used the P-Process.

The P-Process consists of six steps that are followed in sequence to develop and implement effective communication strategies, programs, and activities:

1. Analysis. Listen to potential audiences; assess existing programs, policies, resources, strengths, and weaknesses; and analyze communication resources.
2. Strategic design. Decide on objectives, identify audience segments, position the concept for the audience, clarify the behavior change model, select channels of communication, plan for interpersonal discussion, draw up an action plan, and design evaluation.
3. Development, pretesting and revision, and production. Develop message concepts, pretest with audience members and gatekeepers, revise and produce messages and materials, and retest new and existing materials.
4. Management, implementation, and monitoring: Mobilize key organizations, create a positive organizational climate, implement the action plan, and monitor the process of dissemination, transmission, and reception of program outputs.
5. Impact evaluation. Measure the impact on audiences and determine how to improve future projects.
6. Plan for continuity. Adjust to changing conditions, and plan for continuity and self-sufficiency.

The P-Process is a well-tested framework that specifies the major steps needed to implement a health communication campaign. It provided the framework for SCOPE (Strategic Communication Planning and Evaluation), which is a

CD-Rom–based training tool. It has been applied mainly in developing countries, but is not widely used domestically.

PRECEDE/PROCEED

This framework provides a comprehensive guide to planning and implementing health promotion activities in nine phases; the first five involve diagnosis or needs assessment and the last four involve implementation and evaluation (Green and Kreuter, 1991). Like the P-Process, the PRECEDE/PROCEED framework specifies a needs assessment phase in which the scope and nature of the behavior is documented. Factors that predispose individuals to behave in certain ways or that reinforce them are documented. Once researchers are satisfied that they have a complete picture of the factors that influence the behavior, they can construct interventions to promote better health.

In the PRECEDE/PROCEED framework, there is an implementation phase during which the promotional activity is monitored. The health promotion activity should address predispositions, and reinforcing factors should be identified in the needs assessment phase. An evaluation of the activities should also be conducted to determine whether the behavior changed. These two frameworks, as well as others, specify steps that program planners should follow when creating, designing, and implementing health promotion programs.

The P-Process has been used mostly for implementing international mass media campaigns whereas the PRECEDE/PROCEED framework has been used mostly for U.S. work site programs. Perhaps because the PRECEDE/PROCEED framework has been used more frequently in organizations, it has addressed ecological levels of analysis more explicitly. Both frameworks are useful and both stress the importance of research and evaluation as being integral to health communication and/or promotion. Although these two frameworks have been designed from a campaign planner's perspective, many other frameworks have been developed from the evaluator's perspective.

EVALUATION FRAMEWORKS

Figure 1–1 provides a framework for evaluating a health promotion program. It begins with a needs identification and assessment phase during which the problem to be addressed in the program is specified. The problem may be defined by policy-makers, stakeholders, researchers, or programmers, and based on previous research or a variety of sources (Witkin and Altschuld, 1995). The first step is to determine the magnitude and scope of the problem. The researcher's role is to help define this problem in a manner that makes it amenable to improvement, by documenting how the need is defined and exploring evaluation options. Needs

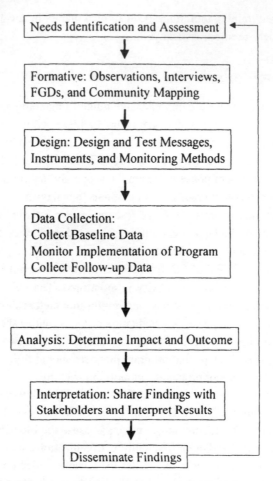

FIGURE 1–1. Framework for evaluation of health promotion programs. FGDs, focus group discussions.

identification is often conducted by funding agencies to help set priorities for their programs.

After the problem has been identified and some sense of its scope and magnitude has been gained, the researcher typically engages in formative research designed to specify its nature more clearly and explain its etiology. Typically, this research is qualitative (see Chapter 3) and the aim is to develop a deep understanding of the causes and consequences of the behavior under study. Importantly, the researchers and program staff can begin to develop a message strategy at this point.

A second stage of formative research entails working with the program staff to understand the scope and character of the intervention being envisioned to address the problem. As the program's design unfolds, possible evaluation strategies and issues are considered so that the evaluation can be linked to the program. Although it may be a long time before the researcher can reap the benefits of the planning and interaction that occurs at this stage, it is essential to be actively involved in formative research to conduct successful evaluations.

At the end of the formative stage and before the program is launched, the researcher will usually collect baseline data. These data provide the quantitative benchmark against which to measure success. The baseline data should be collected before the program is begun; this has the added benefit of providing useful information for program planning. For example, at baseline, to plan the campaign activities, the researcher may collect information on where people get information.

After the program is implemented or the campaign has been broadcast, the researcher typically collects follow-up data. It is generally important that the instruments for collecting follow-up data be identical to those used in the baseline. The follow-up data are then compared to the baseline data as a means of analyzing the effect of the program. Finally, the results are disseminated. The process of analyzing data and disseminating results is referred to as *outcome evaluation,* and it is a major focus of this book.

Although the framework in Figure 1–1 presents evaluation activities sequentially reading from top to bottom, all these activities are interrelated. For example, the way a problem is identified and the formative research conducted depends in part on the objectives set for the outcome evaluation. The ultimate audience for the research results, whether academic or practioners, may influence the researcher's choice of measures at baseline. The sequential framework provides a convenient organizing device, but many evaluations will have nuances that deviate from this general model.

The framework in Figure 1–1 can be condensed into three phases of research as summarized in Table 1–1: *(1)* formative, *(2)* process, and *(3)* summative. Each phase consists of a set of objectives and activities for the evaluator that are distinct yet interrelated. These three phases correspond to three phases in the process of developing an intervention: *(1)* pre-intervention planning, *(2)* intervention implementation, and *(3)* post-intervention impact analysis.

Formative Research

Formative research consists of investigations at the pre-intervention stage designed to aid program development and establish benchmarks for impact evaluation.[1] The pre-intervention planning phase of a health promotion program is

---

[1]Scriven (1972) and Mohr (1992) define formative evaluation as that which is used to inform program modification, and summative evaluation as that which only indicates program impact. I feel that all evaluation should be used to inform programs, thus I do not follow these definitions.

TABLE 1–1. Evaluation Research Stages

FORMATIVE RESEARCH	PROCESS RESEARCH	SUMMATIVE RESEARCH
Activities		
Focus group discussions	Implementation monitoring (viewer logs, broadcast schedule)	Analyze survey data
In-depth interviews		
Secondary analysis		Conduct interviews
Participant observation	Effects monitoring (sales data, visitation data, point-of-purchase interviews)	
Pretest materials		
Objectives		
Understand barriers to action	Frequency of program	Measure outcomes
Learn appropriate language	Potential audience reach	Determine efficiency
Develop conceptual model	Preliminary data on effects	Potential impact
Program stage		
Design and pretest program	Launch and implement program	Terminate and, if successful, replicate program

characterized by a variety of activities that inform its development. Examples include literature reviews, in-depth interviews, focus groups, surveys, and secondary analysis of existing data. These research activities help determine the objectives of the program and the level of outcome needed to be considered significant from a clinical or population perspective. Also during this phase, the researcher can identify potential barriers to implementing the campaign and to promoting specific behavior.

The main objective at this stage is to understand the intended audience in terms of its existing knowledge, attitudes, beliefs, motivations, values, practices, and barriers to behavior. It is also important at this stage to make an inventory of other health promotion activities that have been aimed at this population on this topic in the past. These formative research activities shape the intervention. Formative research should determine at least three things: (1) the level of outcome variables before the campaign, (2) whether that level is low enough to warrant a campaign, and (3) what techniques have been used in the past with what effectiveness to change these outcomes.

One important function of the pre-intervention planning stage is to provide benchmark information for comparison to post-campaign measures. In a study of family planning in Bolivia, for example, we asked respondents to state the methods that a couple can use to prevent pregnancy (see Chapter 8). On average, respondents were aware, when prompted, of 6.3 family planning methods. In the follow-up survey after the campaign, this average increased to 6.6 methods. The baseline information collected during the formative stage was necessary to establish a benchmark measure.

Process Research

Process research consists of investigations conducted during the implementation stage that are designed to document how well the program has been implemented and provide preliminary information about its effectiveness. For communication campaigns, this is when the program is being broadcast or is operating. Process research is often referred to as *monitoring* or *implementation research.*

Such research serves three main functions. First, it documents how the program was implemented, including any decisions made during this phase that altered the program. Was the program conducted as intended or did it deviate from the original purposes? Second, the necessary information is provided to make any mid-course changes in the program. Finally, through process research, information that is critical for replication or expansion of the program is gathered. In Bolivia, we discovered that rural communities had substantively lower levels of campaign exposure—the campaign TV and radio ads were not broadcast as frequently as intended. Consequently, we rebroadcast the campaign to rural areas.

Summative Research

Summative research consists of investigations at the post-intervention stage that are designed to determine the impact on outcomes. Summative research is characterized by collection of data to assess program impact and dissemination of findings. Data collection should occur as soon after the completion of the program as possible (unless the impact assessment is scheduled to be a mid-course assessment). Once the data are collected, researchers must then devote their energy to managing and analyzing the data as quickly as possible to provide results.

Generally, evaluations can be thought of as occurring in at least four steps. First, the researcher does initial analysis to determine the effectiveness of the campaign—among whom and to what degree. Second, these results are shared with the designers to elicit their reactions and get feedback. Third, the researcher provides a report to the funding agencies or stakeholders. This step generally involves writing a report for a lay audience, providing a clear and unambiguous assessment of campaign impact. Finally, the researcher conducts more complex analysis that may be of interest to academic or other communities. This may include the development of new hypotheses or models that can be tested in later interventions. While most evaluations are expected to follow these steps, in practice, few evaluators have the time to follow through on all of these steps.

Summative evaluations may measure both short-term outcomes and long-term impacts (Davis et al., 2000). For example, a campaign designed to increase use of safety belts to decrease deaths due to traffic accidents may include both an outcome and an impact assessment. The outcome assessment measures the extent of safety belt use in a community while the impact assessment measures the rate of traffic fatalities. It is conceivable, though unlikely, that the two assessments would differ, but depending on the type of program, both assessments may be needed. With safety belts, the link between use and traffic fatalities is clear, but in other examples this may not be the case. The advantage of outcome assessment is that it can usually be conducted more quickly than an impact assessment, so that changes in policy can be made in a timely manner.

Some fields may refer to short-term assessments as impact evaluation and long-term ones as outcome evaluation. Consequently, it is often helpful to indicate the time frame when specifying the evaluation such as immediate outcomes and long-term impact. Many programs may consist of both immediate outcome assessments and longer-term impact assessments. In other words, a program may be designed to change certain indicators that are thought to influence other outcomes that occur much later. The evaluation needs to track the short-term outcomes and make appropriate adjustments because waiting for the long-term impacts to change often takes too long. This text will focus on methods for outcome assessment.

Consider, for example, programs designed to increase awareness of contraceptives so that couples can use appropriate methods of fertility control to achieve their desired number of children. It would take at least 5 to 10 years to know whether this change came about. Thus, evaluating a campaign on this criterion after 1 or 2 years would be unwise. Instead, evaluators can measure the campaign's effect on awareness of methods and reported contraceptive use.

This text concentrates on how to conduct outcome assessment of health promotion programs and health communication campaigns. Integral to this process, however, is an understanding of how the various research methods and activities fit together. Competent evaluators use a variety of research methods, and they know how these methods complement one another.

Methodology Mix

The mix of research methods used in an evaluation is a function of several factors, including the type and scale of the program, the evaluation budget, and the

project size. Typically, qualitative methods such as in-depth interviews and focus groups are used in the formative phase to develop messages and pilot-test
materials (Chapter 4). In contrast, quantitative methods such as survey data analysis are used in the summative phase to estimate a campaign's effect. A mix of
both qualitative and quantitative methodology is often employed for monitoring.

Many exceptions to this pattern exist, however, and it is not uncommon for
researchers to rely on qualitative data to determine the outcome of an intervention. It is also common for researchers to conduct considerable quantitative survey analysis to determine potential market sizes and the demographic characteristics of intended audiences. In sum, evaluators are encouraged to become familiar
with many research methods and to integrate them into their evaluation designs.
Evaluations are best when they consist of multiple methods and measures.

Program Stages

One of the reasons that evaluators must be so versatile is that they are called on
to evaluate many different types of programs at different stages of implementation. Some campaigns may be pilot projects or innovative attempts to disseminate information, whereas others may be ongoing campaigns where the evaluation is designed to test a new message or refine an old one. The program stage
influences the level of effort and the technical procedures undertaken during the
evaluation. Specifically, mature programs that have been tried and tested in the
past may require fewer resources to evaluate than novel ones since there is more
uncertainty when evaluating the latter.

SUMMARY

This chapter has provided an introduction to the topics covered in this book. It
outlined a framework for organizing evaluation activities (Fig. 1–1) that can be
classified into formative, process, and summative research. The skills needed for
each research phase vary considerably, and the evaluator must be well versed in
all of them. Conducting an evaluation requires that investigators know and anticipate the need for all of these research activities and that they find the right
people to perform them. The activities are interrelated, and comprehensive evaluations require competency in all of them.

The general framework provided here is a guide to determining which activities typically occur at what time; it entails a partial checklist of the many data-
gathering and analysis activities that are possible in an evaluation. It is by no
means exhaustive. Good evaluators are always looking for evidence to document
program success. Often casual conversations with taxicab drivers or astute ob-

servations of people on the street provide important insights for an evaluation. These data-gathering activities may not be described in detail in journal articles, but they can contribute to an interesting and insightful evaluation.

It might seem to the reader that conducting evaluation is difficult, and it can be. The remaining chapters attempt to clarify the tools and skills needed to facilitate the evaluation process. Our first challenge is to understand the range and scope of communication and health promotion activities that have been used to promote healthy behavior.

Chapter Two

Health Promotion Interventions

The purpose of health promotion program evaluation is to determine the effectiveness of interventions designed to promote healthy behavior. This chapter describes these interventions, their scope, and their terminology. A wide variety of health promotion programs have been conducted in many settings over the past four decades. This chapter provides a description of these different intervention strategies, and the conditions that must be met for them to be successful.

INTERVENTION STRATEGIES

There are at least eight intervention strategies, each requiring different skills, often targeted toward different populations. The evaluation methodologies used in one type of intervention are often not those used in another type of intervention. Whenever possible, the interventions described here are accompanied by a discussion of evaluation design. The first section of this chapter describes these eight strategies, presented in the order of the size of the audience they reach.

Provider Training

These interventions are designed to improve the way providers communicate with clients or patients. Provider training programs usually occur in health-care facilities and are accompanied by dissemination of print materials or other communication aids. This strategy consists of training providers in better interpersonal communication (verbal and nonverbal) and use of aids such as flip charts, wall charts, posters, cue cards, flyers, and brochures. Providers include physicians, counselors, nurses, social workers, receptionists, and anyone else who has contact with clients.

Evaluation of provider training is important because of the increasing emphasis on quality of services. Most evaluations are conducted by interviewing clients before and after they have received services using a checklist of recommended practices; this provides a consistent recording tool. Service statistics collected over time may also provide evidence of training effectiveness. These studies should be supplemented with trained ethnographic observations and transcript analysis of the provider–client interaction.

Theories of interpersonal communication and persuasion are used to evaluate provider training programs (Roter and Hall, 1988; Bruce and Jain, 1989; Bruce, 1990; Kim et al., 1992). Provider training is expected to change behavior in at least three ways: first, by making providers better communicators with their clients; second, by making providers appear more competent; and third, by providing materials such as flyers and brochures that clients can use later.

Community-based Distribution or Outreach

In this strategy, outreach workers convey health information at home or in public locations, going door-to-door to disseminate information or distribute products and recruit new acceptors. Outreach can be effective because prospective acceptors meet directly with someone who can answer questions about the product and who may be similar to the prospective acceptor and has experience with the product. In some cases, the outreach workers are satisfied users and thus highly credible sources. This strategy is popular in developing countries where labor costs are low, and it has been used in the U.S. to great advantage by Avon and Tupperware.

The principal advantage of community-based outreach is that personal contact reassures the prospective acceptors that others have already tried the behavior and support its adoption (Fisher and de Silva, 1986). Prospective acceptors can question the outreach workers about their concerns. Outreach workers can compile these questions and relay them back to management. Finally, outreach workers can have the product with them and demonstrate its use and perhaps sell it.

There are several disadvantages to outreach programs. First, the workers need to be trained. Second, even when trained, they will vary considerably in their ability to sell the product. Third, they may not be able to reach many households over a large distance. These limitations aside, outreach programs can be an effective means to recruit new adopters.

Community-based distribution (CBD) is similar to community-based outreach, as workers visit households and sell the product. Here, specific depots or homes have supplies of the product. For example, some international family planning programs provide CBD workers with supplies of pills, condoms, and diaphragms that they can sell to clients from their homes.

Outreach programs can be evaluated by comparing rates of new acceptors in areas with and without workers, or with trained and untrained ones. In addition to recruitment rates, user satisfaction and return rates can also be compared. Thus the number of new clients or the satisfaction of these clients is often the dependent variable used to evaluate the success of outreach workers.

Health promotion programs often use outreach workers as a supplement to mass media programs. Outreach workers provide an interpersonal reinforcement to the mass media messages. Health promoters can supplement outreach activities by providing materials, such as flyers, for workers to use. They can also use mass media to raise awareness of the outreach programs. In this way, people will be aware of the outreacher's goals when he or she visits them. In community-wide cardiovascular disease trials (North Karelia, Stanford, Minnesota, and Pawtucket), both mass media and community outreach were used to promote health. Evaluation results showed that the mass media and outreach workers each served different purposes—the mass media raised awareness and the outreach workers provided support.

Outreach has been particularly useful for substance abuse prevention and treatment programs (Needle et al., 1995). Since many substance abusers have little contact with, and may be distrustful of, the health-care system, outreach is one of the best ways to reach them. These programs can be implemented and evaluated using network analysis techniques to track who is connected to whom (Latkin et al., 1995; Levy and Fox, 1998; Valente and Davis, 1999; Kincaid, 2000). These study designs may consist of determining who recruits whom to get medical services. For example, outreach workers can be given incentives to recruit substance abusers into treatment who in turn recruit others (Broadhead et al., 1998).

Community Mobilization

In this strategy, community leaders identity the community's needs and create programs to address them. Community events such as fairs, street theater, and advocacy events may be part of this strategy. Community mobilization projects are usually geographically limited and often serve as pilot programs for later efforts scaled up to a larger area. Community mobilization and participation rely on residents becoming actively involved in identifying and solving their own problems. Ownership and responsibility for the program lie with community members, so that they become empowered to be agents of change.

Community mobilization interventions can take many forms, but most often they consist of town hall meetings to solicit community involvement. Local committees are usually established to determine community concerns and develop programs to address them. Although community involvement takes many forms, the process of soliciting community participation and action can be replicated in many settings.

To some extent, these programs focus on community rather than on individual behavior, and hence require evaluations to shift the focus from individual to community. Evaluations need to document changes in participation by community residents via participatory research. To date, narrative forms of documentation have been the main technique used to evaluate community mobilization projects. The development of quantifiable community-level indicators poses a new challenge for program evaluators. This may be possible using network methods designed to document changes in community structure (Wickizer et al., 1993; Stoebenau and Valente, 1999).

Social Marketing

In this strategy, business marketing principles are used to promote prosocial goods and services (Wiebe, 1951; Kotler and Zaltman, 1971; Kotler and Roberto, 1989). Products acquired at a subsidized price are promoted and sold, and extensive communication interventions such as brand-name advertising, point-of-purchase promotion, and various public relations activities are undertaken. Some people use the term *social marketing* for any promotion of health and social behaviors, regardless of whether there is a product to sell.

Social marketing programs are evaluated by measuring the distribution of products to retailers on a monthly, quarterly, or annual basis. If possible, sales data are recorded and analyzed as well. These data are accompanied by point-of-purchase interviews with customers and sales clerks. Evaluations may also include cost-effectiveness, by subtracting the costs of the social marketing from sales receipts.

Social marketing programs are evaluated less frequently because their advocates are more willing to "let the market decide." As in the promotion of commercial products, success is measured by sales volume. Consequently, many social marketing campaigns are evaluated primarily by tracking sales data, which is often more reliable, rather than through survey or experimental research.

Mass Media Advertising

In this strategy, television, radio, and print are used to disseminate commercials produced in short, 30-second or 1-minute spots to large audiences. Typically, these campaigns have a variety of spots linked together conceptually and disseminated over a finite time period. Advertising campaigns create brand identification and attempt to link specific images to specific products. Although they are not expected to change the behavior of many people, they are important for a variety of reasons. First, they raise awareness of the product or idea, making it widely known. Second, they can establish a positive image for the behavior, making it desirable. Third, they can generate interpersonal communication about the behavior, leading to subsequent behavior change. Thus, although mass media advertising may not be sufficient for behavior change, it is often necessary.

Advertising campaigns are evaluated by means of many methodologies, but the most common is a simple before-and-after survey. Sometimes comparisons are made between regions where one received the campaign and the other did not. They are also evaluated with sales data, point-of-purchase interviews, and even laboratory studies.

Entertainment-Education

Often referred to as *Enter-Educate,* this strategy uses entertainment to educate audiences about health issues (Piotrow et al., 1997; Singhal and Rogers, 1999). Entertainment programs include drama, film, radio and television soap operas, music and variety shows, and talk shows with audience participation (Church and Geller, 1989). Television, radio, and film dramas have been the most common form of entertainment–education, primarily in developing countries to promote family planning, reproductive health, and female empowerment (Singhal and Rogers, 1999). Entertainment dramas can achieve more audience involvement than simple commercial advertisements since the audience can identify with the characters and become emotionally involved.[1]

The evaluation of entertainment–education campaigns poses special challenges, but also creates many opportunities. Some people may watch a few episodes of a TV soap opera while others may watch every episode and identify strongly with the characters. This variation should be measured and linked to any potential outcomes. Factors that motivate watching and involvement need to be considered.

Street theater, fairs, puppet shows, and carnivals provide a localized form of entertainment–education (Valente et al., 1996; Valente and Bharath, 1999). Street theater can be a very effective intervention strategy because it is entertaining and immediate. Furthermore, street theater is public and can be supplemented with interpersonal counselors who stay after the performance to answer questions.

---

[1]Entertainment programming for social change originated in Britain with *The Archers*, a radio drama about agricultural practices in Britain, first broadcast in 1951 and still on the air today. Although *The Archers* no longer attempts to provide educational programming, many believe the show still has an educational agenda.

Evaluation of street theater programs is usually done by interviewing people before and after they watch the performance. These studies can be biased unless the sample is appropriately selected. Evaluations of street theater provide useful information on audience reaction and message comprehension, as well as changes in knowledge and attitudes. More long-term studies need to be conducted to determine if watching street theater can change behavior.

Interactive Health Communication

In this strategy, computer and other telecommunication technologies are used to deliver health-related information through the Internet, telemedicine, kiosk systems, and any computer-based system. These new technologies provide interactivity and flexibility not previously available in communication media (Rice and Katz, 2001).

Some groups evaluate the accuracy and quality of Internet sites that provide health information. Currently, there are private companies that attempt to be the source for health and medical information, some linked to larger health care providers, others not. Government agencies are also active in supplying health information over the Web.

Since interactive health communication is new, most studies of it have been conducted in laboratory settings. In these studies, users complete a survey and spend time interacting with a computer-based health program and then complete a follow-up survey. Evaluations measure whether users learned something from the program and how they interacted with it.

Multimedia or Community-wide Programs

This strategy uses a variety of media, enlists community support through opinion leaders, and trains provider personnel. These programs are comprehensive, attempting to change community norms regarding health and the system that provides it (Box 2–1). Multiple media strategies such as mass media advertising, outreach, and store-based promotion are coordinated to deliver consistent messages. Many scholars believe that the best approach to behavior change is a multimedia approach that reaches the largest possible audience through as many different channels as possible.

Several large and extensively evaluated community-based, multimedia, health promotion projects have been conducted in the last few decades (Shea and Basch, 1990a, 1990b). These community-wide health programs, designed to reduce the prevalence of heart disease, include the Northern Karelia Project in Finland, the Stanford (California) Heart Disease Prevention Program, the Minnesota Heart Health Project, and the Pawtucket (Rhode Island) Heart Health Project (see Box 2–1). Although these programs were usually effective, the gains in the intervention communities were soon matched by those in the comparison ones.

Box 2-1. COMMUNITY-WIDE PROGRAMS

The best known examples of community-wide programs (CWPs) include the following (see Shea and Basch, 1990a, 1990b; Freimuth and Taylor, in press, for reviews):

- North Karelia project (Puska et al., 1985, 1986)
- Stanford Three-City project and Stanford Five City project (Maccoby and Farquhar, 1975; Maccoby et al., 1977; Maccoby, 1988; Farquhar et al., 1990; Flora et al., 1989; Fortmann et al., 1995; Winkleby et al., 1996).
- Pawtucket Heart Health Program (Lefebvre et al., 1987; Lasater et al., 1990; Wells et al., 1990).
- Minnesota Heart Health Program (Mittelmark et al., 1986; Finnegan et al., 1989; Perry et al., 1992; Weisbrod et al., 1992).
- Midwestern Prevention Project (Pentz et al., 1989, 1990).

The community-wide approach to health promotion was first developed in the early 1970s in North Karelia, Finland. The project was initiated because the government of Finland discovered that it had the highest rate of death attributable to cardiovascular disease in Europe, and the North Karelia region had the highest rate in Finland.

Cardiovascular disease (CVD) was related to a Finnish diet high in fat and low in fresh vegetables or fruits. Finland also had high rates of smoking and vodka consumption. The Finnish people and government agreed to undertake measures to reduce CVD nationwide. The program used community volunteers as change agents and mass media advertisements to promote better eating habits. The North Karelia project reduced CVD (Puska et al., 1985).

The Stanford programs were launched in northern California and were also designed to reduce CVD by promoting healthier eating habits, smoking cessation, and exercise. The North Karelia and Stanford projects were followed by the Minnesota and Pawtucket projects. All four projects attempted to use comparison cities that did not receive the treatment, and all four included (1) mass media promotion, (2) point-of-sale promotion, (3) use of volunteers, and (4) panel and independent samples for the evaluation. All four study investigators had difficulty saying that their projects were successful (although North Karelia demonstrated its impact more conclusively) because trends in the comparison communities eventually matched those in the intervention ones.

Although the community-wide programs were not as successful as hoped, some important evaluation lessons have been learned: (1) the value of different strategies for data collection, (2) the importance of measuring contamination between intervention and comparison communities, and (3) the way societal trends and factors may overwhelm project goals.

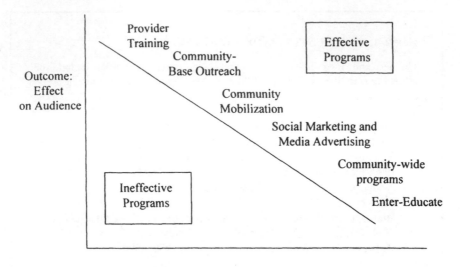

Reach: Percent of Audience Exposed to Message

FIGURE 2–1. Conceptual model of tradeoff between program reach and outcome.

Evaluating the effectiveness of community-wide programs can be challenging since it is difficult to identify the role any particular intervention has on the outcome. Since behavior change is often a result of a complex interaction at many levels, it is hard to isolate one program component that may have been responsible for any observed changes. When policies, training, and service facilities are all being improved, many or all of these interventions may be responsible for programmatic effects.

Summary of Communication Interventions

These eight strategies represent a hierarchy of health interventions from small to large audiences. That is, provider training is usually face-to-face whereas community mobilization involves groups, and mass media programs attempt to reach a large audience. Some health promotion projects use only one of these strategies, while others use a combination. Figure 2–1 presents a conceptual model of the trade-off between program reach and outcome. The Y-axis represents outcome, the degree of change in behavior expected by the program; the X-axis represents reach, the size of the audience reached by the program. As reach increases, the degree of behavior change expected by the intervention decreases. Provider training, for example, can be effective since it is specific to the individual but does not reach a large audience. Programs that change few people's behavior and reach a small audience (lower left quadrant) are ineffective, while those that change many people's behavior and reach a large audience (upper right quadrant) are considered effective. These generalizations concerning the effectiveness and reach are subject to debate.

These eight types of health promotion intervention have been used to change a variety of health behaviors among different audiences. Most programs will consist of an intervention similar to one or a combination of these eight types. Some, such as mass media advertising, have been used more often than others, but all can be effective. The choice of intervention type depends, in part, on available resources, characteristics of the behavior, and the population. Although the characteristics of the programs are interesting, the question always asked of these interventions is: were they successful?

PROGRAM IMPACT CONDITIONS

Evaluations of health promotion programs are numerous and span a variety of academic disciplines. Perspectives concerning program effects in the communication field range from large effects, such as the hypodermic needle hypothesis, to minimal effects (Klapper, 1960), to no effects (see McQuail, 1987). The literature on communication campaign effects began in the 1940s with an influential paper by Cartwright (1949), which argued that campaigns to sell War Bonds during World War II were successful.

Rogers and Storey (1987; also see McQuail, 1987) divided campaign effects research into three historical research eras. Campaigns were thought to *(1)* have minimal effects during the 1940s and 1950s, *(2)* be very successful during the 1960s and 1970s, and *(3)* have moderate effects during the 1980s and 1990s. Each era was marked by a seminal publication that set the tenor for its era. In the minimal effects era, many researchers cited the work of Lazarsfeld and colleagues, as they tried to determine whether mass media messages influenced voting behavior (Lazarsfeld et al., 1948; Berelson et al., 1954). They found that mass media campaigns swayed few voters directly. Voting preferences changed little during the course of a campaign, and those voters who did change their attitudes relied primarily on the attitudes of their friends and colleagues (Katz and Lazarsfeld, 1955; Katz, 1957, 1987; Eulau, 1980; see Gitlin, 1978, for critique). Two other studies contributed to the perception that campaigns have only minimal effects: Hyman and Sheatsley's (1974) review of campaigns to promote public affairs knowledge, and Star and Hughes' (1950) evaluation of a campaign to promote support for the United Nations in Cincinnati. These studies painted a rather pessimistic view of a media campaign's ability to influence audiences.

More optimistic researchers (Cartwright, 1949, 1954) persevered, attempting to draw lessons from the failures in order to make campaigns more effective. A second era focusing on conditions under which campaigns could succeed emerged in the 1960s and was summarized by Mendelsohn (1973), who argued that campaigns can succeed when their designers do four things: *(1)* conduct formative research, *(2)* set reasonable goals, *(3)* segment the audience, and *(4)* use interpersonal channels. Positive results from programs such as the children's TV show *Sesame Street* led researchers to reconsider the ability of a media campaign to create social change. Another prominent campaign success was the significant drop in smoking behavior when anti-smoking ads were aired on television (Flay, 1987a, 1987b; Wallack, 1981).

Today, many researchers believe that health communication campaigns can have modest effects on behavior. The nature of these impacts, however, is still debatable. For example, McQuail (1987) distinguishes between media effects by categorizing them according to two dimensions: whether the effects are intentional or not, and whether the effects are long or short term. Media campaigns are thought to have short-term, intentional effects while multimedia, community-level campaigns are thought to have long-term ones. Currently, campaigns are believed to have effects under certain historical, cultural, political, or sociological conditions (McQuail, 1987; Finnegan et al., 1989; Piotrow et al., 1997; Valente and Saba, 1998).

Research on health communication campaigns and health promotion programs has shown that four conditions—situational, programmatic, theoretical, and methodological—need to be met for programs to be successful. The importance of these four conditions may vary by health topic and by population. Each condition, however, needs to be assessed before a program is launched.

Situational

The program needs to address a need that can be satisfied by adopting a specific behavior (Hornik, 1989; Hornik et al., 1992). Successful programs should address behaviors that can be changed, which implies that the audience is willing to change and that there are no significant barriers to changing their behavior. This also implies that the program will not hit ceiling effects in which there is already a high percentage of adopters.

The situational condition may imply that the benefits to changing behavior will outweigh the costs. Programs are not likely to be successful when they ask people to change behaviors for which the costs outweigh the benefits. Some people will change their behavior when the costs are greater than the benefits, but there are not many behaviors or people for which this is true. The situational condition is fundamental yet often overlooked. Needs assessments are conducted to determine whether the situational condition is met.

Programmatic

The program must reach its intended audience and appeal to it. The programmatic condition contains at least 16 components concerning its design and dissemination.

1. The program should reach a significant percentage of the audience, and reach them frequently and over a period of time. Optimal values for program exposure will be discussed in Chapter 11. Program impact is often directly related to the degree of exposure.

2. The program should appeal to the audience by creating a program that the audience likes. The program's appeal will be a function of the production quality, such as good use of graphics, actors, and scripts.

3. Program messages should be tailored to and culturally appropriate for the audience. For example, successful adolescent smoking prevention programs send the message that smoking is odorous and hence a turnoff to members of the opposite sex, rather than trying to convey information about the long-term adverse health effects of smoking.

4. Program media should be appropriate. People use different media for different purposes. Program designers need to match their message to the audience's media preferences.

5. Program messages should match the needs of the audience. For example, some situations will require that programs disseminate information about how a product works, while for others it will be about where to get it.

6. The program should coordinate the supply of the product so that it is available for potential adopters. Some programs have been judged unsuccessful because the product was not available for purchase when the campaign increased demand for it (Valente, 1997).

7. Program logos and slogans should be repeated at service sites and sales locations to reinforce the message (Valente and Saba, 1998).

8. The source attributable to the program should be perceived as credible by the intended audience (Hovland et al., 1953). Credibility varies by audience and topic. For example, white, middle-class audiences may perceive the government as a credible source for health information while other ethnic and economic groups may not. Credibility can sometimes be enhanced by using data to support a message.

9. The source attributable to the program should be perceived as trustworthy by the intended audience. Trustworthiness, like credibility, varies by topic and audience, and is hard to create.

10. Programs that are replications should be implemented in the way they were intended to be implemented.

11. The program should contain a specific call to action that tells the audience what to do and how to adopt the promoted behavior (Piotrow et al., 1997). If the program does not make a specific behavioral recommendation, the audience cannot be expected to know what to do.

12. Programs should be part of a continuous process of involvement with the audience to bring about change. One-time interventions are rarely effective.

13. Programs should use interpersonal communication by using outreach workers. If the program is being broadcast, then messages should ac-

knowledge that interpersonal communication is important by using people similar to the audience as spokespersons. Programs can also use opinion leaders as spokespersons.

14. Programs should have mechanisms for feedback so that the audience can
communicate with program designers. For example, enter–educate soap
operas encourage the audience to write letters to their favorite characters
or the show's writers (Singhal and Rogers, 1999).

15. Programs should promise a reward for adopting the behavior. There must
be some benefit to the behavior, and this benefit should be communicated.

16. Programs should avoid fear appeals unless they have been shown to be
effective (Hale and Dillard, 1995; Monahan, 1995; Stephenson and Witte,
2001). Rational appeals are sometimes effective but most scholars feel that
emotional appeals are the most effective, especially those that emphasize
the positive benefits of a health behavior.

These programmatic conditions are extensive and situation-specific. The effectiveness of programs, however, rests on whether these conditions can be met.
Crafting messages and creating interventions is both an artistic and scientific process. The evaluator rarely has much control over the situation and programmatic
conditions. The final two conditions, theoretical and methodological, however,
are the primary responsibility of the evaluator.

Theoretical

Factors that influence or inhibit behavior include socioeconomic status, demographic characteristics, attitudes, values, perceived norms, and so on. Behavior
change theory specifies how these factors relate to one another by constructing
a conceptual model of the process of behavioral change. By using theory to guide
program design, the messages can target factors thought to influence behavior.

For example, many adolescents smoke because they believe "everyone" does
it. Perceived norms for smoking thus lead to smoking. Programs can be created
to change this perceived norm and hence reduce adolescent smoking. In this example, theory about the cause for a behavior is used to design the program's
message.

Theory is also used to inform the evaluation by indicating what needs to be
measured. The variables in the conceptual model should be measured so that the
model can be tested. In the adolescent smoking example, perceived norms needed
to be measured since the program was aimed at changing them.

Choosing a theory and constructing a conceptual model is the topic of Chapter 3. In short, it is the product of three activities: knowledge of existing theories, knowledge of their past use, and conducting formative research. The theo-

retical condition can determine the success of a program and its evaluation as much as the situational and programmatic conditions. The methodological condition, on the other hand, does not affect program success but does affect the ability to measure it.

Methodological

The program's evaluation provides an accurate description and interpretation of how it did or did not influence the audience. The challenge for evaluators is tailoring it to the program. The variety of intervention strategies covered in the first part of this chapter demonstrates that programs take many forms. The evaluation needs to match the program and no one evaluation design will work for all programs. Evaluators thus need to know the study design options in Chapter 6.

The methodological condition requires that the evaluation demonstrate the degree of change attributable to the program, ruling out other plausible explanations. Most of this text addresses the logic and mechanics of evaluation, thus they need not be covered here; however, three factors that contribute to the failure of many evaluations warrant mention here.

First, many studies have not allocated enough time for behavior change to occur. Change takes time, yet most program evaluations are conducted over a short time interval, not allowing for long-term effects to be measured. Second, program designers often have too high an expectation for the degree of effect achievable by a program. These expectations drive study sample size and hence study conclusions (Chapter 7). Third, many evaluations measure outcomes poorly or measure the wrong ones (Chapters 8 and 9). This book is designed to address these and other issues that affect the success of an evaluation.

Many health promotion programs and their evaluations have not met these four conditions. It is thus tempting to say that the program did not work when in fact the conditions for success were not met. To be sure, many programs fail, but it is important to understand the reasons for these failures so that investigators have a better chance of success in the future.

SUMMARY

This chapter has provided a description of different types of health promotion programs used to change health-related behavior. The eight strategies range from provider training to community mobilization and mass media approaches. Each strategy was accompanied by a short discussion of the evaluation issues relevant to that strategy. Figure 2–1 presented a conceptual graph of the relationship between expected program reach and impact.

The second section described four conditions necessary for a successful program evaluation. These conditions—situation, programmatic, theoretical, and methodological—are often not met, and hence programs are often incorrectly determined to be unsuccessful when, in fact, the conditions for success were not in place. Consideration of these conditions may lead some designers to delay or avoid launching programs altogether. It is hoped, however, that specifying these conditions will result in better programs and improved evaluations. The next chapter presents behavior change theories to guide these endeavors.

Chapter Three

Behavior Change Theory

Some people think evaluation is an applied activity, lacking theoretical richness. The evaluation process is improved, however, when conducted with a theoretical perspective. Theory helps establish program goals and objectives, and provides guidance on how to measure them. A theoretical perspective should be explicitly stated to guide the program and its evaluation. It may sometimes be necessary for the researcher to disentangle this theoretical perspective if it is not explicitly stated. Theory attempts to explain people's behavior and the factors that motivate changing it. Thus, theory provides the basis for effective program development and meaningful program evaluation.

The traditional view of evaluation was that designers implemented a program and evaluators determined whether it was effective. Evaluator objectivity was preserved by a lack of contact with and knowledge of the program. Early work in which evaluators did not know a program's characteristics is referred to as *black box evaluation* (Chen and Rossi, 1983; Weiss, 1997). Black box evaluation has given way to theory-based evaluation in which the designers and evaluators use theory to inform their activities. Evaluators thus know how the designers intend to change behavior and they may actively participate in program planning and implementation.

Theory-based evaluation is the use of theory to explain how an intervention is expected to change outcomes. Theory can provide the basis for constructing

33

an intervention and it increases the likelihood that the intervention will be successful. For some interventions, theory is implied and not explicitly stated. In these instances, evaluators must work with program designers to determine the theoretical basis for their programs. Theory influences every aspect of an evaluation, including study design, instrumentation, and interpretation of results.

This chapter presents some of the theories developed to explain human behavior that are useful in evaluating health promotion programs. The choice of which theory to use in a program evaluation depends in large part on the topic, goals, and priorities of the program. Additionally, the resources committed to a program may determine the expectations for it. A modest intervention may be intended to raise awareness without attempting to change attitudes or behavior. Consequently, the evaluator should concentrate on documenting change in awareness and not on change in behavior. A more ambitious program might be expected to change behavior and hence the evaluator needs to document such impacts.

This chapter summarizes seven theories and four perspectives on behavior change, then distinguishes between program and research success and failure, and closes with a discussion of theory selection. Choosing an appropriate theory of behavior change to guide a health promotion program can be difficult. Evaluators need to know theories and how to apply them in diverse settings. The motivation for selecting a theory comes from its appropriateness to answer the research questions posed; it can also come from formative research or past experience. The main difference between theories and perspectives is that theories provide specific testable hypotheses, whereas perspectives more often suggest variables to be measured or strategies to be considered.

THEORIES

There are seven theories about human behavior that are useful in evaluating health promotion programs: diffusion of innovations, hierarchy of effects and steps to behavior change, stages of change, the transtheoretical model, theory of reasoned action, social learning theory, and the health belief model. Each of these is discussed below.

Diffusion of Innovations

Most promotion programs are designed to inform the public, change their attitudes, and promote specific behaviors. Diffusion of innovations is a theory that describes how new ideas, opinions, attitudes, and behaviors spread throughout a community (Ryan and Gross, 1943; Katz et al., 1963; Valente, 1993, 1995;

Rogers, 1995; Valente and Rogers, 1995). "Diffusion is the process by which an innovation is communicated through certain channels over time among the members of a social system" (Rogers, 1995, p. 5). Diffusion theory has been used to study the spread of new computer technology, educational curricula, farming practices, family planning methods, medical technology, and many other innovations. Diffusion theory has five major components: *(1)* diffusion takes time, *(2)* people pass through stages in the adoption process, *(3)* they can modify the innovation and sometimes discontinue its use, *(4)* perceived characteristics of the innovation influence adoption, and *(5)* individual characteristics influence adoption.

In diffusion theory individuals are classified in terms of their time of adoption relative to a community or population. The first people to try a new practice are called *innovators* or *pioneers*. The second group to adopt are called *early adopters*. These first two groups constitute the first 16% of adopters. The next 34% of the population to adopt are the *early majority*, followed by the *late majority* and then *laggards*.

Diffusion theory specifies five stages in the adoption process: knowledge, persuasion, decision, trial, and adoption (Rogers, 1995). Before individuals adopt a new practice they must be aware that it exists, and many programs are created to increase this awareness. After people become *(1)* aware of a new health idea or practice, they *(2)* learn more about it, then *(3)* make a conscious decision to try or not try it, then *(4)* they must obtain it, and finally, *(5)* the new behavior becomes incorporated into their normal way of doing things (see Table 3–1).

Once individuals adopt a new behavior they may modify it by using it in ways not originally intended. For example, telephone answering machines were designed to answer calls when the owner was away, but are now also used to screen calls or leave messages for other members of the household.

Diffusion theory states that the way people perceive a health behavior affects whether they will adopt it. For example, people who think eating fresh vegetables is consistent with their cultural values are more likely to eat them. Five types of perception influence this adoption (Fliegal and Kivlin, 1966): relative advantage, trialability, compatibility, observability, and simplicity—all of which are associated with earlier adoption. Another is the degree of radicality in the innovation. Radical innovations represent dramatically new ways of doing things, thus they take longer to spread.

Finally, there are numerous individual characteristics associated with earlier behavior change. For example, more educated, cosmopolitan, and wealthier individuals are usually earlier adopters of innovations. Associations between individual characteristics and behavior change are dependent on the type of innovation and the community within which the innovation diffuses. Some behaviors are easier to adopt and thus spread more rapidly, and some communities are more receptive to change and thus innovations spread more rapidly in them.

TABLE 3–1. Comparison of Stages of Behavior Change

DIFFUSION OF INNOVATIONS (ROGERS, 1995)	HIERARCHY OF EFFECTS (MCGUIRE, 1989)	STEPS TO BEHAVIOR CHANGE (PIOTROW ET AL., 1997)	STAGES OF CHANGE (PROCHASKA ET AL., 1992)
1. Awareness	1. Recalling message	1. Recalls message	1. Pre-contemplation
	2. Liking message	2. Understands topic	
	3. Comprehending message	3. Can name source of supply	
	4. Knowledge of behavior		
2. Persuasion	5. Skill acquisition	4. Responds favorably	2. Contemplation
	6. Yielding to it	5. Discusses with friends/family	
	7. Memory storage of content	6. Thinks others approve	
		7. Approves oneself	
		8. Recognizes that innovation meets need	
3. Decision	8. Information search and retrieval	9. Intends to consult a provider	3. Preparation
	9. Deciding on basis of retrieval	10. Intends to adopt	
		11. Go to provider	
4. Implementation	10. Behaving in accordance with decision	12. Initiates use	4. Action
		13. Continues use	
5. Confirmation	11. Reinforcement of desired acts	14. Experiences benefits	5. Maintenance
	12. Post-behavior consolidation	15. Advocates that others practice behavior change	
		16. Supports practice in the community	

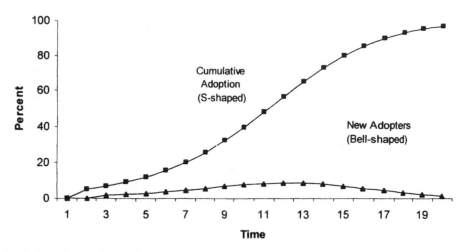

FIGURE 3-1. Typical diffusion curve.

Diffusion theory states that a new behavior is initially adopted by a few mem-bers of a community; over time the percentage of adopters increases until the po-tential audience is saturated. A typical diffusion curve is graphed in Figure 3-1 and shows how initially only a few people make the change. Over time, more individuals adopt the new practice until all (or almost all) members have done so. At some point, the innovation ceases to be advantageous and is replaced by a different practice or some modification of the existing one.

The attitude and practice curves generally conform to a logistic growth curve, or S-shaped pattern, reflecting the cumulative percentage of people who have adopted the behavior over time. The curve is S-shaped because adoption is ini-tially slow and then it takes off, often reaching a maximum rate about the time half the population has adopted the new behavior. After the halfway point, there are fewer non-adopters left in the population so the adoption rate slows and the curve eventually levels off. Critical mass is achieved when diffusion generates its own momentum and is self-sustaining (Valente, 1993, 1995; Rogers, 1995). Numerous explanations have been postulated for the S-shaped curve of adoption, including profitability, persuasion by peers, cost–benefit calculations, and media influence.

Diffusion theory has been developed by studying a variety of innovations in various fields, such as hybrid seed corn (Ryan and Gross, 1943; Griliches, 1957), medicine (Coleman et al., 1966; Greer, 1977; Anderson and Jay, 1985), educa-tion (Carlson, 1964), policy innovations among states (Walker, 1969), fluo-ridization adoption among cities (Crain, 1966), and many more topics (see Ham-blin et al., 1973; Rogers, 1995, for reviews).

Figure 3–2 displays growth curves for the spread of knowledge, positive atti-tude, and practice of a behavior. These three variables—knowledge (K), attitudes

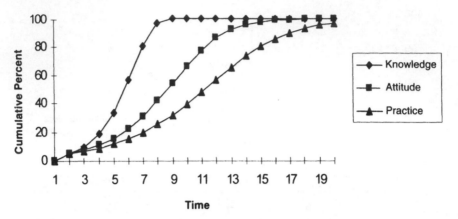

FIGURE 3–2. Knowledge, attitude, and practice curves.

(A), and practices (P)—are often referred to as *KAP*. The percentage of the population aware of the innovation increases most rapidly. It can take somewhat longer for that same percentage to have a positive attitude, and still longer for the same percentage to adopt it. The KAP graph serves to *(1)* demonstrate the existing or expected percentages for each variable at any point in time, and *(2)* show the expected gap between knowledge and practice, indicating the time it takes a population to move from knowledge to practice (the so-called KAP-gap).

Figure 3–2 shows that awareness spreads rapidly, but as time passes, fewer new people become aware as the proportion of non-knowers decreases. This pattern has been demonstrated most frequently in research on news diffusion where the information is usually simple (Deutschmann and Danielson, 1960; DeFleur, 1987). Awareness diffusion often occurs via mass media since they reach many people.

Media campaigns can accelerate demand for a product. Figure 3–3 shows two adoption curves, one with and one without a promotional media campaign. The bottom curve represents the pattern of behavior change in the absence of a mass media campaign, where adoption is driven by word-of-mouth communication—which can be quite slow, especially for seldomly discussed topics (although see Rosen, 2000). In contrast, the top curve shows how a media campaign can accelerate adoption, where some individuals were persuaded to adopt by the media campaign. The increase in adopters also occurs because the media campaign has put the topic on the public agenda and thus increased the amount of word-of-mouth communication.

The area bounded by the two curves represents the degree of increased behavior change due to the media campaign. At each time interval (years or months, whatever is relevant) researchers can measure impact by the difference between the level of adoption with and without the media campaign. Mathematical mod-

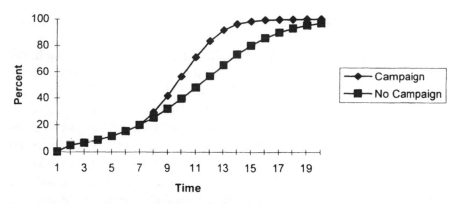

FIGURE 3–3. Campaigns can accelerate behavior change.

els to make projections and other evaluation techniques can be found in Valente (1993).

Diffusion of innovations theory is probably one of the most widely used theories of behavior change (Glanz et al., 1997). Diffusion has been useful for forecasting future levels of behavior and providing insights into cultural change. Moreover, diffusion theory has shown which attributes of innovations influence the rate of adoption, and has provided the basis for opinion leader and change agent interventions (Valente and Davis, 1999). A major limitation to the use of diffusion theory, however, is that campaign evaluations rarely involve the diffusion of a behavior from its inception to saturation. Usually behaviors are promoted in the middle of the growth curve when there is already a significant minority of users and the campaign attempts to increase the percentage to a majority. In this situation, behavior change can be approximated with linear models.

Researchers are advised to pay close attention to the baseline level of their indicators. Since many behavior change processes are thought to grow as in Figure 3–1, the baseline percentage of adopters can affect the level of impact expected. If the baseline level is too low, then the diffusion process may not have started and change may be minimal. If the baseline level is too high, then there are ceiling effects indicating that most individuals have already adopted and not much more behavior change can be expected. If baseline levels are in the middle of the curve (25%–75%), then more change can be expected.

A second limitation to diffusion theory concerns the stages of behavior change. The stages have not been measured consistently and hence conflicting results can be obtained. For example, the definition of a positive attitude toward a behavior can vary considerably. Secondly, the stages are in some sense redundant since, for most innovations, awareness has to precede having a positive attitude, which has to precede adoption. Individuals have to know about an innovation before they can form an attitude about it and have to feel positively about it before they are willing to try it.

A third limitation is that, although the KAP model is a useful guide for health communication campaign evaluation, it is a limited model. Six behavior change sequences can be derived from the KAP variables: KAP, KPA, AKP, APK, PAK, and PKA (Valente et al., 1998b). In an empirical test, data from a campaign evaluation conducted in Peru showed that individuals did not follow the KAP sequence of behavior change, but rather most followed a practice–knowledge–attitude (PKA) or practice–attitude–knowledge (PAK) sequence. Others (Chaffee and Roser, 1986; McQuail, 1987) have argued that variables such as audience involvement or characteristics of the behavior are likely to influence the sequence of behavior change. Thus, researchers should use caution when adopting a KAP perspective and be sure that it is an appropriate model for the behavior under study.

Hierarchy of Effects and Steps to Behavior Change

McGuire (1989) and Piotrow and others (1997) expanded the stages of adoption into a hierarchy of behavior change that is more specific to health promotion evaluation. In the hierarchy-of-effects and the steps-to-behavior-change (SBC) models, the five stages of adoption (see Table 3–1) are expanded to include numerous substeps (McGuire 1989; Valente et al., 1996; Piotrow et al., 1997): the rows in Table 3–1.

The hierarchy steps are useful for two reasons: *(1)* they denote a more active audience in terms of information-seeking and advocacy of the behavior, and *(2)* they provide 12 or 16 specific, measurable steps in the process of behavior change. Expanding and relabeling the stages of adoption clarifies some of the characteristics associated with each stage in the process of behavior change. Through the hierarchy model, a rate at which individuals progress through each stage of the change process can be proposed (Box 3–1).

The central challenge to the hierarchy and other stage models is to specify how each step is measured. There are at least three ways: *(1)* ask respondents whether they are aware of the behavior, have a positive attitude toward it, and/or practice it; *(2)* ask respondents whether the program influenced their awareness, attitude, and/or practice; and *(3)* compute the change in scores between baseline and follow-up surveys for the questions asked in *(1)* and/or *(2)*. While the hierarchy model makes predictions about the levels of change expected at each step in the process, it does not indicate how the steps should be measured. Moreover, it is unclear whether individuals are expected to progress steadily through the steps in behavior change. For example, it may be that progression between earlier steps is more rapid than progression through later ones.

Box 3-1. THE HIERARCHY MODEL

The hierarchy of effects model has been used extensively by the Center for Communication Programs to evaluate its health communication programs. McGuire (1989) stated in his formulation of the model that one could posit a rate of effectiveness and then use it to calculate the percentage of individuals that would be expected to progress through the steps in behavior change. This hypothetical example assumes 12 steps, an 80% effectiveness rate (the rate that the campaign moves individuals between steps), and calculated percentages at three different levels of exposure—80%, 60%, and 40%.

	LEVEL OF EXPOSURE (%)		
HIERARCHY VARIABLE	VERY HIGH	HIGH	MODERATE
1. Recalls message	80.0	60.0	40.0
2. Likes message	64.0	48.0	32.0
3. Comprehends message	51.2	38.4	25.6
4. Knowledge of behavior	41.0	30.7	20.5
5. Discusses with others	32.8	24.6	16.4
6. Considers it important	26.2	19.7	13.1
7. Positive image of behavior	21.0	15.7	10.5
8. Intends to get information	16.8	12.6	8.4
9. Intends to practice behavior	13.4	10.1	6.7
10. Gets information on behavior	10.7	8.1	5.4
11. Begins practice	8.6	6.4	4.3
12. Experiences benefits of practice	6.9	5.2	3.4

To use the hierarchy model to estimate the percentage of behavior change and each intermediate step, the exposure and effectiveness must be specified and the percentages computed. For example, a high exposure of 80% and effectiveness of 80% result in 7% of the population being expected to experience the benefits of the behavior (7% was calculated by multiplying 0.8×0.8 to get 0.64 and then 0.64×0.8 to 0.512 and so on, until we reached 0.086×0.8 to get 0.069). Future applications of the hierarchy model can vary the effectiveness rates along with exposure levels and vary the effectiveness rates by step.

The diffusion/hierarchy process is seen as a general model of behavior change. Other researchers have also created stages-of-change models. Indeed, few researchers expect a direct and massive behavioral conversion of a population due to an intervention. *Change takes time and it is wise to classify this process in terms of stages both for individuals and communities.*

Stages of Change and the Transtheoretical Model

Prochaska and colleagues (Prochaska et al., 1992; Prochaska and Velicer, 1997) created the stages-of-change model in which people are classified in one of five stages—precontemplative, contemplative, preparation, action, and mainte-nance—each representing a mental shift toward adoption of behavior change (see Table 3–1). Health messages are expected to be more effective if they are tar-geted at people's particular stage of change. In the precontemplative stage, peo-ple do not intend to take action. In the contemplative stage, they intend to change in the future, and in the preparation stage they intend to change in the near fu-ture (immediately). In the action stage, people have made some behavioral mod-ification, and in the maintenance stage they have made the behavior change for some period of time (usually 6 months or longer).

Prochaska and others' (1992) stages-of-change model has been used to mea-sure the effects of health promotion programs such as the Centers for Disease Control and Prevention's (CDC's) multisite AIDS community demonstration project (CDC AIDS Community Demonstration Projects Research Group, 1998). In that study, the key dependent variable measuring program effectiveness was the participants' score on a five-point scale representing the stage of behavior change. Holtgrave and colleagues (1995) outlined this model's use in designing health messages and Maibach and Cotton (1995) added social cognitive theory components that also suggested avenues for message design.

There are three distinctions between the stages of change and the diffusion/ hierarchy stages. First, the diffusion/hierarchy stages were derived from studies designed to determine attributes associated with early or later adoption of new techniques, whereas the stages-of-change model was derived initially from stud-ies intended to get people to quit smoking. The emphasis in stages-of-change model was to understand how people quit a behavior (smoking), not how they adopt a new one. Second, this model measures cognitive states and shows how these change during adoption, whereas the diffusion model focuses more on how information sources and knowledge vary during adoption. Finally, the diffusion model has a much more extensive history and application than that measuring stages of change, and so has been tested in multiple settings. Nonetheless, the stages-of-change model is used much more today.

There are at least three reasons for the frequent use of stages (or steps) in eval-uation. First, they provide a way to group people and compare these groups in terms of factors that affect behavior. Second, progression between stages can be used as an outcome rather than relying exclusively on behavior. Third, change is not continuous, but rather, marked by distinct events, steps, or stages that sig-nify progression to adoption of change. Most behavioral theory accepts that change occurs in stages and that it is possible to identify distinct events in the process so that stages can be delineated. Most theorists acknowledge that a change in attitude can be an important step toward change in behavior.

Theory of Reasoned Action (Attitudes, Intentions,
Motivations, and Beliefs)

Another often-used behavioral theory is the theory of reasoned action (Fishbein and Ajzen, 1975; Ajzen and Fishbein, 1980; Fishbein et al., 1994) which posits that individual behavior is driven by beliefs, attitudes, intentions, expectations, and social norms. The theory of reasoned action states that individuals hold attitudes and beliefs that shape their intentions to engage in a behavior that in turn influences their actual behavior. To change behavior, health promotion programs have to first change attitudes and beliefs about the behavior (Petty and Cacioppo, 1981). For example, a smoking cessation program will be effective to the degree that it can change attitudes toward smoking and beliefs concerning quitting, and increase intentions to quit.

Increasingly, the theory of reasoned action has included perceptions of community norms as an influence on behavior. The theory of reasoned action says that attitudes and intentions are influenced by subjective interpretations of the norms, social influence, and social pressure regarding the behavior. Returning to the smoking cessation example, intentions to quit smoking may be based partly on whether individuals perceive that their friends support smoking (Ennett and Baumann, 1993; Alexander et al., 2001). Indeed, it is not surprising to find that individuals are often influenced by those whom they interact with, and many researchers feel that people learn primarily from their interactions with others. A leading framework for studying how individuals learn from others is known as *social learning theory.*

Social Learning Theory and Self-efficacy

Bandura (1986) has developed a social learning theory, arguing that individuals learn behaviors from those around them by imitating role models. Health promotion programs should present role models that the audience can identify with so that the modeled behaviors will be imitated. Bandura has argued that self-efficacy influences an individual's ability to imitate modeled behaviors. People with self-efficacy, who believe in their own ability to change, are better able to relate to, understand, and hence imitate modeled behaviors (Bandura, 1986). Those without self-efficacy can develop it vicariously by watching role models. According to Bandura's social learning theory, role models should *(1)* be similar to the audience, *(2)* demonstrate the behavior, and *(3)* be rewarded for practicing it.

If the audience identifies with the role model, they can vicariously experience the behavior and the rewards of adoption. Bandura has conceived of this process as occurring in four stages: attention, retention, reproduction, and motivation. *Attention* refers to getting the audience to watch and become involved in the program. *Retention* refers to presenting the models and behaviors in such a way that the audience remembers them when confronted with a decision to adopt the behavior later. *Reproduction* refers to presenting the behaviors repeatedly, perhaps in different contexts. *Motivation* refers to the expectation that positive feedback and reinforcement will come from practicing the behavior.

By applying social learning theory, health promotion programs can use role models to demonstrate appropriate health behaviors. For example, in *Fakube Jarra,* a radio soap opera broadcast in The Gambia about three working-class families living in a fictional village of The Gambia, Fakube Jarra is the village wise man whom everyone turns to for advice. Of these three families, one does everything wrong, one balances their actions between right and wrong, and one family does everything right. The bad and good families make bad and good decisions, while the family in between sees the conflicting influences and often turns to Fakube Jarra for advice, who encourages them to make the right choices.

In one episode, for example, a married woman has difficulty getting pregnant after the husband becomes infected with a sexually transmitted disease (STD) during an extramarital affair. The husband blames the wife for their inability to have a child and threatens to leave her. On the advice of Fakube Jarra, the husband gets treated at a health center and the couple's infertility problem is solved. The clear message is that the man's STD infection caused the couple's infertility, and the behavior of the characters becomes the models that the audience can imitate.

The *Fakube Jarra* soap opera thus used social learning theory by providing role models that the audience could identify with and showed them adopting appropriate behaviors. Social learning theory offers a theoretical framework for designing health-related soap operas and other health communication programs. The last theory presented here focuses on individual beliefs about one's susceptibility to and perceived severity of a disease or illness.

Health Belief Model

The health belief model (HBM) (Becker, 1974; Rosenstock, 1974, 1990; Strecher and Rosenstock, 1997) states that behaviors change when people think that *(1)* they are at risk for contracting a disease, *(2)* it is severe, and *(3)* proposed remedies are cost–beneficial. The health belief model also states that "cues to action" can trigger health-related behavioral change. The health belief model is tested by measuring perceived severity, susceptibility, and cost–benefits, and then hypothesizing that those with higher scores on these variables will more likely change their behavior. The intervention is a cue to action to engage in the behavior.

Communication campaigns and information reported through the mass media or via word of mouth can provide a cue to action. Saba and others (1994) reported on a study that tested a communication campaign's ability to provide a cue to action for condom use as a measure for HIV/AIDS prevention in Peru. This study showed that individuals with high scores on the health belief index (the sum of the three perceptions mentioned above) were more likely to be influenced by the campaign than those with low scores on the index. Thus, the campaign may have provided a cue to action.

PERSPECTIVES

The seven theories discussed above are used frequently in health promotion, and are often supplemented with four perspectives, discussed below. These perspectives usually do not provide a set of testable hypotheses by themselves, but rather provide important information on the contexts of and influences on behavior. Theories often need to be applied with these perspectives in mind.

Ecological Perspectives

Most theories of behavior change focus on individual-level attributes and behaviors. Increasingly, though, researchers are focusing on communities, organizations, or groups as influences on behavior. This shift in focus from individuals to different levels of analysis has been termed an *ecological perspective,* which argues that individual behavior is understood better when viewed in the context of communities, organizations, policies, and societal norms (McElroy et al., 1988; Green et al., 1996; Stokols, 1996). These contexts are often beyond personal control, yet they influence behavior. The ecological perspective shifts the emphasis from individuals to a broader understanding of the environmental and social context of behavior and in so doing sometimes identifies barriers to behavior change.

In studies from the ecological perspective the following levels of analysis are typically considered: (Fig. 3–4): *(1)* individual (intra-individual) characteristics, *(2)* interpersonal, *(3)* institutional, *(4)* communal, and *(5)* societal. By including analyses at these levels, researchers can examine and incorporate various sources of influence on behavior in addition to an individual's attributes. Taking an ecological perspective on health behavior might lead researchers to look at governmental or organizational policies that present barriers to good health.

Sometimes health promotion programs will need to change the environment before individuals can change (Green et al., 1996). For example, nutrition promotion programs should ensure that nutritious food is available to be purchased or is offered in schools. From the ecological perspective, individuals may influence their environment, particularly when they organize into groups and organizations that engage in health promotion. Hence the ecological perspective is consistent with efforts to create programs that encourage individual and community empowerment (Green et al., 1996). When individuals feel empowered to change

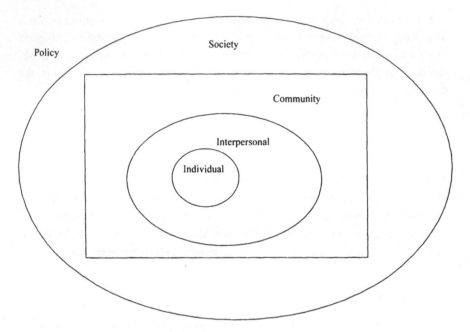

FIGURE 3–4. Ecological models specify multilevel influences on behavior.

their environments they gain control over the conditions that influence their behavior, leading to a sustained change in behavior. From an ecological perspective, self-efficacy, motivation, values, beliefs, and attitudes are important determinants of behavior change.

The limitation to the ecological perspective is its complexity. There are numerous ecological levels and interconnected systems that influence behavior, and measuring them in any one study seems problematic at best and nightmarish at worst. Few studies have been able to include ecological analysis and fewer still have been able to understand ecological levels well enough to create interventions to change them. Although many large programs attempt to change factors at other ecological levels, such as at the material, social, and human capital levels, all too often the evaluation is conducted only at the individual level of analysis.

Social Network Analysis

In the seven theories described, some attribute of individuals is specified as an important component to be changed by an intervention. In contrast, a paradigm has emerged that focuses on social networks and how they influence behavior.

By shifting the focus from individuals to networks, programs can create messages aimed at social networks. For example, a program designed to promote smoking cessation among adolescents might encourage a group of friends to quit together.

Network analysis provides the tools needed to assess the level and type of interpersonal communication about a new (or existing) product both before and after the program (Valente, 1996). Network indices offer a means of assessing whether the program was successful at increasing interpersonal communication and thus provide a measure of success, even though it may take years to change behavior. The outcome is determining the interpersonal communication about the targeted behavior; it thus becomes important to study what people said.

Network analysis provides techniques for measuring whether network characteristics influence behavior. For example, a study was conducted in Cameroon among women in voluntary associations to determine the factors that influenced their decision to try contraceptives. It was found that women who used contraceptives were more likely to report that they *thought* their close friends used contraceptives regardless of whether those friends reported that they used them (Valente et al., 1997).

One advantage of the network perspective is that it can be used to evaluate effects of health promotions on individuals, groups, and communities. In addition to determining whether interpersonal communication changed for individuals, network analysis shows whether the program affected communication patterns within a community or organization. For example, it may be that members of a rural community turn to their friends for information about proper nutritional habits. A promotional program could change this pattern of interpersonal communication so that individuals would seek out those who were knowledgeable about nutrition. The network analysis would reveal whether the program changed the pattern of whom people turned to for advice on nutrition (Stoebenau and Valente, 1999).

Although most researchers acknowledge a link between mass media influence and interpersonal communication, the integration of these approaches remains a challenge for scholars in the communication field (Chaffee and Mutz, 1988; Hawkins et al., 1988; Barnett and Danowski, 1992). Network analysis techniques can be incorporated into health promotion research by providing measures for interpersonal influence. For example, in an evaluation of a campaign in Bolivia designed to promote family planning and reproductive health, individuals who adopted use of contraceptives, with a *minority* of their close friends being contraceptive users, reported higher campaign exposure than those who adopted use with a *majority* of their close friends being users. It was speculated that the campaign substituted for interpersonal sources of information (Valente and Saba, 1998).

Social Marketing Perspective

Many health promotion programs use marketing principles to guide their activities. Social marketing, the use of marketing principles for promoting social goods, was launched when Wiebe (1951) wrote: "Why can't you sell brotherhood like you sell soap?" Wiebe (1951) reviewed successful and not-so-successful World War II era campaigns—one using Kate Smith to sell War Bonds, and one to recruit civil defense volunteers as well as others. Wiebe showed that marketing principles helped show why some campaigns succeeded and others did not.

Kotler and Zaltman (1971) expanded Wiebe's analysis by applying more fully marketing principles and theory. According to Kotler and Zaltman (1971), many early campaigns were based on what policy-makers perceived the needs of society to be. They state: "The marketing concept . . . calls for most of the effort to be spent on discovering the wants of a target audience and then creating the goods and services to satisfy them" (Kotler and Zaltman, 1971, p. 5). Unfortunately, with social products, determining those wants is not always easy. "*Social marketing* is the design, implementation, and control of programs calculated to influence the acceptability of social ideas and involving considerations of product planning, pricing, communication, distribution, and marketing research" (Kotler and Zaltman, 1971, p. 5).

Marketing theory provides a planning process useful for introducing and promoting new (and old) products (Kotler and Roberto, 1989). Social marketers are encouraged to conduct formative research (see Chapter 4) to understand the intended audience, conduct a market analysis to determine the optimal price at which the product should be offered, and then develop a brand strategy for the product that includes naming it and developing feasible distribution channels.

The four P's are central to social marketing: *(1) p*roduct (what is being sold), *(2) p*rice (at what cost both monetary and otherwise), *(3) p*lace (where and how it can be purchased), and *(4)* promotion (how consumers learn about and are persuaded to use it) (Kotler and Roberto, 1989). Social marketing strongly emphasizes research during each step in the planning process to inform decision-making. For example, when contemplating distribution channels, it is advised to research and test them beforehand. If problems occur during the campaign, marketers should be prepared to change the distribution strategy.

A major contribution of marketing research to the evaluation of health campaigns is the concept of *audience segmentation,* or the partitioning of an audience into distinct groups based on the audience's psychosociodemographic characteristics. The advantage of audience segmentation is that the population can be divided into smaller groups that are more cohesive and hence easier to understand. In most populations there is considerable variation in attitudes, beliefs, practices, and, importantly, media use. Consequently, groups differ in terms of the best ways to reach and persuade them. For example, a program promoting the benefits of exercise should be tailored to different age-groups.

Common audience segmentation variables are gender, age, education, socioeconomic status, geographic location, ethnicity, occupation, language, media preferences, and so on. Many of these variables overlap with one another and many different techniques are used to segment an audience. Audience segmentation typically occurs during design of the campaign so that the designers can target it for specific groups. Audience segmentation also occurs during the evaluation to determine if the campaign was more or less effective among specific groups.

The main difference between social marketing and health communication campaigns is that social marketing often concentrates on one product or service, whereas communication programs are often concerned with an entire class of products or ideas. Social marketers try to establish a strong market share for a particular commercial product within a domain, whereas a communication strategy may try to change the conception of that domain within the culture. For example, in the field of family planning, there may be social marketing campaigns to promote specific brands of condoms or pills, whereas a health communication campaign would promote the use of contraceptives—any contraceptive—to reduce unwanted fertility. The campaigns may complement one another and coordination of their messages is strongly encouraged; when messages are not clear or consistent, or where promotion of one product depends on disseminating negative information about another (e.g., condoms versus oral contraceptives), the audience can become confused, and probably neither program will be effective.

A second difference between social marketing and a health communication campaign is that social marketers devote as much attention to the distribution channels of the product as they do to the promotional campaign. Naturally, communication specialists tend to focus on the promotional campaign and concentrate on how to increase demand for a product and deemphasize the need to ensure that the product can be delivered to appropriate sales or other distributional outlets. From a communication perspective, if the demand is strong enough the market will provide the distributional mechanisms. While this may be true in the long run, it is wise to ensure that the audience can actually purchase or otherwise obtain the product being promoted. The social marketing perspective makes explicit the relationship between supply and demand factors in health behavior change.

Supply and Demand

Health promotion programs are often designed to generate demand for a product rather than to increase the supply of that product. *Supply* refers to the components of a product or service that involve making it available for consumption. For example, the supply side of family planning is the provision of contracep-

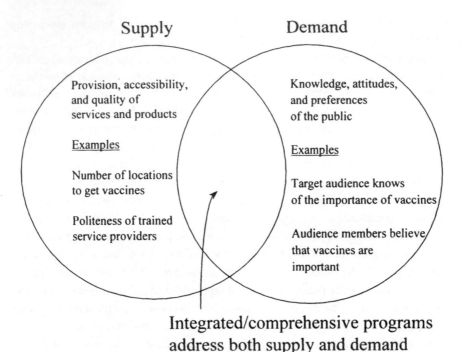

Supply   Demand

Provision, accessibility,   Knowledge, attitudes,
and quality of   and preferences
services and products   of the public

Examples   Examples

Number of locations
to get vaccines   Target audience knows
                                     of the importance of vaccines
Politeness of trained
service providers   Audience members believe
                                     that vaccines are
                                     important

Integrated/comprehensive programs
address both supply and demand

FIGURE 3–5. Supply and demand variables and interventions.

tive counseling and devices used to regulate fertility. The availability of condoms is a supply-side variable (Fig. 3–5), as is the availability of quality counseling and services.

Demand refers to the characteristics of the consumer population in terms of their desires and preferences for the service or product. For example, the degree to which a given population chooses to use contraceptives is their demand for them. Supply and demand factors interact in a dynamic way, each affecting the other. It is unwise to generate demand for products and services that cannot be supplied, and inappropriate to supply products for which there is no demand. An ideal program integrates supply and demand factors to obtain a synergy in supplying the services and products that are demanded. Programs implemented to increase demand should ensure that the supply of quality services are available to meet this demand.

USE AND SELECTION OF THEORY

The theories and perspectives presented here provide a brief glimpse of the theoretical landscape, yet many theories have been omitted. For example, some re-

TABLE 3–2. Theories of Behavior Change

THEORY	REFERENCE
Diffusion of innovations	Rogers, 1995
Hierarchy of effects	McGuire, 2001
Steps to behavior change	Piotrow et al., 1997
Stages of change	Prochaska et al., 1992
Social learning theory	Bandura, 1977
Theory of reasoned action	Fishbein and Ajzen, 1975
Health belief model	Becker, 1974
Perspectives	
Ecological factors	McElroy et al., 1988
Social networks	Valente, 1995
Social marketing	Kotler and Roberto, 1989
Supply and demand	

searchers argue that socioeconomic factors are the most important determinants of behavior. Smoking in the U.S., for example, tends to occur at higher rates among blue-collar workers than among the wealthy. Researchers should consult multiple theories (see Table 3–2) and not rely on only one behavior change theory or perspective. The world is complex and no one theory can be expected to explain fully the many factors that influence human behavior.

Theory is useful for describing behavior change and specifying the mechanisms thought to influence individual decision-making. Theory often plays a crucial role in the early and later stages of the evaluation because it informs design of both the program and evaluation. Theory is used in at least four different evaluation activities: *(1)* specification of goals and objectives,[1] *(2)* program design, *(3)* variable measurement, and *(4)* statistical analysis of data.

Program Design

Behavior change theory is used to design program strategies and messages. If research shows that individuals do not practice a health behavior, theory helps explain why. If research shows that people lack sufficient knowledge to adopt a specific behavior, then an information campaign can be launched to change that. Suppose individuals lack the self-efficacy needed to try a new practice. Using social learning theory, soap operas can be created in which characters model the desired behavior. Individuals who identify with these role models might develop increased self-efficacy to perform the behavior, thus facilitating behavior change.

[1]As discussed in Chapter 7, this directly influences the sample size and sample selection strategies.

In settings where individuals think they are not at risk for a disease, the health belief model may be used to design a campaign to communicate susceptibility.

In some cases, research has shown that interpersonal persuasion was necessary to change social norms regarding behaviors. For example, Lomas and others (1991) studied birth delivery practices and found that doctors automatically performed cesaeran births for mothers who had a previous cesaeran. The researchers wanted doctors to follow guidelines recommending that they try natural labor first before automatically performing C-sections. Lomas and others (1991) recruited local opinion leaders (other doctors) to be advocates for vaginal birth after C-section (VBAC). The intervention was successful, resulting in a 142% increase in VBAC. In this case, theory influenced the campaign strategy (using opinion leaders) rather than the campaign message. In addition to informing campaign strategy and messages, theory is used in variable measurement.

Variable Measurement and Survey Design

Theory is used to specify how variables should be measured by providing definitions and prior experiences. Definitions indicate how a variable should be measured by describing it. Prior studies provide examples of previous measurements. For example, anti-smoking program evaluations have a standard set of questions that are used to measure smoking frequency (Kovar, 2000). Smoking can be measured as any puff on a cigarette during a lifetime or whether the respondent has smoked a cigarette in the last week or month. Measurement is important since it influences the interpretation of study results. By reviewing other studies, evaluation results can be compared with those that have been conducted in other settings or on other populations.

Theory is also used to determine the variables to include in the study by indicating which ones should act as controls. So even though an evaluator may not be interested in a concept, if other studies have shown that it influences behavior then it should be measured. For example, studies among adolescents have shown that smoking by peers is associated with smoking and although an anti-smoking program may not address this specifically, the evaluator still needs to measure perceptions of peer smoking to control for it. After deciding on measurement techniques, evaluators use theory to set program goals and objectives.

Setting Goals and Objectives

Goals are general statements about what is to be achieved. For example, a goal for a communication campaign might be to inform the public about contraceptive options so that individuals can make informed decisions about reproduction. Goals set the general direction and intent of the campaign. *Objectives* are specific operational definitions within the goal. For example, a contraceptive cam-

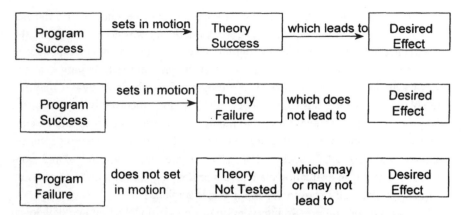

FIGURE 3–6. Weiss's view of program versus theory failure.

paign may set an objective to increase awareness of the availability of condoms to control fertility from 75% to 85%. Objectives should be SMART: *S*pecific, *M*easurable, *A*chievable, *R*ealistic, and *T*imely (Piotrow et al., 1997).

Objectives can be absolute or relative. Absolute ones are the difference between follow-up and baseline; relative ones are the difference divided by the baseline. The above example specified that the campaign would increase awareness from 75% to 85%, which is a 10 percentage point (absolute) increase, but is a 13.3% (relative) increase (10/75 = 13.3). When a percentage change is absolute, then it is a percentage *point* change, whereas if it is relative to the baseline measure, then the increase (or decrease) is a *percentage* change.

Goals and objectives are important for at least three reasons. First, they provide a benchmark for determining program success. Second, they provide incentives for staff to work toward, helping to focus activities on achieving them. Third, they provide a way to determine the sample size needed for the evaluation (Chapter 7). After a program has been designed, instruments developed, objectives set, and the program conducted, theory is used to conduct the evaluation.

Theory versus Program Failures

Weiss (1972) distinguished theory versus program failures. Figure 3–6 (Weiss, 1972, p. 38) shows three scenarios of program and theory success or failure. In the first scenario, a successful program sets in motion a theoretical process resulting in the desired outcome. In the second scenario, theory fails and the successful program sets in motion a process that did not result in the desired outcome. Here we have a successful intervention but do not detect an impact because the behavior change theory failed.

In the third scenario, because of a program failure, the intervention did not start an expected causal sequence; therefore, the theory was not tested. Thus, the congruence between theory and program is very important. A correspondence between the two increases the likelihood that the program will be judged a success by avoiding theory failures. If the program fails, the investigator may not be able to test theory, but if the theory fails, one may incorrectly conclude that the program failed. To avoid program failures, audience research should be conducted and community involvement elicited in the strategic planning process (Dignan and Carr, 1992; Backer et al., 1992; Andreason, 1995; Siegel and Donner, 1998). Also, an evaluation plan should be developed for monitoring program implementation and exposure by the intended audience.

To avoid theory failure, an intervention or impact model should be developed that translates study concepts into hypotheses (Baumann et al., 1991; Rossi and Freeman, 1993). The *impact model* consists of causal hypotheses that specify the behavioral change expected from the campaign and any covariates that influence the process. The model can be diagrammed by showing how the concepts, including the campaign, relate to one another.

Theory Selection

There are many theories of behavior change, much disagreement on what constitutes theory, and a pressing need to use theory in program evaluation. How does an evaluator select a theory? The choice depends partly on the behavior being targeted, as some behaviors can be studied with certain theories that are used repeatedly. Repeated use of the same theory or perspective can result in a research area becoming fallow and of little interest to new investigators (Kuhn, 1970). Consequently, consideration of new and novel theories and perspectives is encouraged.

Theories are often selected because they were developed for a particular behavior or used in the past, or because the researcher is familiar with it. There are at least four influences on theory selection: *(1)* formative research conducted on the topic, *(2)* literature reviews and meta-analyses, *(3)* prior experience or training, and *(4)* influence from peers. Although formative research is often the best reason to select a theory, prior experience and precedent are also good justifications. If a theory was used in the past, the evaluator has experience to guide the measurement and anticipated effects as well as plausible interpretations of how the program influenced the audience. If a theory is chosen because the researcher is experienced with it, then at least the researcher can be confident that it was used wisely. Indeed, as this chapter has shown, there is a limited array of theories to choose from. Once a theory or theories are selected to guide the evaluation, the components are put into a conceptual framework that outlines how the variables relate to one another. The researcher then extracts from the conceptual framework the specific causal hypotheses to be tested.

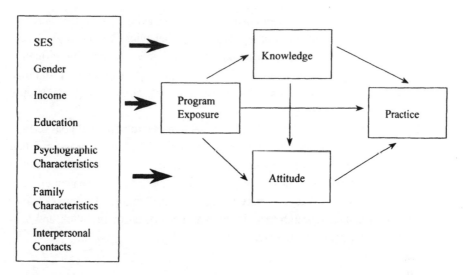

FIGURE 3–7. Conceptual model of program impact. SES, socioeconomic status.

Figure 3–7 depicts the general theoretical framework used in this book. This program impact model posits that sociodemographic variables, such as socioeconomic status, gender, and so on, influence program exposure and knowledge, attitudes, and practices (KAP). The exposure variable, along with knowledge and attitudes, interact with each other and perhaps lead to a change in behavior. Campaign exposure directly influences KAP; knowledge influences attitudes; and attitude influences practice. Figure 3–7 is a simplified depiction of the expected evaluation results—a linear model with no feedback loops. The conceptual framework specifies the variables to be measured in the model and expected relationships between them. While there are certainly exceptions to this model that would contain recursive links (Chaffee and Roser, 1986; Valente et al., 1998b), it is a general model that can be used to evaluate health promotion programs.

SUMMARY

This chapter surveyed some theories used to evaluate health promotion programs. Space constraints limit the number and scope of theories that can discussed, but the intention was to familiarize researchers with behavioral theories and explain their role in evaluation, not to provide a comprehensive review. The major theories discussed were diffusion of innovations and the hierarchy of effects, both of which specify a sequence of steps in behavior change. Also briefly discussed were Prochaska's stages of change, theories on attitude and behavior linkages, and the health belief model.

Four perspectives were presented that are not behavior change theories, but describe important influences and constraints on behavior. The ecological perspective focuses on community, organizational, and policy factors that influence behavior and should not be ignored when developing and evaluating programs. Other perspectives discussed were social networks, social marketing, and supply versus demand.

The use of theory for program design, variable measurement, and goal setting, was also discussed. Theory can sometimes distinguish whether the program failed because of a program or a theory failure. The factors that influence the selection of a theory were also presented. For each theory, there are different interpretations and perspectives that can make using them challenging. The next chapter introduces formative research techniques that are qualitative in nature and useful for designing program messages.

Chapter Four

Formative and Qualitative Research

Formative research is conducted before a program is designed in order to understand a population's existing knowledge, attitudes, beliefs, values, motivations, norms, expectations, and practices. It ensures that *(1)* a promotional program is necessary, and *(2)* the messages created are appropriate for the need
identified. Although formative research does not necessarily have to be qualitative, it usually is. This chapter discusses how qualitative research is used to design programs and, in some cases, evaluate them. The perspective advocated here
is that program designers should actively involve the audience in program creation and message development.

Researchers should conduct appropriate formative research to improve their
chances of success. If program designers listen to the needs and desires of the audience, use them to help design the program, and then pretest it with them, it is
more likely to be successful. Thus, formative research makes the impact evaluation easier because the program addresses needs in a way understood by the audience. Furthermore, formative research provides the opportunity to pilot-test evaluation instruments so that they provide the necessary information. It is wise to
conduct considerable formative research and may even be unethical not to do so.

Mody (1991) argues by analogy for the audience participation approach in the
field of development communication: "What would we say about physicians who
prescribed medicine without examining their patients? Are development media

producers doing something similar as they work to promote the health of their nations?" (Mody, 1991, p. 49). No matter how talented the media producers and campaign designers, if the campaign does not resonate with the audience and meet their needs, it will not be effective.

In some cases, qualitative research is used to evaluate programs and in many cases it is used to redesign or refocus program messages or strategy. This is particularly true in longitudinal studies in which there is time to change a program on the basis of formative research that has been conducted during the program (Rice and Foote, 1989). Qualitative research is an essential component to health promotion program evaluation and should be conducted by trained qualitative researchers.

Guba and Lincoln (1981) argue that qualitative tools such as unobtrusive observation provide the opportunity to measure the real-life context of social programs, how they are implemented, and how they affect people's lives. *Observation is particularly important for programs that have direct contact with the intended beneficiaries of the program.* Programs with direct client contact may be highly variable, depending on the program implementers and the settings in which programs are executed. Guba and Lincoln (1981) refer to this as *naturalistic inquiry,* concentrating on understanding the implementation and impact of a program in its "natural" setting.

Good qualitative research has four characteristics: *(1)* systematic, *(2)* iterative, *(3)* flexible, and *(4)* triangulate (SIFT). It is systematic because the same procedures are followed in a variety of settings. It is iterative because analysis is ongoing, including new information and results as they are discovered. It is flexible because the researcher can adapt to new information that emerges during data collection. It should triangulate by using at least three different measurement techniques so that multiple methods are used to provide answers (Miles and Huberman, 1994; Bernard, 1995).

These advantages to qualitative research make it preferred over quantitative methods for formative research. This chapter discusses four kinds of qualitative research: *(1)* in-depth interviews, *(2)* intercept interviews, *(3)* focus group discussions, and *(4)* observational studies. Other types of qualitative methods that bridge qualitative and quantitative methods are also presented. The chapter ends with a discussion of other data sources, such as TV ratings, that should be considered when designing a campaign evaluation.

QUALITATIVE METHODS

In-depth Interviews

In-depth interviews represent probably one of the richest sources of information available to researchers. In-depth interviews are semi-structured interviews between researchers and members of the audience or intended population. They can take as little as one-half hour or can last for 1 to 2 hours, and be extended in repeated encounters. The researcher should prepare a list of open-ended questions before conducting the interview and this guide should be fairly consistent throughout all the interviews conducted on a particular topic.

In-depth interviews should be open-ended so that the respondent is free to give opinions on topics that may be tangential to the topic of the interview. Allowing the respondent freedom to answer questions in this way provides the opportunity to learn about the topic in unanticipated ways. By engaging in an open-ended dialogue, the conversation between the researcher and subject can wander to topics that are salient. In-depth interviews also identify the words and phrases that people use to describe their behavior.

For example, in a study of the factors that influence injection drug users to use a needle exchange program, it was discovered that many did not use it because they could buy clean needles on the street at locations that were often more convenient. Hence, it was discovered that the needle exchange program provided a valuable service to them, but it did so through intermediaries referred to as satellite exchangers (Valente et al., 1998a). Although the satellite exchange activity was known at the time, it was the in-depth interviews that revealed its importance.

An important aspect of successful in-depth interviews is rapport between the researcher and the subject. One means of establishing rapport is for the interviewer and respondent to have similar characteristics. For example, it is usually recommended that the researcher and subject have similar ethnicity, gender, and age. In studies of contraceptive use, for example, same-gender interviews are likely to be preferred while in studies of automobile safety belt use it may be much less important.

There are many techniques used for successful interviewing. First, it is helpful to start the interview with casual conversation about non-controversial topics to begin to build rapport and develop a conversational rhythm. The interviewer should introduce him- or herself and provide a general background on the purpose of the interview. This can be somewhat scripted. The interviewer should note the time, location, and environment of the interview.

In the second phase, the interviewer explores the topic, using a set of open-ended questions. The interview should help determine attitudes and feelings about the behavior being discussed, prior experiences with it, how and when the respondent first became aware of it, and so on. The interview may wander across a variety of topics. Good interviewers know how to explore seemingly tangential topics and probe the respondent to provide rich information.

In the third phase, closure, the interviewer asks any important questions that have not yet been answered or discussed. These questions are asked because they are important, yet were missed or not answered fully. This phase should also provide the opportunity for any other comments that were not mentioned. At the end of this stage, the interviewer thanks the respondent and asks if there are any other questions.

Once the interview is completed, the researchers should review their notes and expand them from memory. If the interview was recorded, the tape should be checked immediately so that it can be partially reconstructed if there was a recording problem. Interviews should be recorded whenever possible, since note-taking can be a distraction.

In-depth interviews should be conducted among enough respondents to get a coherent picture of the audience's knowledge, attitudes, and beliefs. Quantitative information is usually not collected during the interview since generalization and tabulation are not the goals. Subjects, however, should be stratified according to gender, age, and other relevant variables so that some variation among the interviews is available. Variables pertinent to the audience segmentation (Chapter 3) should be included in the segmentation of the qualitative interviews.

There is no magic number or formula that determines the number of interviews to conduct. Many researchers conduct interviews until they become repetitious. Others conduct two to four interviews per relevant audience segment. For example, for a campaign targeted to men and women ages 15–34 interviews among both men and women and among various age-groups such as 15–19, 20–24, 25–29, and 30–34 would be needed. If 2 interviews per group were conducted, then 16 interviews (2 genders × 4 age-groups × 2 per group) would be required.

Intercept or "Person-on-the-Street" Interviews

Many formative research studies are conducted by interviewing people in public locations such as shopping malls, movies theaters, and city plazas. Researchers determine locations for the intended audience and then choose times and places to conduct the interviews. For example, an audience of married women with children might be interviewed at toy stores.

Intercept interviews are useful for getting a sense of public perceptions about a product or issue. Although the data will have some bias, since the respondents. who happen to be shopping on that particular day and in that particular location are likely to be different from randomly selected persons from the population, this method can be useful for pretesting instruments, messages, and materials.

To improve the quality of intercept interview data, a number of steps should be taken: (1) approval of all relevant persons should be obtained (e.g., from the mall owners and shopkeepers); (2) the survey should be pretested so that it reads properly, and changed on the basis of early results; and (3) the days, times, and interviewers should be varied so that a broader sampling of respondents is obtained. One of the main limitations of intercept interviews is that interviewers select whom they approach for an interview. The interviewer will often loiter until they see someone who looks approachable. This selectivity will bias the results from intercept interviews and should be controlled by establishing randomization procedures. For example, every tenth person who enters a mall might be interviewed, thus minimizing the sample bias.

Focus Group Discussions

Focus group discussions (FGDs) are "a carefully planned discussion designed to obtain perceptions on a defined area of interest in a permissive, non-threatening environment" (Krueger, 1994, p. 18; also see Debus, 1990). The basic procedures for FGDs were introduced by Merton and colleagues (1956) and have not changed much over the years. These discussions are used widely in marketing and advertising research to test new concepts and products and pilot-test advertising campaigns. The FGDs can provide informative, valid, and reliable results in a timely and cost-effective manner.

Participants should be recruited at least 2 weeks before the focus group convenes. They should be similar to one another so that they feel comfortable with one another (Krueger, 1994). For example, a FGD on smoking should be conducted among smokers. Participants should not know one another. They are asked to come to a place reserved for the focus group and offered an incentive to participate. Researchers should recruit more participants than needed, since some cancel at the last minute (a 30% cancellation rate is common).

Each group should have 4 to 12 people, and ideally between 8 and 10 (Krueger, 1994). The discussions should be conducted by a trained moderator who follows a scripted guide, consisting of open-ended questions designed to generate discussion. The moderator facilitates and guides the discussion. The FGDs can be very successful when there are specific information needs that respondents can speak knowledgeably and openly about.

The focus group begins with an introductory icebreaker to get participants relaxed. Sometimes participants are invited to introduce themselves before beginning the discussion. The moderator should encourage a free flow of ideas, attitudes, opinions, and experiences, but should not appear to be asking a predetermined series of questions. The discussions generally last about 2 hours.

Focus group discussions have a number of advantages and disadvantages (Krueger, 1994). They are socially oriented, flexible, cheap, and quick and have face validity. Their disadvantages are that they can be difficult to organize and analyze, they require trained moderators; and their results can be unpredictable. As Krueger states, "focus groups are valid if they are used carefully for a problem that is suitable for focus group inquiry" (Krueger, 1994, p. 41).

Focus group discussions are often used by program designers to understand the audience's perspective on a particular behavior. For example, a program for smoking cessation might conduct FGDs among quitters to learn how they quit. The data can then be used to design the program and the accompanying evaluation instruments. The FGDs are also used to test the program before it is implemented. This pilot test provides a check to see if the program is understandable and appealing.

Through FGDs designers can learn the language the audience uses to discuss a topic, which is useful for message development. For example, FGDs of the intended audience for Viagra revealed that men did not like the word "impotence," but instead preferred the medical abbreviation "ED," which stands for erectile dysfunction. Subsequent ad campaigns promoting Viagra advertised it as a cure for ED without mentioning impotence.

Focus group discussions are also used to evaluate programs both during and after their implementation. Participants can be asked about a behavior and any information they may recall about it. In other cases, the program is shown and group members provide their opinions about it.

Focus group discussions work because humans are social animals. The FGDs provide the opportunity for people to listen to others and then react to these opinions. The give-and-take established in an open-ended group discussion can be illuminating and people often find that they have attitudes and opinions that they did not realize they had. It is the creation of the dynamic exchange of ideas and opinions that signifies an excellent FGD. While FGDs are not a panacea to all research needs, they are used extensively and can provide rich information.

The chief drawback to FGDs is that they can provide misleading information in three ways: *(1)* the group may be overly influenced by one or a few people, *(2)* people may be reluctant to voice opinions that deviate from what is normative, or *(3)* the topic may not be of sufficient interest for participants to generate opinions. These drawbacks are sometimes unavoidable but can be offset by a trained moderator who can recognize and minimize them.

Many programs use both FGDs and in-depth interviews to understand attitudes, norms, and beliefs about an issue before designing a program. This is strongly recommended when the topic consists of a sensitive topic that may be influenced by community norms. For example, in a study of adolescent attitudes toward sexuality and premarital sex in Malawi, researchers collected data both from focus groups and through in-depth interviews (Helitzer-Allen et al., 1994). The authors "found that the FGDs elicited more socially "correct" answers and produced good data on social norms, but not very good data on deviations from those norms. By contrast, in-depth, one-on-one interviews were necessary for eliciting good data on actual knowledge and experience" (Helitzer-Allen et al., 1994, p. 80).

Observational Studies

Observational studies are obtrusive and unobtrusive measures in which researchers watch and record behaviors in their natural settings. Observational studies are often used to understand barriers to behavior change and the real-life conditions that influence behavior. Observational studies can be declared or undeclared. In a *declared* study, researchers let subjects know that they will be observed. For example, researchers may tell nurses and receptionists at a hospital that they are studying in-take procedures and will observe the way clients are admitted. In *undeclared studies*, notification is not made and the researcher observes behavior often without subjects' knowledge.

One type of undeclared observational study is a *mystery client study,* which is conducted by researchers posing as clients for the product being promoted. For example, in a study of pharmacy distribution of clean needles for injection drug users, researchers posed as drug users trying to purchase syringes in pharmacies. The researchers discovered that many pharmacists did not want to sell syringes to them even though the pharmacists were required by law to do so. In family planning studies, researchers can pose as individuals interested in getting family planning information or obtaining family planning methods (Huntington and Schuler, 1993). It is also possible to hire non-researchers to pose as clients and have them collect the data. Such studies can be used to determine whether service providers are polite and sympathetic, provide accurate information, and give clients the products they want. Another variation of this technique is for providers to act as clients at other facilities so that they can experience firsthand the client's perspective.

Quantitative Analysis of Qualitative Data

Several techniques are available to quantify qualitative data. For example, interview transcripts can be analyzed to find links between different concepts. Many people may mention fear and cancer together, indicating that many people are afraid of getting cancer.

To analyze text from in-depth interviews and other sources, computer programs such as NVIVO can be used. This program allows the researcher to highlight text phrases and assign codes to them. The researcher can then determine how certain elements in the interviews relate to one another and try to construct a model of the textual data. Typically, a researcher reads through all transcripts and develops initial categories. Then he/she will code the text into these categories, refining them during the coding process. NVIVO constructs a diagram of concepts nested within one another, and depicts how they relate to one another (see Appendix A for website information to get qualitative data analysis software).

Although this type of qualitative research is challenging and time consuming, it provides a rich, in-depth understanding of the data. Like quantitative research, it requires considerable training, and researchers are constantly developing new methods to improve it. There are also numerous techniques such as free-listing and pile- or Q-sorting that can be used as aids in in-depth interviewing (Bernard, 1995, 2000; Gittelsohn et al., 1996).

Recording Technology

In-depth interviews and FGDs should be audio recorded. The audio recording provides a record that can be reviewed later and shared with other researchers. Audio recording is cheap and is a wise investment. Moreover, recording alleviates the need to take copious notes during data collection and instead enables the researcher to focus on what's being said. Detailed analysis usually requires transcripts.

Experience has shown that recording is unobtrusive, as subjects generally ignore the tape recorder. More than one interview has been lost because a researcher mistakenly believed it was being recorded; the LED lights were on, flickering according to the volume in the interview, but the pause button had been pressed. Tape recorders should be checked and re-checked before, during, and after a session, and back-up batteries, tapes, and recorders should be readily available. Someone other than the moderator should take notes.

MESSAGE/MATERIALS TESTING

Focus group discussions and interviews are often used to pretest messages and materials. After a program has been designed, it is essential to pretest it on the audience. The pretest shows whether the audience will understand, like, and/or be motivated by the materials. Pretesting is crucial to the program and should indicate whether (1) the program should be changed, (2) some aspects should be modified, or (3) it can be implemented as is.

Pretesting should be conducted at multiple stages, when (1) the concept is being developed, (2) the first materials, such as the storyboards, are developed, and (3) the program is ready for implementation. Conducting pilot tests during stages one and two is difficult since there are few materials to use for the subjects to react to. Nonetheless, small pilot tests at this stage can ensure that the program designers are on track and can save considerable expense later.

The most critical pilot test is that before the program is launched, when designers have the first spots, episodes, or materials ready to be disseminated. A small sample of respondents can be recruited and exposed to the materials. Afterwards, they should be interviewed and asked whether they liked it and understood it, and whether it would motivate them to perform the desired action. It is also possible to develop different versions of the materials and have them select which one they prefer.

Pilot testing can be conducted both as in-depth interviews and FGDs. Researchers can disguise the materials to determine whether it appeals to the audience under more life-like conditions where it will compete with other messages. For example, TV commercials can be embedded in a stream of other programming to disguise them. Researchers will then ask about the other programming as if it were the object of study, and then casually ask about the commercials.

Researchers can vary the type and quantity of the program that the pilot-test audience is exposed to. These data can then be analyzed to determine whether the program was effective under laboratory conditions. It is important that researchers get reactions from the target population before the program is launched to avoid implementing an unappealing or misinterpreted one.

Siegel and Doner (1998) add that sometimes professionals should review materials before they are disseminated so that *(1)* the materials are accurate and in accordance with expert opinion, and *(2)* the researchers can testify to their veracity should controversy emerge later. In addition to these qualitative research techniques, there are quantitative techniques that are sometimes used at the formative stage. Three research techniques—simulations, ratings data, and content analysis—provide quantitative data that can be used to inform program development or monitor its implementation.

QUANTITATIVE FORMATIVE RESEARCH

Simulations

Simulations are systematic hypothetical scenarios extrapolated from existing conditions to process "what-if" scenarios. The advanced processing capabilities of computers has resulted in a growth in the number and variety of computer simulations used to develop theoretical models. Simulations can be used to think through theoretical models of behavior. However, the process of creating simulations can draw researchers away from collecting empirical data. The important test of a simulation is how well the assumptions and rules built into the simulation represent to reality.

Researchers use simulations to study the process of behavior change. For example, a simulation might try to estimate the amount of time it takes for particular information or behavior to flow through an organization. The parameters would include the rate of interpersonal communication conversion and the acceleration expected from a promotional program. The simulation would show how long it would take for everyone to become aware of and adopt the new behavior.

Simulations can also be used to extrapolate information from existing findings. For example, suppose a researcher finds that a small pilot program increases a behavior by 10% in one community. The researcher can extrapolate that finding to a larger population and estimate the degree of impact expected if the program were to be expanded. Simulations are rarely used to study health promotion since there are already many real-world experiences to study.

Ratings and Coverage Data

Evaluation research often entails documenting the amount of media coverage and advertising on a topic, regardless of whether it is part of a campaign. Ratings and coverage data track what's out there in the media marketplace. *Ratings and coverage data* represent the type, reach, and frequency of media attention on an issue. Ratings data are the size of audience for a particular program, advertisement, or channel, usually presented as a proportion of all households or people and then separately as a proportion of all relevant households. For example, a TV show rating is the percent of all households that watched it, while the share is the percent of viewers who were watching TV at that time. Ratings data thus provide a measure of campaign *reach*.

Frequency is the number of exposures, on average, each individual received. Interviews are conducted to measure frequency, which includes the number of different commercials each person recognized and estimates of how many commercials each person saw. For example, ratings data for a TV advertising campaign promoting safety belts in a 3-month period would indicate how many people were watching TV when the ads were broadcast. Subsequent interviews would determine how many people the ads reached and the average number of times they were exposed to the ads.

There are a variety of services available for collecting ratings and coverage data, most being available electronically. Siegel and Doner (1998) provide a list and the websites of the most prominent U.S. tracking services by medium: for radio, Arbitron; for magazines, Mediamark; for television, Nielsen; and for newspapers, Standard Rate and Data Service (see Appendix A for website addresses). Campaigns that use mass media should get ratings data for the programs or advertisements aired as one means of ensuring that the campaign reached the audience. The reach and frequency data obtained through a ratings or other monitoring service can then be compared with that reported by the surveys.

Many campaigns, however, do not rely simply on their own programs, but rather interact with the media in such a way that media coverage of a topic may not be controlled. In such cases, researchers should scan the media coverage to determine what is being communicated to the public. Scanning should occur before, during, and after a campaign is broadcast to document competing messages and determine whether the campaign generated additional media coverage.

Content Analysis

Content analysis is a technique used to quantify programs and messages communicated via the mass media and can be performed on TV programs, films, newspapers, radio, letters or other written documents, or just ab . ' any communication. Content analysis can be used to determine how the media portray and cover issues and verify that a campaign was conducted in the manner intended.

Content analysis is an unobtrusive research technique (Webb et al., 1966) used to study phenomenan without interacting with the population being studied. Content analysis typically consists of the following steps: (1) deciding on the universe of messages or units to be studied (e.g., the number of newspaper stories, TV shows, etc.), (2) selecting a sample from that universe, (3) constructing a coding scheme to quantify the messages, (4) coding the content, and (5) analyzing and interpreting the data. It generally requires a team of researchers to conduct content analysis since the volume of material is usually quite large. It is also necessary to have at least one person and perhaps more people code at least some of the same text so that intercoder reliability can be established.

Construction of a coding scheme for content analysis is difficult. For example, a study of alcohol consumption portrayal on daytime TV soap operas would require an enumeration of the universe of all daytime TV soap operas. First a random sample of shows would have to be taped, then the coding scheme would be used to collect data to test hypotheses concerning the portrayal of alcohol consumption.

The coding scheme should be taxonomic to allow researchers to capture as much data as possible about each program. Coding sheets should record the show's name and time of broadcast, and when and under what conditions a drink was taken. They should capture information surrounding the drink event: who did it, where, what the person drank, how many drinks accompanied the one just taken, who was with the person when he or she took the drink, and so on. There is a considerable amount of data concerning the event that could and should be recorded.

Theory and the hypotheses guide the data collection procedures. Since there is a lot of information in any show, the data needed for hypothesis tests and, hence, coding should be specified in advance, otherwise the researchers will be coding a lot of useless information. In the alcohol consumption example, testing a hypothesis on the relationship between alcohol and stress would require data on the type and degree of stress that accompanied all drinking, but not necessarily data on alcohol costs.

Data analyses and reporting typically consist of frequency counts and comparisons. The alcohol study would report the amount and variety of drinking associated with the demographic characteristics of the characters. A significant association between drinking and stress would indicate support for the hypothesis. The data may also be used to report time trends or more complicated associations between constructs identified in the analysis. For additional information on content analysis, consult Berelson (1952) and Krippendorf (1980).

A recent study by Roberts and colleagues (1999) used content analysis to determine the degree of substance abuse in popular movies and music. The study showed that consumption of illicit drugs, alcohol, tobacco, and over-the-counter/prescription medicines was ubiquitous. "Alcohol and tobacco appeared in more than 90% of the movies and illicit drugs appeared in 22%" (Roberts et al., 1999, p. 1).

Case Studies

A *case study* is an in-depth description of the activities, processes, and events that happened during a program (Yin, 1989). Case studies are used both to inform the program design and to evaluate it. They are appropriate when the program is unique and generalization is unlikely. A series of related case studies, however, may lead to some generalization.

Case studies are conducted using three primary means of data collection: *(1)* observation, *(2)* interviews with key personnel, and *(3)* document review. In a typical case study, the researcher becomes familiar with the organization or coalitions implementing the program. As it unfolds, observations and interviews with key participants are conducted. Program documents, such as memos, reports, background documents, are identified and catalogued. Most case studies describe a unique program at one place and time. Some researchers specialize in case study methodology and may conduct numerous related cases to develop a body of research.

Case studies are used when a program *(1)* is unique and unrelated to other activities, *(2)* is complicated and other data collection unwieldy, *(3)* addresses a small and/or unique population, *(4)* does not have a clear goal or objective, or *(5)* consists of multiple sites in which context, environment, or approach differ. Case studies can be useful for evaluating programs that address unique or short-term problems. For example, a campaign might be created to inform a community about a temporary problem with the water supply. A complex study design may not be appropriate given time and resource constraints, but an evaluation is still desired. A case study that documents campaign development, implementation, and effectiveness may be the most appropriate methodology.

Case studies are also used when the program and/or the evaluation data needed are too complex (GAO/PEMD, 1991a, p. 40). Complex programs that may require individuals to visit many sites to receive the information and services needed to ensure program success may have to rely on case studies as the only methodology. For example, suppose a treatment plan required that patients visit different offices accompanied by certified assistants. Interviewing patients about which offices they visited and when and how they visited them would be burdensome to the clients, but a case study that followed several clients through the system would provide a good evaluation.

A third use of case studies is when a program serves few people, but an evaluation is still warranted. In such cases, sampling and data collection may not feasible or practical, but some determination of program implementation and impact is desired. For example, suppose a lobbying organization created materials for legislatures of a state government. Interviewing the legislators would be difficult, but a case study of how a few legislators used the materials would be feasible.

A fourth use of case studies is evaluation of a program without clear objectives or goals (Yin, 1989). Some programs are created or modified in such a way that the goal of the program is unclear, even though it may be widely claimed to be a good and effective program. A case study can document the program's activities and may help set new objectives.

Finally, case studies can be used to evaluate a program being implemented in multiple sites in which the approach, environment, or context is different. In such situations, it may not be possible to quantitatively characterize differences in environment such as quality of staff implementation. A case study of the context of the various implementation environments may provide a more valid evaluation of the program.

USING FORMATIVE TECHNIQUES FOR OUTCOME EVALUATION

The qualitative techniques discussed in this chapter provide the depth of understanding needed to develop a program that will appeal to the audience and motivate changes in behavior. Qualitative techniques are also used to pilot test messages and materials. Quantitative techniques, discussed in later chapters, are then used to determine impact or changes in outcomes to document the percentage of behavior change. It is possible, and indeed recommended, to also use qualitative data to supplement the quantitative data. In some cases, qualitative data can be used for impact evaluation. The reasons include *(1)* cost constraints, *(2)* the program is small, *(3)* quantitative data are impossible to get, *(4)* the qualitative research is a complement to the quantitative data, and *(5)* to collect anecdotal data that may be more persuasive and compelling in the media or policy arena than the quantitative analysis.

The costs associated with quantitative research can be high when one considers the cost of instrument development, data collection, and analysis. Consequently, small programs with limited budgets may conduct FGDs or in-depth interviews to get feedback on the program. These data may provide some lessons learned and some sense of effect. The value placed on qualitative evidence varies greatly since some designers, policy-makers, and evaluators prefer qualitative and narrative presentations whereas others exhibit an almost religious zeal on quantitative results.

Small programs not expected to have a large effect may also lend themselves to qualitative evaluation. Such programs may be a pilot test or one in a series of activities cumulatively expected to bring about the desired behavior change. Although not expected to cause behavior change itself, proper implementation still needs to be documented.

Qualitative impact evaluation is also used for programs that address sensitive issues, such as abortion, where it may be difficult to collect valid or reliable data on pertinent attitudes and behaviors.

The best use of qualitative research techniques for outcome evaluation is to complement an existing quantitative outcome evaluation. Researchers are encouraged to conduct interviews and focus groups that can be used to "tell the story" that the quantitative data document. Moreover, the qualitative research may uncover aspects of the program's effect that are not discernable from the quantitative study. Finally, qualitative data can be used to understand quantitative results that may be anomalous or counterintuitive.

Qualitative data often provide anecdotal evidence of a program's impact. Anecdotes are often surreptitious, but provide unexpected evidence that may be seen as more credible by policy-makers or outside agencies. Anecdotes may be gathered formally during an interview or focus group and informally during chance encounters in everyday life. Precisely because the anecdote is unsolicited, a policy-maker may give credence to it. For example, suppose a policy-maker hears from a friend at a dinner party that the friend was influenced by a radio program. The policy-maker may feel that the campaign was a success.

Qualitative research has many strengths and is an important element in any research endeavor. Many people feel that qualitative research is easier to conduct than quantitative research. This is not true. Qualitative research may be more difficult to conduct than quantitative research because the quantitative researcher has carefully specified rules that dictate data collection, management, and interpretation. Qualitative research, on the other hand, is more interpretive and takes more experience. Like evaluation itself, qualitative work is sometimes as much art as science and therefore sometimes depends on intuition and creativity.

SUMMARY

This chapter reviewed qualitative and non–survey-based methods used in health promotion and evaluation research. Many of these techniques are used primarily in the formative stage of program development to understand behavior. The main techniques presented were in-depth interviews and focus group discussions. These two qualitative methodologies can provide rich, detailed information on when, why, how, where, and with whom people engage in behaviors.

More importantly, these qualitative techniques can provide data that are easily understood, and provide it in a timely manner. The researcher can communicate the research to other project teams with little delay. Often the program designers understand the data clearly since it is presented in non-technical language. The amount of qualitative research and number of interviews or focus groups can be adjusted to fit available budgets.

This chapter also discussed the use of qualitative techniques for pilot testing. Researchers can arrange focus group discussions to test messages and materials by showing them to the intended audience and getting their reactions and suggestions. Finally, other research techniques (simulations, content analysis, case studies) and data sources (ratings) useful for comprehensive program evaluation were discussed. The chapter closed with a discussion of the use of qualitative research for outcome evaluation. Naturally, most evaluations will not involve all of these research techniques and data sources, but a well-trained evaluator needs to be aware of them and know when to take advantage of opportunities that increase the accuracy and strength of the evaluation. The various techniques outlined in this chapter will often complement the process and outcome research presented in the next two chapters.

Chapter Five

Process Evaluation

Process evaluation is the research conducted to understand a program's creation, dissemination, and, in some cases, effects. Process evaluation is also referred to as *implementation research, utilization research,* and/or *program monitoring.* Process evaluation collects data to *(a)* document program implementation, *(b)* make mid-program revisions, *(c)* conduct outcome analysis, and *(d)* replicate the program. In sum, process evaluation "is concerned with documenting and analyzing the way a program operates, to assist in interpreting program outcomes, and to inform future program planning" (Dehar et al., 1993, p. 211).

There are few studies on process evaluation because evaluators often treat programs and campaigns as black boxes, with emphasis on whether they are effective rather than on the reasons for their success. Evaluators assume that programs were implemented as intended and with little variation across settings. Process evaluation is often overlooked in program evaluation because researchers assume that everyone will get the same message. This logic, however, neglects some critical factors. First, it ignores the importance of documenting how a particular program was produced and the decisions that influenced message production. Some programs contain messages that are inappropriate for the audience; documenting how they were created helps avoid such problems in the future.

Second, programs often consist of more than just one message. Programs use many media to reach different audience segments. Documenting which media reach which individuals with what frequency is critically important to understanding how the program did or did not reach its objectives. Also, different individuals process messages differently. Although a program may disseminate its messages in such a way that everyone can be exposed to them, people vary greatly in the degree to which they pay attention to these messages.

A third reason that process research is overlooked is that it is most useful when programs fail or are implemented poorly. Implementation data are less useful when a program is implemented as intended since the data simply confirm expectations. In contrast, when a program is implemented poorly, process data are useful as an explanation for why it failed. These barriers to process research have given way to a recognition that process research should be conducted to document program implementation.

This chapter defines terms and issues important in process research. Six points at which to conduct it are presented, followed by sections on how to conduct it. The chapter closes with a discussion on the distinction between process and impact research.

Two common measures used in health promotion program process research are fidelity and dose. *Fidelity* refers to the degree to which a program is implemented as planned. Fidelity may determine a program's success, since many programs lose their fidelity over time or when implemented in diverse settings. As programs expand and are replicated, they often change in unexpected ways, making them less effective. Conversely, many programs are successful because implementors can adapt them to local needs. These adaptations may be replicated in other settings, creating successes instead of failures. Thus implementation fidelity has an inherent contradiction: there is value in adaptation, but there may also be costs and decreased effectiveness.

Dose is the degree of program exposure or intensity of its delivery. Dose is likely to vary directly with effect. Dose should be measured during program implementation to document the amount of program material being created and disseminated.

Researchers should monitor the program during its implementation to measure fidelity and dose. These monitoring activities include viewing and inspection of the materials as they are produced, pretesting of materials with the intended audience, analysis of broadcast logs, analysis of viewer diaries, and exit interviews with the target population.

In general, the longer the program, the more important the process evaluation. When programs are implemented over a long period of time they change for a variety of reasons: *(1)* the resources available for the program can change; *(2)* the implementing agencies can change; *(3)* unanticipated problems with program delivery may (and do) occur; and *(4)* unanticipated problems may occur in the evaluation. Process research documents these problems so that they can be addressed.

The basic research question driving process research is the following: Is the program operating and being implemented as designed? Process research provides fine-tuning of operational systems, assessment and reassessment of resource allocations, and identification of programmatic and operational alternatives. By monitoring a health promotion program, investigators can determine whether it is disseminated and received as it was intended. It is possible that the intended audience will not be exposed to the program or exposed in ways that render it ineffective. For example, a mass media campaign designed to reduce substance abuse may be broadcast during times or shows that are not popular among the intended audience and so does not reach them.

For health promotion programs, process evaluation documents "reach and freq": How many people did it reach and with what frequency? Although process evaluation has many components, it can be divided into six areas. First, process evaluation documents how a program was created and designed. Second, it documents the dissemination, channels, and times of broadcast. Third, it is used to determine whether the intended audience was exposed to the program and interpreted it appropriately. Fourth, process evaluation is used to monitor whether the program is having the desired effect. Fifth, it helps determine whether the product or service is available. Finally, it can be used to monitor the interorganizational coordination of service sectors.

SIX POINTS FOR PROCESS EVALUATION

Process research can be conducted at any of the following six points in a program's development: (1) message production, (2) dissemination, (3) audience comprehension, (4) audience reception and interpretation, (5) monitoring supply, and (6) interorganizational relations. Documenting a health promotion program's implementation at each of these points has implications for achieving the goals of the process evaluation. Figure 5–1 illustrates the major focal areas for process evaluation for each perspective.

Message Production

Process evaluation at this stage documents program creation. It includes how a creative agency was selected (if one was used), how logos or slogans were created, which people produced the spots or programs, and how the process unfolded. These data can be gathered by observing the individuals and agencies involved in the process.

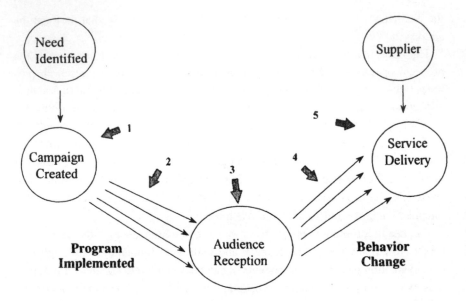

FIGURE 5–1. Process evaluation can be conducted at five points in the health promotion process.

Data might also come from documents such as memos, contracts, and meeting notes. For example, to select an ad agency for a campaign, researchers may solicit proposals and bids for the contract. The materials used for these activities provide valuable process data. In addition, notes from meeting and planning sessions can be used to document how ideas were created and developed into message strategy. Examples of early drafts or discarded program ideas provide fodder for the process evaluation.

Program Implementation

Process evaluation of program implementation consists of monitoring the volume, channel, and schedule for program dissemination. For example, monitoring a mass media advertising campaign consists of recording the time and duration of campaign spots. Monitoring these data also consists of counts of how many posters, flyers and other media were produced and how they were disseminated.

In health promotion programs that use mass media, researchers can contract with media monitoring companies to track when spots or programs are broadcast. These tracking systems record the broadcast days and times and an estimate of the ratings and audience share. Ratings–share data are an estimate of the number of of households that watched specific programs, which provides an estimate of campaign exposure. Unfortunately, these data will not indicate audience attention or comprehension, but they do provide a preliminary indication of exposure. Further process evaluation is required to measure audience comprehension.

Audience Comprehension

Monitoring of audience comprehension consists of activities designed to determine the degree of exposure and comprehension. Although similar to the monitoring of message dissemination outlined above, monitoring audience comprehension differs in that it consists of collecting data directly from audience members rather than from professionals. For example, an anti-tobacco campaign comprehension study would measure audience awareness and comprehension of the spots during the campaign.

Monitoring of audience comprehension is usually conducted with surveys that are distinct from those designed to measure program effects in three ways. First, they do not necessarily need to be conducted on a random sample of respondents because the goal is to measure comprehension, not whether there are effects generalizable to a population. Second, the interview is short, since it is not necessary to measure attitudes and behavior. Third, the survey is designed for rapid turnaround so that the results are communicated to campaign designers immediately in case changes need to be made.

Audience Effects

The fourth point for process evaluation is monitoring program effects during implementation. Audience effects can be monitored more easily if the program promotes a product or service that can be purchased. For example, campaigns designed to promote contraceptives use sentinel sites to monitor the volume of clients during the campaign. These sentinel sites provide a "real-time" check on whether the campaign is recruiting new users.

Effects monitoring provides a preliminary assessment of the short-term outcomes of a program. For example, monitoring a condom promotion campaign might consist of measuring the number of condoms sold at pharmacies each week. The data might indicate that sales increased during the months of the campaign. The chief difference between effects monitoring and outcome evaluation is that effects monitoring merely indicates whether the campaign changed behavior but does not provide the opportunity to test behavior change theory or determine among whom the program was more or less effective.

Effects monitoring is particularly useful in longer programs; effects can be estimated before the program is completed. In a program spanning one or several years, it is wise to monitor effectiveness so that changes can be made if it is not effective. It does not make sense to implement a promotional campaign for a substantial period of time (more than a few months) without an estimate of effectiveness.

Adequate Supply

Some health behaviors require people to buy or access a product. For example, condoms have to be purchased or otherwise obtained. Process evaluation research documents the supply of products being promoted. In a successful condom promotion campaign, pharmacies need to monitor their stock of condoms so that they don't run out.

Process research at point-of-sale locations monitors supply to avoid stock outages or to inform potential customers that they are temporary. Through monitoring of supply, barriers can be detected, such as difficulties that people have when trying to buy a new product. For example, if a vaccination promotion program advertised locations that are difficult to access, the supply monitoring would indicate differences in use rates despite people being aware of and intending to get vaccines.

Interorganizational Climate

An additional arena to be monitored is changes in interorganizational climate. Health promotion programs can energize agencies to work together in new ways. Often a program signals a new era in health-care delivery and agencies will take the opportunity to redefine their roles.

Process data can be collected on these interagency relationships and coordination activities that occur during the program (Wickizer et al., 1993). The interorganizational relationships affect how services are delivered and access to care (Kwait et al., 2001). Poor interagency referral practices, for example, can negatively affect the public's health, and even the best program won't be able to overcome this barrier.

Not all programs require all six types of process research; the scope and extent of the process evaluation plan will depend on the scope and nature of the program. The larger and longer the program, the greater the need for process research. Whether that research should focus on message development, dissemination, or effects depends in large part on the programmatic and theoretical needs of the evaluation.

USES OF PROCESS EVALUATION DATA

Process evaluation data serve a number of specific functions. First, they can be used to document and fix problems with the implementation. This is probably the most significant function, as waiting until the campaign is completed to learn of a problem with implementation is avoided. The implementation problems encountered, documented, and fixed can occur at any of the six points specified in Figure 5-1.

The process data should indicate whether the program is reaching its audience. If not, then designers can take corrective action by changing the program's dissemination or message strategy. It may be that the program was originally designed to air TV spots during particular programs thought to be popular among the target audience. If the ratings of those programs changed between program design and dissemination stages, however, then the spots might not be seen by the audience and hence a new strategy is needed.

A second use of process evaluation in health promotion programs is that it can alert researchers to other programs or activities that may interfere with the its message. When people are bombarded with health-related messages from the media, their communities, family, and friends, it can be hard to single out messages from one particular program. Process evaluation documents the "information environment" at the time of campaign broadcast. The data should describe other programs that appeared and other messages that may have competed with or complemented the program.

A third use of process evaluation is to detect the degree of message diffusion. This is particularly important in studies comparing a program's effect to a control group that did not receive the program. Unfortunately, messages often diffuse to control communities, invalidating comparisons between them. A good process evaluation documents this diffusion and thus explains the lack of program effects. In this sense, the process evaluation provides a measure of contamination.

Process evaluation is also particularly useful when replicating a program by repeating an existing campaign or creating a new one on a similar topic. Process data are used to inform the replication because they document the thinking and decision-making processes for the original program. This will help accelerate the replication and improve the likelihood of success.

In an advertising campaign to promote contraceptives in Bolivia, it was discovered that the smaller urban areas had lower program exposure than the larger cities (Valente and Saba, 1998). Consequently, the campaign was rebroadcast in these smaller urban areas. Although the data were collected as part of the outcome evaluation, they were used in a "process" manner (Box 5-1). Process data collected while the program is broadcast can be used to make mid-campaign corrections.

This illustrates the chief challenge to process evaluation: collecting and reporting data in a timely enough fashion to be useful. Most of the studies that report process evaluation results come from community-wide programs that were implemented over a number of years (e.g., McGraw et al., 1989). Collecting

Box 5-1. EVALUATION RESEARCH FOR CAMPAIGN DESIGN:
TWO CASE STUDIES

Classifying research as formative, process, or summative is useful, but can be
limiting. The following two case studies were initially summative evaluation
studies, but became formative and process research experiences.

BOLIVIA GENDER SERIES

In June 1994, a Bolivian TV series titled *Naked Dialogue* was designed as a
man-on-the-street talk show that addressed gender issues in Bolivian society. In
twelve 1-hour episodes aired at 9:00 pm on Saturday nights, *Naked Dialogue*
addressed topics such as domestic violence, alcohol abuse, machismo, reproductive health, and homosexuality. Six organizations were involved in the planning and implementation of the program, which was to be produced on a small
budget of $12,000 for 1 year. Research and evaluation costs were also to be
charged to this budget, and some of the collaborating institutions thought that
since there was so little money, the research should be canceled. Conflict
emerged; half of the team wanted evaluation, half did not.

The pro-research faction prevailed by *(1)* developing an inexpensive research plan, *(2)* soliciting input from everyone on the survey and study design, and *(3)* contributing matching funds from another source. A market
research firm was contracted through competitive bid to conduct 200 randomly
selected household interviews midway and at the end of the broadcast period.
In addition, 4 focus groups and 42 in-depth interviews were conducted with
low-income Bolivians before and after the series was broadcast. Much of the
cost of the analysis and interpretation of the research was assumed by Johns
Hopkins University/Population Communication Services since the research
budget of $3000 only covered the quantitative data collection. The 12 episodes
of *Naked Dialogue* were broadcast from March 1996 through May 1996 and
data were collected at mid-term, April 1–5, 1996, and follow-up was May
15–17, 1996.

Results showed that Bolivians liked *Naked Dialogue* because it addressed
relevant issues, but they did not like its format. Furthermore, the promotional
strategy to advertise the show had not been effective since the target audience, adolescents ages 15–19, were not aware of it. Changes were made, and
in 1997, *Naked Dialogue* was renamed *Moon Skin* and became the second-
most popular program on TV. The show reached 1,045,480 people, and it
won the first prize in the 1998 Latin American Video Festival Directed by
Women. Those who were initially opposed to evaluation became enthusias-
tic supporters.

ECUADOR CLINIC STUDY

APROFE is a nongovernmental organization that provides reproductive health
services to lower- and middle-income Ecuadoreans at 12 family health clinics

primarily in the city of Guayaquil (Ecuador's second largest city). In September 1994, to launch a radio campaign, researchers conducted interviews with women ages 15–40 at randomly selected households within easy walking distance to a clinic (50 meters). Results indicated that people *(1)* thought APROFE was government owned and operated, *(2)* would be willing to pay for services, and *(3)* were not aware of the range of services offered by APROFE. Data also showed that people who visited APROFE in the past were satisfied with the quality and cost of services. The main reason that clients did not come to the clinic or encourage their friends to come was that they thought that it was government owned and operated and therefore of poor quality, even though they themselves had had good experiences there. APROFE had an image problem.

The radio campaign emphasized its non-governmental status and that individuals could make appointments or be seen on a walk-in basis. Data analysis showed that clinic attendance increased 30% after the program, from a monthly average of 3120 clients before the campaign to 4072 after the campaign. Clients who came for services other than family planning increased as well (580% in one clinic, from 88 to 599 clients).

DISCUSSION

The first lesson from these studies is that research enabled designers to create effective strategies to improve behavioral outcomes by providing information on appropriate messages and media. The research was practical, convincing people of its utility.

Second, the research was both quantitative and qualitative and conducted before and after the campaign. It did not fit into a static evaluation framework of only providing impact assessment, rather it was integral to campaign planning and implementation. Although both program and evaluation staff initially conceived of the research as summative rather than formative or process, the data were used in all three ways.

Finally, the research techniques, instruments, and procedures were not particularly complex. Although perseverance and talent were needed, the procedures were not high-level statistical calculations. The respondent selection was random, but not based on a census enumeration of households and the analysis consisted primarily of univariate and cross tabulations.

Campaigns often fail to reach their objectives because they are poorly implemented or they target the wrong behaviors (or moderating/mediating factors). Conducting research to create and implement programs reduces the likelihood of these failures and increases the likelihood of success. These studies were designed initially to document program impact. The research results, however, provided important information for program redesign and reformulation.

process data in a 6-month media campaign and using it to inform program decisions during that period can be difficult since it takes months to collect, process, and interpret the data. Consequently, most process data are used to supplement interpretation of outcomes rather than to inform strategic decisions during broadcast.

HOW TO DO PROCESS EVALUATION

One means of conducting process evaluation is to collect information on the costs of program activities. Cost data indicate the importance of program components and provide a record of activities. Cost data can also be used to determine the cost-effectiveness of the program and estimate the expenses for other programs.

Aside from cost data, there are at least four sources of process data: (1) direct observation, such as watching individuals as they are exposed to the program; (2) service statistics, such as the volume of attendance at health centers (note that a few items of data gathered consistently and reliably are generally better for monitoring purposes than a more comprehensive set of information of doubtful reliability); (3) service provider data, such as record logs of how many clients were seen each day; and (4) program participant data, such as records of who attended which event when.

Process evaluation is conducted by trained researchers or by members of the public trained for such purposes. The personnel needs for process research depend on the type of process research being conducted. For example, viewer logs created to monitor campaign broadcasts can use people from the target audience, whereas ethnographic observations of the implementation of a new curriculum will require trained researchers.

Trained observers can conduct participant observation to measure campaign materials dissemination and their use. For example, a health campaign that disseminates brochures for counselors or pharmacists can use trained observers to determine if they are being used in the way intended in natural settings. The role of trained observers will vary depending on the type of campaign and the needs of the evaluation.

In some instances, process research may be more akin to contemporaneous history (King et al., 1987). In this sense, evaluators use primary documents such as memos, meeting notes, and other historical traces to construct a narrative of the program's creation and implementation. This type of process research relies less on counting activities and more on describing how the characteristics of the implementation affect program goals.

Process research is also conducted with population-based surveys to measure campaign reach and outcomes. These interviews are conducted while the campaign is broadcast and serve to alert researchers to any problems in implementation. This can be crucial if the campaign changed or historical events occurred between the pretest and implementation.

DISTINCTION BETWEEN RESEARCH TYPES

Although formative, process, and summative research are explained in separate chapters in this book, researchers should realize that these activities are not necessarily always distinct. There have been instances in which formative research becomes an evaluation of past activities (summative), which results in immediate recommendations for new practices (process). An illusion of this is in Box 5–1, which describes a project in Bolivia where a TV talk show evaluation was designed to address important public health issues such as domestic violence, sexually transmitted diseases, and attitudes toward sexual orientation. A small-scale summative evaluation was planned to determine whether the program achieved its objectives. The results indicated that Bolivians very much liked the topics of the show, but they did not like the format of man-on-the-street interviews. Consequently, the show was changed dramatically to an in-studio talk show host format and became the second-most popular show on Bolivian TV.

The point here is that evaluators are encouraged to use all of their research to its best advantage to improve health promotion programs. Often the evaluation research can serve formative, process, and summative roles at the same time, thus increasing its value and emphasizing the degree to which evaluation research is a critical component of programs.

SUMMARY

Programs can fail because they do not reach their intended audience, the message was not right for them, or it varied considerably among individuals (Rossi et al., 1999). Process evaluation documents these variables so that researchers understand the conditions for program success and whether the program can be replicated in other settings. This chapter provided an explanation of process evaluation research, which documents a program's implementation. Process evaluation identifies factors that influence a program's success and information needed for its replication. Figure 5–1 identified six points for conducting process evaluation: program creation, dissemination, audience impressions, product supply, audience effects, and interorganizational relations.

Although the literature on process evaluation and program monitoring is sparse for health promotion programs, it is an important part of an evaluation study. Researchers are advised to plan process research, particularly for long (over 6 months) and complex programs. To determine the effect of a health promotion program, researchers need to design and implement outcome studies that involve numerous components, including study design, data collection, and data management—all of which are covered in the next section.

Part Two

Methods

This section covers study design, data collection, management, and preliminary analysis. Chapter 6 discusses study design, specifying intervention and control groups, and the timing and collection of data. Chapter 7 explains how to decide on the sample size, and Chapter 8 provides guides for questionnaire construction. Chapters 9 and 10 cover the fundamentals of describing and analyzing data. Researchers may return to this material frequently as they design evaluations in various settings.

Chapter Six

Study Design

A *study design* specifies the number, timing, and type of data measurements relative to the intervention. Understanding study designs is crucial to conducting effective evaluation studies, since these designs specify the logic needed to determine program impact. This chapter discusses study designs, with an emphasis on intervention and control (or comparison) groups, and conveys the logic of study designs. Chapters 7 through 9 present the computer and statistical tools needed to implement them.

The goal of a health promotion program evaluation is to determine whether a program caused a change in the outcome. The first section of this chapter presents the conditions for showing causality. Study designs are then explained through examples to illustrate their strengths and weaknesses. The chapter then presents hypothetical study scores to explain how to interpret study results and hence how study designs attempt to control for threats to validity. Finally, some guidance on selecting an appropriate study design is given.

BACKGROUND

Study design and logic are rooted in the scientific method, which consists of procedures for testing hypotheses and making inferences from study results. Study design terminology and methodology have grown considerably over the years, in part because studies are not conducted exclusively in the physical and lab sciences (as was the case before the twentieth century). Evaluation studies are conducted in a wide variety of settings, among diverse populations, and hence require a variety of approaches.

In the early part of the twentieth century, the first major study design lessons were learned from agricultural studies and psychologists studying human behavior. After World War II, major social transformations occurred in the U.S. and elsewhere, at which time sociologists, educators, and economists began making contributions to evaluation practice and methodology. The evaluation activity across these different topic areas has created a substantial literature spanning numerous disciplines with often confusing terminology and different traditions. Adapting evaluation techniques from the biological and physical sciences to the social sciences remains a major challenge, and sometimes a source of tension.

The central challenge to designing studies is that they must be rigorous enough to make conclusions about program impact, yet face constraints of time, resources, program staff, and the willingness and protection of human subjects. These constraints often reduce the number of available study design options. This chapter presents study design techniques so that researchers can appropriately yet creatively, cope with these challenges.

The first requirement of a study design is that it be practical, which often prevents use of the best study design that might be theoretically possible. It is important, however, to construct the best study possible, given the available resources, and to plan that study well. Planning a study meticulously from the beginning saves time that is often wasted in unnecessary data collection, analysis, and conjecture (GAO/PEMD, 1991a, p. 9). *Researchers should know all study designs and their strengths and weaknesses so that they can create the best one, given stakeholders needs, populations affected, and available resources.* Since evaluation studies are often conducted to determine whether a program caused some change in an outcome, it will be helpful to first discuss causality.

CAUSALITY

One of the chief goals of an evaluation of a health promotion program is to show that the program caused an increase in knowledge, attitudes, or behaviors in some health-related domain. For example, an ideal program and evaluation concerning diabetes screening would be able to conclude that it caused an increase in the number of persons screened for diabetes. *Causality* is the determination that one event, action, state, or behavior is responsible for another (Gordis, 1996; Salmon, 1998). The criteria for showing causation are as follows (see Table 6–1):

TABLE 6-1. Conditions to Be Met to Show Causality

ISSUE	DESCRIPTION	MEANS OF CONTROL
Change	Outcome variable varies over time	Measure variable before and after campaign
Correlation	Intervention exposure and outcome vary together (dose-response relationship)	Demonstrate correlation between program and outcome
Time–order	Exposure to intervention occurred before outcome change	Use panel data Use time-sensitive measures
Specification	Other confounding factors are controlled	Measure other factors
Theoretical link	A theoretical explanation links the intervention and the outcome	Explore alternative theories

1. Change. The outcome variable varies over time.
2. Correlation. Exposure to the program and the outcome variable co-vary together (when one changes the other changes). The correlation criterion can be conceptualized as a dose–response relationship such that an increase in the dose of the program is associated with an increase in the outcome.
3. Time–order. Exposure to the program occurred before the outcome changed.
4. Specification. The correlation between program exposure and the outcome cannot be explained by other variables that have been omitted or improperly measured. If these variables are omitted from the analysis, then there is a specification problem. Proper model specification indicates that all relevant variables have been properly measured and included in the model.
5. Theoretical link. There is a theoretical (and logical) explanation that explains how and why the program caused the change in outcome, and other explanations are less plausible.

Meeting the conditions for causality is difficult and not to be undertaken lightly. Conditions 4 and 5 above specify that the researcher examine alternative explanations for any impact that is detected in a program evaluation. Considering alternative explanations is difficult since the inclination is to demonstrate effects rather than disproving them. Ruling out alternative explanations is done by eliminated or minimizing threats to validity.

STUDY VALIDITY

Validity is the degree to which a study or measure is accurate. There are at least four types of validity. *Study validity* is the degree to which the study design accurately measures program impact. *Measurement validity* is the degree to which

TABLE 6–2. Types of Validity

STUDY VALIDITY		MEASUREMENT VALIDITY	
EXTERNAL	INTERNAL	DIMENSIONALITY	REPRESENTATIVENESS
Generalizable measures	History	Uni-versus multi-dimensional	Criterion
Representative sample	Maturation	Orthogonal versus oblique	Content
Generalizable results	Selection Sensitization Testing		Construct

a variable represents the concept it is intended to measure. *Statistical validity* is the degree to which appropriate statistical methodology is used to analyze data. *Program validity* is the degree to which the intervention was delivered in sufficient quantity and quality to have an expected effect (Sechrist et al.,1979). Program validity was discussed in Chapter 5 (process evaluation), measurement validity is explained in Chapter 9 (where the related topic of reliability is also addressed), and statistical validity is addressed in Chapter 10. In this section, study validity is contrasted with measurement validity, since the two are sometimes confused.

Table 6–2 shows that validity is used to describe study and measurement characteristics, both of which have subcomponents (e.g., external versus internal for study validity). Validity refers to whether something is true or accurate. Consequently, it is important in evaluation research, because an evaluation must be valid for it to be useful.

Study validity is the degree to which program impact is accurately and truly measured. There are two types of study validity: external and internal. *External validity* is the degree to which results can be generalized to a larger population and often depends on whether samples were properly constituted. Externally valid studies can be extrapolated to a larger population or to other settings.

Internal validity is the degree of certainty in the results. Internal validity is determined by a study's rigorousness—its ability to measure what truly happened during the study. Are the results an accurate representation of the program's effect? Researchers have confidence in results from internally valid studies.

There are a number of threats to internal validity that evaluation studies try to control for, including history, maturation, testing, instrumentation, and sensitization. *History* is the occurrence of uncontrollable factors during the study. In health communication campaigns, history occurs when unanticipated events get on the media agenda. For example, suppose a celebrity was hospitalized with a drug overdose during an anti–drug use campaign. This event would be widely reported in the media and raise awareness of substance abuse issues. Consequently, the campaign may attract more attention and hence be more effective than if the overdose had not occurred. History cannot be controlled, and so researchers need to monitor the environment to measure historical effects.

Maturation is the effect of time that cannot be controlled, typically because study subjects age during the study. Maturation is not usually a threat in heath promotion programs since they are often implemented in a relatively short time period. Researchers can test for maturation by including age variables in the statistical analysis and conducting attrition analysis.

Testing is the effect of taking a test or survey on subsequent responses. For example, repeated administrations of a knowledge scale will have higher scores at later times because people get better at taking the test. Testing effects are usually controlled by comparison with control groups not pretested.

Instrumentation is the effect of data recording procedures on results, as subjects react to instruments differently. For example, a survey might measure communication campaign exposure by asking respondents whether they recall any TV ads concerning substance abuse. The survey measure is not the same as observing respondents' TV viewing behavior. People with the same campaign exposure may respond to the survey differently. The best safeguard against instrumentation bias is to pilot-test instruments and use multiple instruments (such as a survey complemented with observations).

Sensitization is the interaction between the pretest and intervention. Sensitization occurs when a pretest makes the respondent more aware of the program and hence more influenced by it. Sensitization is a major concern for program evaluators, because surveys can make individuals aware of topics and issues that they would not normally have paid attention to. For example, completing a baseline survey on substance abuse may incline respondents to pay attention to a media campaign about it.

These five threats to validity may cause changes in outcomes, thus they need to be controlled so that the changes attributable to a program can be determined. Ruling out these threats to validity strengthens the internal validity of the study. After internal validity is assessed, the researcher can consider external validity, the degree to which findings can be generalized.

Many studies are conducted in settings conducive to change and hence are more likely to have positive findings. These study settings may have, for example, a cooperative staff, a culture that accepts change, powerful leadership, and access to expert sources of opinion. In these cases, the study may be internally valid because it accurately measured program impact at that site. However, the study may lack external validity because the site chosen was not typical and hence the program may not be effective when replicated in other sites. The factors that influence access and selection of study sites should be documented.

In sum, study designs provide measures for these threats to validity so that the evaluation can claim that a program caused a change in an outcome. Study designs are used to control and measure these threats to validity. Before presenting study designs, two important distinctions in data collection and analysis need to be presented.

Panel versus Cross-sectional Samples

The first is whether the sample is panel or cross-sectional. The data management and statistical procedures are quite different for panel and cross-sectional data.[1] In a *panel* sample, the same respondents are interviewed at multiple points in time. The initial sample is selected (Chapter 7) and re-interviewed at each point in time, typically after a program is implemented. The data are merged with each previous time period's data (Chapter 8). The variables from each time period are given unique but similar names. For example, the variable age at three time points might be called age1, age2, and age3. The identification numbers for observations in a panel dataset need to be the same for the same people so that they can be merged.

In a *cross-sectional* sample different respondents are interviewed at multiple points in time. A new sample of respondents needs to be selected at each point in time, typically before and after a campaign. The data are appended (added to the bottom) to data from the previous time period. A new variable indicating time of interview (whether pre- or posttest) is created. For cross-sectional data, the variable names are the same at each time (age is called age in both pre- and post-test).

The distinction between panel and cross-sectional data determines: *(1)* data management procedures, *(2)* selection of appropriate statistical tests, and *(3)* inferences from these tests. Data management procedures, such as naming variables, combining survey waves, and constructing new variables, differ between the two. The statistical tests for panel and cross-sectional data are similar, save for a few important differences. First, panel studies may calculate change scores by subtracting pretest from posttest, whereas cross-sectional studies cannot, since the data come from different individuals. Second, panel studies may use lagged variable analysis—the same variable measured at a prior time period—whereas cross-sectional studies cannot. In terms of inferences, cross-sectional studies make comparisons at the population level to show change, but not at the individual level. These differences have advantages and disadvantages.

The advantages of panel over cross-sectional data are that panel data *(1)* measure change with difference scores, *(2)* indicate exactly which individuals, with what characteristics, changed behavior, *(3)* require smaller sample sizes, and

---

[1] The distinction between panel and cross-sectional designs is sometimes referred to as within (panel) versus between (cross-sectional) studies, since panel studies make comparisons within individuals whereas cross-sectional ones compare differences between them.

TABLE 6–3. Trade-offs Between Panel and Cross-sectional Designs

PANEL DATA		CROSS-SECTIONAL DATA	
ADVANTAGES	DISADVANTAGES	ADVANTAGES	DISADVANTAGES
Measure change with difference scores	Hard to follow up	Usually generalizable	Cannot create difference scores
Measure exactly which individuals changed behavior	Attrition can bias results	Larger samples can be collected	Need to collect larger samples
Require smaller sample sizes	Can lack generalizability		Require more intensive data
Are easier to analyze	Create sensitization		

(4) are associated with easier statistical analysis. The disadvantages of panel data are that *(1)* follow-up with respondents may be difficult, *(2)* attrition can bias the results, and *(3)* generalizability is less. In contrast, cross-sectional studies are often more generalizable, require data collected from larger samples, and require more intensive data analysis to control for confounding factors (see Table 6–3). Cross-sectional studies may be less risky to implement than panel ones.

Cross-sectional studies are conducted when *(1)* generalizability is important, *(2)* testing a new theory, *(3)* the population is mobile or otherwise hard to contact, and *(4)* follow-up with respondents will be difficult. When generalizability is important, a cross-sectional study may be preferred since pretest interviews may sensitize respondents to the program. Hence results from panel studies can be hard to generalize to a population that was not sensitized. Testing a new theory or novel application of an old one should use cross-sectional data also because of sensitization effects. Since attrition is non-random, factors that affect it are also related to the behavior, so panel samples may be biased in ways that cross-sectional ones would not. Furthermore, panel studies are hard to conduct when the population is mobile or otherwise hard to contact such as migrant workers, homeless people, or rural developing country households that lack addresses.[2] Sample loss due to attrition may invalidate study results. Finally, cross-sectional samples are preferred to panel ones when study respondents are reluctant or unable to be interviewed in later surveys. For example, studies conducted over a long time period such as 10 years, when many subjects will relocate, may have too much attrition to be worth collecting.

An alternative is a rolling sample (Kish, 1965, 1987)—a panel sample is collected and those lost to follow-up are replaced by new subjects selected in the same way. This provides a rejuvenated panel sample throughout the study pe-

[2]It is possible to conduct such studies by including numerous identifiers, such as place of employment and residence of other family members, in addition to drawing a map for future interviewers.

riod. Rolling sample implementation can be complicated by the need to identify who was added to the sample and when.

Panel samples are more useful than cross-sectional ones at documenting the process of behavior change. Since interviews are conducted with the same people, determining exactly who changed behavior and by how much can be measured. The degree of program exposure can be linked to these changes. Panel studies are used extensively in laboratory studies of program effects but less often in field studies, primarily to avoid testing and sensitization threats.

Statistical inferences depend on whether the samples are panel or cross-sectional. Panel studies measure behavior of specific individuals whereas cross-sectional ones measure it for populations. In a panel study, we can say that individuals who were exposed to the program changed their behavior; for cross-sectional ones, we may only say that there was an association between seeing it and changing behavior.

Study designs have been created for panel data, and in some ways, they are more rigorous than designs for cross-sectional data. Researchers are more likely to be able to make causal claims with panel rather than cross-sectional data. Both types, however, have strengths and weaknesses, and the choice of which to use depends on the substantive issue at hand, the population under study, and the availability of sampling frames. Many evaluations use both cross-sectional and panel data to capitalize on the strengths of each.

Unit of Assignment

A second study design option is whether to assign the intervention at the individual or group level. Many studies randomly assign subjects to treatment and control conditions. For example, clinical trials on the effectiveness of a drug randomly assign people to receive the intervention (a pill) or the control (a placebo). This option is often not available for community-based programs in which random assignment to conditions is not possible. This is particularly true for health communication campaigns, which tend to use mass media to inform and persuade audiences, hence everyone has the opportunity to be exposed to the intervention.

To address this problem, researchers use the community as the unit of assignment and analysis; some communities get the intervention, and others act as controls. Data are still collected on individuals, but they are acknowledged to be clustered within communities. Impact is measured by aggregating the data, computing averages for the communities and comparing them. For example, if 10 communities received a campaign and 10 did not, the researcher could compute average outcome scores for the 20 communities and compare the averages. This analytic technique provides a test of program impact at the community level. Community-level assignments make quasi-experimental studies experimental ones.

Experimental versus Quasi-experimental Designs

In the classic experimental design, study subjects are randomly assigned to intervention (also known as treatment or experimental) and control groups, with the expectation that outcome variables will be better for those in the intervention group. Random assignment is expected to eliminate any differences of individual characteristics between groups (i.e., on average, they will have the same education, gender, income, age, etc.). Data from experimental designs can be relatively easy to analyze because of this randomization.

Experimental methodology was originally developed in fields such as agricultural science, where it is possible to assign a plot of land to a treatment condition such as adding fertilizer and another plot to control (no fertilizer). The key feature of experiments is that subjects are assigned to groups randomly so that individual biases regarding who gets the intervention are controlled. Experimental designs are only feasible when the program being evaluated can be limited to certain groups or individuals. As mentioned above, in the case of communication campaigns, it can be difficult to perform an experiment because it is hard to restrict them. Consequently, although the experimental methodology is ideal for evaluating interventions, it is not appropriate for all health promotion program evaluation (Cook and Campbell, 1979). As mentioned above, experiments can only be used when programs can be limited to a group of people and random assignment is possible. Random assignment to conditions is hard when evaluating mass media campaigns because broadcasts cannot be restricted.

Experimental methodology may also be misleading when evaluating a new or evolving program, as the program will probably change during implementation. Sometimes evaluations are conducted to determine whether and how a program should be modified before it is expanded to other communities. So the evaluation results will apply to the provisional program, but probably not to the one that is eventually implemented on a larger scale. Finally, some experiments have low generalizability or external validity since they are conducted in artificial settings, such as a laboratory. Because people act differently in these settings than at home, the study results will be biased.

The experimental methodology is rigorous and is an ideal to strive for in designing quasi-experiments. These experiments approximate true ones to the degree that uncontrolled differences between the intervention and control groups are minimal (Cook and Campbell, 1979; Rossi and Freeman, 1993). These study designs may require restricted dissemination of promotional materials, and although some investigators argue that it is unfair to withhold programs from people who might benefit from them, others contend that their impact should be known before disseminating the programs to a larger audience.

In Campbell and Stanley's (1963) informative book on experimental and quasi-experimental designs, they treat many field studies as quasi-experimental since the researcher cannot control which respondents or subjects will receive the intervention. Many of the examples in this book are quasi-experimental because assignment cannot be controlled.

To summarize, this section presented *(1)* the conditions needed to show causality, *(2)* classification and definition of validity threats, *(3)* the distinction between panel and cross-sectional data, *(4)* the distinction between individual and group levels of assignment, and *(5)* the distinction between quasi-experimental and experimental designs. These distinctions are important for understanding study designs.

STUDY DESIGNS

Table 6–4 describes six study designs, using the following terms:

X = the intervention, a health promotion program or communication campaign.

O = the data collection observation, a survey questionnaire.

Subscripts can be used to distinguish different X's and O's. For example, X_1 and X_2 might refer to two interventions: X_1, a media campaign; and X_2, a media campaign plus interpersonal counseling. For observations, scripts are used to distinguish observations for intervention and control groups and before and after a campaign.

Table 6–4 lists common study designs in increasing order of complexity for one intervention. Researchers can create as many intervention and observation

TABLE 6–4. Study Designs

DESIGN	BASELINE	INTERVENTION	FOLLOW-UP	CONTROLS
Post-program only	—	X	O	None
Pre- and post-program	O	X	O	Selectivity
Pre- and post-program with	O	X	O	Testing
post-only control group	—	—	O	
Pre- and post-program with	O	X	O	History and
control group	O	—	O	maturation
Pre- and post-program with	O	X	O	
control group and	O	—	O	Sensitization
post-only program group	—	X	O	
Solomon four-group	O	X	O	
	O	—	O	All of the
	—	X	O	above
	—	—	O	

O, observation, such as a survey; X, intervention/program; —, no observation or intervention.

conditions as needed for an evaluation. A program with many different interventions may have many conditions.

Post-program Only

The simplest study design is a measurement after the program. The survey should measure program exposure and behavior. The correlation between program exposure and behavior provides some measure of effectiveness, provided all possible demographic and situational variables are controlled. This study design provides data on how many people were exposed to the program and their reaction to it, by reporting reach and frequency. These data can also be used to measure the appeal and attractiveness of the program and for future program planning.

The main advantages of post-only designs are that they are cheap and easy to do. The disadvantage is the lack of information on behavior before the campaign. Without a baseline with which to compare the follow-up, changes in knowledge, attitude, and practice cannot be calculated. To demonstrate a causal link between the program and behavior, change in the behavior has to be measured. Consequently, the minimum study design requirement is a before-and-after design.

Pre- and Post-program

A pre- and post-program study design measures outcomes before and after the program. It is expected that outcome scores will improve between the pre- and post-program measures. For example, evaluating an exercise promotional campaign should show that exercise increased between the pre- and posttests. This design is also known as "before–after" or as an "advertising model," since it is often used to evaluate advertising campaigns (Flay and Cook, 1989).

This design can be used with both panel and cross-sectional data and at both individual and community levels of analysis. It reduces some threats to validity since it provides a baseline against which to compare the post-program scores and is often used when creating a control group is not feasible. A cross-sectional comparison of pre- and post-program scores consists of selecting two comparable independent samples before and after the program and making population-level comparisons. For example, 400 randomly selected respondents in one region of The Gambia were interviewed before and after a 9-month radio soap opera. Analysis showed that family planning knowledge, attitudes, and practices increased significantly between administration of the two surveys (Valente et al., 1994a). The shortcoming of this cross-sectional methodology is that there may be fluctuations in sample characteristics that account for differences in outcomes between the two surveys, despite statistical controls.

A panel design eliminates this problem because the same people are interviewed and changes are measured for individuals, not solely at the population level. For example, in an evaluation of a street theater's effectiveness at reducing family planning misinformation, people passing by the performance were interviewed about their family planning knowledge before and after the drama (Valente et al., 1994b). The study showed that the drama reduced misinformation by 9.4%. Since a very short time elapsed between pre- and post-intervention measures (1 hour), other factors that may have caused this change in knowledge can be ruled out.

The trouble with the pre–post design is the lack of a control group, and hence it is hard to know what would have happened in the absence of the program. If the program is a short one and there are few contaminating events, this design may be sufficient. A second problem with the pre–post design is the inability to measure the influence of survey-taking on the scores (testing effects).

In sum, this design provides a baseline comparison and meets the causal conditions of change and time-order. However, it cannot rule out other explanations, such as testing in panel surveys or sample fluctuations in cross-sectional ones. Consequently, many researchers add a post-only control group, which is easy to create and implement in real-world settings.

Pre- and Post-program with Post-only Control

In the study design of pre- and post-program measures with a post-only control group, a survey is conducted before the program and then a second group is surveyed only after the program. The post-only control group can be those not exposed to the program (as shown in Table 6–4) or those who could have been exposed, but did not recall it (discussed below). This design is often used in the evaluation of health communication campaigns because it is easy to implement in real-world settings in which a true control condition cannot be created.

When a true control group cannot be created, a quasi-control group is created from the post-program survey. This quasi-control group consists of those respondents who reported not being exposed to the program. Program exposure is measured in the post-program so that respondents can be divided into those exposed and those not exposed (or into those with low and high exposure; or no, low, medium, and high exposure, and so on). The exposure variable is used to create three groups: *(1)* pre-program, *(2)* post-program not exposed (or low exposure for programs that have high reach), and *(3)* post-program exposed (or high exposure). In a successful program, outcome scores for the three groups should increase, with group 1 being the lowest and group 3 the highest, or they should be the same for groups 1 and 2, but be statistically higher for group 3 (posttest exposed).

One problem with this design is that successful programs have high reach and so the unexposed group is often too small or too different from the rest of the sample to be comparable. In such cases, the post-only sample can be divided into those with low and high exposure or scaled along a continuum. It is important to compare the post-only exposed and unexposed (or high and low exposure) groups on all relevant sociodemographic variables (age, education, income, media access, cultural background, etc.) to be sure that the non-exposed and exposed groups are comparable. Note that in this instance, it may be advisable to increase the sample size for the post-program sample since it functions as two groups (follow-up treated and follow-up control).

Rossi and Freeman (1993) state that any program that reaches >80% of the audience should not be partitioned into exposed and not-exposed groups, because the two groups will be too different. In other words, if as much as 80% of the sample reports being exposed to the program, then the 20% not exposed is probably too different from the exposed group to represent a reasonable control group. Since many factors affect exposure to a campaign, researchers should be cautious when comparing exposure groups. As a guide, a 60/40 cutoff should be used for comparing dichotomized exposure groups, and at least 20% in each group of a three-group comparison.

The Gambia radio soap opera study mentioned above used a pre–post program study with post-only control (Valente et al., 1994). Two cross-sectional samples of residents of one region were interviewed before and after the broadcast. After a change in outcomes was demonstrated, the post-drama sample was divided into those who reported listening to the drama and those who did not. Outcome scores were higher for those who reported listening to the drama than for those who did not, lending support for an interpretation of program effects.

In panel studies, this design has a post-only group that is exposed to the program, but not pre-tested. This control group would be created in studies using panel data to test for the effects of sensitization. For example, Valente and Bharath (1999) interviewed 100 randomly selected people at 10 different 3-hour dramatic performances designed to improve knowledge about HIV/AIDS transmission. The same 100 people were interviewed immediately after the performances, and an additional 100 people were interviewed after the performance only. Results showed that the drama increased knowledge by 26 percentage points. Comparison of the post-performance scores between those interviewed before and those not interviewed before the performance provided an estimate of the effect of taking the pretest (3 percentage points in this case). This design does not determine how much of this difference was due to the pretest alone or to a pretest/ intervention interaction known as *sensitization*.

The main limitation of the three designs discussed above is that they cannot measure the degree of change due to history and/or maturation—threats to validity that happen over time. The longer the time between measurements, the greater the threats of history and/or maturation. These designs cannot measure how much of the correlation between program exposure and outcomes is due to other events or activities that happened while the program was implemented.

Indeed, the researcher can say little about what would have happened in the absence of the program, and hence a control group is desired.

Pre- and Post-program with Control Group

This design includes a predetermined control group that is interviewed before the program, and not subsequently exposed to it. The scores for the intervention group are compared to those of the control group to determine if changes occurred in the intervention group relative to what happened without the program. For cross-sectional data, this design reduces to a pre- and post-program with post-only control, unless it is a community-level study.

There are some good examples of the pre- and post-program with control group. Reger and colleagues (1998) evaluated a campaign in West Virginia that promoted low-fat milk as a substitute for regular or 2% milk. They interviewed randomly selected respondents from two communities—one exposed to the campaign and the other not. Results showed that the campaign-exposed community reported more switching from high-fat to low-fat milk than in the control community.

In Tanzania, Rogers and colleagues (1999) evaluated a soap opera that promoted HIV/AIDS prevention and family planning practices. The 2-year program was broadcast nationally except for one region, which broadcast a different program at the time of the soap opera's broadcasts. They found that knowledge, attitudes, and practices regarding HIV/AIDS prevention and family planning increased significantly in the intervention communities, but not in the comparison area.

In Guatemala, Bertrand and others (1987) evaluated a radio campaign that promoted vasectomy as a form of family planning. They broadcast the campaingn in one community and used outreach workers in another. They found that the mass media were effective, compared to the comparison area (no intervention), and that the effects of the outreach workers were, in part, dependent on the quality of the outreach workers.

Implementing this design can be difficult since restricting broadcasts from the control regions is not always possible. All the examples discussed above had assignment at the community level. The payoff, however, is that data analysis and interpretation are easier, since the control group measures what happened in the absence of the campaign. This study design controls for most threats to validity, provided that the intervention and control groups are comparable for all relevant characteristics. Indeed, selecting control groups that match the intervention groups is the central challenge of using this design.

With panel data, this design can be used to subtract pretest scores from posttest ones in both intervention and control groups, and then these differences can be subtracted from one another (difference of differences). This value provides a measure of program effects; it does not, however, control for testing and sensitization effects. The net change may be an effect of the intervention, the pretest, or pretest sensitization making the groups aware of the program. Thus, additional control groups are needed to measure these threats to validity.

Pre- and Post-program with Control and Post-only Program Groups

This design has five measurements: two pretests (one for the program group), and three posttests (two among the program groups). This study design has a group that received the program, but was not pretested (as discussed in pre- and post-program with post-only group) and so was not sensitized to it. This study design is only used with panel data or community-level studies, since group 3 is the same as group 1 in a cross-sectional study.

As a hypothetical example, suppose a campaign was launched to improve knowledge of the harmful effects of substance abuse, and during the study, a historical event such as the death of a famous person from a drug overdose occurred. The post-only intervention group could be used to determine whether the outcome changed as a result of the pretest or as a result of the combination of the historical event and the campaign.

The post-only intervention group controls for the sensitizing effect of the pre-program measure. Cross-sectional surveys do not have this bias. Sensitization can be a strong factor in a program's impact, so cross-sectional designs are often used. Some researchers use laboratories to disguise the program, which can solve the sensitization problem but may detract from the program's impact. This design controls for most threats to validity, but it is not complete because every group has either been pretested or received the intervention. The final study design adds a post-only control group.

Solomon Four-Group

The Solomon four-group design is named for Solomon's (1949) article that demonstrated the need for two non-pretested control groups in experimental designs. The Solomon four-group design is the most complete study design, since it controls for most threats to validity. This design has four conditions with six different observations: two pre-program ones (one exposed) and four post-program ones (two exposed). The four-group design can only be implemented with panel samples or community-level studies.

The Solomon four-group design measures impact relative to the control group that measures history and maturation effects. The non-pretested groups provide measures of the effect of (1) testing (the effect of the pre-program survey), and (2) sensitization (the effect of the pre-program survey on attention to the program).

It can be difficult to use a four-group design in a health communication campaign evaluation, and most examples come from school- or community-based health promotion programs (e.g., Kvalem et al., 1996), since it is easier to restrict the program to schools or organizations.

Comparison of Study Designs

Each of these six study designs has strengths and weaknesses. Although the four-group design is the gold standard, it is rarely feasible for evaluation of a health communication campaign and is not appropriate for many health promotion programs. The trained evaluator knows the function of the control and intervention groups and develops an appropriate study design. The evaluator needs to decide which design is feasible, given the study circumstances, and how to implement a design that controls for threats to validity.

Simpler designs can be easier to conduct because they do not have to be defined beforehand. The results from more complex designs, however, are often easier to analyze and interpret. A design that creates a control group from the post-program data will require considerable analysis to determine the right exposure and control variables. Conversely, a Solomon four-group design requires only that the researcher compare outcome scores to determine whether the intervention groups have better outcomes than the controls—a much simpler data analysis task. Furthermore, the more complex study designs may enable researchers to make more confident statements concerning program effects.

Study designs determine the data management, analysis, and kind of inferences to be made from the data. There are numerous factors that influence the type of study design, and every program evaluation will have unique characteristics that demand some trade-off between threats to validity that can be controlled and the inferences made from the study. The following section presents hypothetical data to illustrate how to interpret evaluation data.

HYPOTHETICAL SCORES

Table 6–5 reports hypothetical scores for a four-group panel study to illustrate the interpretation of study results. The scores represent the hypothetical results from a program to improve SAT scores. The scores presented here are hypothetical correct scores out of a 1600 maximum. In this study, students were randomly assigned to the four groups. Random assignment is important, since the researcher assumes, in this case, that the pretest scores in the groups that did not get pretested would have been the same as those in the groups that did. The hypothetical scores are (Table 6–5):

1000 for the pre-course categories

1400 for the post-course trained and pretested

1100 for the post-course trained and not pretested

1200 for the post-course not trained and pretested

1050 for the post-course not trained and not pretested.

The difference between the post- and pretest scores was computed by simple subtraction and the results are also shown in Table 6–5. The differences for groups not pretested were computed by using the average from the groups that were pretested. For example, if the pretest scores were 1100 and 900, the average of these two scores would be the estimate for the pretest score in the non–pretested groups. The difference between pre- and posttest scores for the pretested groups was 400 and 200 for the program and non-program students, respectively. These change scores can be computed with a panel sample since they represent changes in individual scores, but could not be computed at the individual level if the data were cross-sectional. The difference scores for the non-pretested groups, 3 and 4, were 100 and 50 for the program and non-program groups, respectively.

The difference scores can be used to measure the degree of change attributable to the program and threats to validity. The 400-point increase between the pre- and posttest program is attributable to pretest sensitization, the program, and time-related threats to validity, such as maturation and history. This 400-point increase is compared to that in the other groups to measure impact.

The 50-point increase for group 4 is the easiest to understand since the post-only group did not receive the program or a pretest. Hence, this 50-point increase (1050 − 1000) can be considered the effects due to time only—either maturation or history (from these data one cannot distinguish which). The 100-point increase for group 3 is a result of time and the program. Since time accounted for 50 points, 50 points are attributable to the program.

The 200-point increase between pre- and post-campaign scores for the non-program group is attributable to the pretest and time. Since time accounted for 50 points, the remaining points (150) are attributable to the pretest effect. The

TABLE 6–5. Hypothetical Study Outcome Scores (Panel Study)

	RECEIVED PRETEST	PROGRAM	POSTTEST	DIFFERENCE	EFFECT OF
Group 1	1000	Yes	1400	+400	Program, pretest, and time
Group 2	1000		1200	+200	Pretest and time
Group 3		Yes	1100	+100	Program and time
Group 4			1050	+50	Time

400-point increase between pre- and post-test program scores for the program group is attributable to the pretest, time, and the program. Since time accounted for 50 points, the program accounted for 50 points, and the pretest accounted for 150 points, which leaves 150 points being attributable to sensitization (the pretest improved the effectiveness of the program).

Many studies strive to obtain data like this. Each of the four study groups contributed information needed to understand the factors that influenced the posttest scores. The post-only group without intervention measured the effects of time; the pre- and post-program without intervention group measured the effects of time and the pretest. Few real-world studies provide such clear data and interpretation, but these hypothetical data illustrate the purpose of the various study groups.

These hypothetical numbers provide an illustration of estimating program impact. In an actual study, a variable is created to represent each group and this variable is used in statistical analysis of the data (Chapters 9 and 10). The aim of this chapter has been to present study designs and their strengths and weaknesses, and to emphasize the importance of selecting the best study design possible given the constraints of the study.

SELECTING A STUDY DESIGN

Four practical issues face researchers when deciding on a study design (Fisher et al., 1991). First, respondents should be randomly assigned to intervention or control group conditions, whenever possible. Inferences of program effectiveness are greatly facilitated when respondents do not self-select to the program or control group. Second, if random assignment is not possible, then comparison groups should be formed so that they are as nearly equivalent to the intervention group as possible. Third, data should be collected at multiple time points, especially before the program. Fourth, multivariate statistical techniques should be used to control for confounding factors. These four guidelines will help evaluators create the best study possible within given constraints.

Good research designs provide an ethical and accurate assessment of program impact with the most valid and reliable data. The goal is to avoid inaccurate descriptions of the intervention and how it affected the population being studied. A good rule for researchers is to collect data (1) through multiple sources, (2) at multiple points in time, and (3) with multiple replications.

Evaluators constantly make trade-offs between rigor and practicality, and rarely have the flexibility to establish multiple control groups. Consequently, they need to be aware of the limitations of their designs and attempt to develop mechanisms for measuring or controlling threats to validity. For example, a short mass media campaign may not need to be evaluated using control groups because the threats to validity that the control group measures, such as history and maturation, will be minimized. Evaluators need to know the campaign's characteristics, its anticipated effects, and the threats to validity that are counterarguments to concluding program impact. Then the researcher can design an appropriate study.

Experience has shown that a small amount of data collected rigorously is more valuable than a complex study implemented poorly. There is a tendency to create study designs that use large samples without properly controlling for threats to validity that are unique to or inherent in a program evaluation. Rather than spending resources on a series of large cross-sectional samples, an evaluator might consider following a small cohort over time and supplementing it with unobtrusive measures such as sales data, foot traffic, and so on. The point here is to consider the aims and objectives of the program, the evaluation study, the theories that guide it, and the possible threats to validity that need to be controlled to make claims of causality.

BLINDED STUDIES

While rarely used in health promotion program evaluation, many epidemiological studies and clinical trials are conducted using a *double-blind study*, a study in which neither the subjects nor the researchers know which group is receiving the intervention and which is the control. Thus, both the subjects and researchers are "blind" to the assignment.

Double-blind studies are conducted to control for the reaction that subjects might have if they know they are in a study. For example, if there is a treatment being tested to ease arthritic pain, study subjects might report less pain if they think that they are taking a medication for it. Blinding the researchers is done to minimize the bias researchers might introduce into the study or the data. For example, if the researchers know which subjects are given the medication, they may treat them differently by trying to detect subtle differences in their behavior.

Conducting blinded studies is impractical in most health promotion evaluations because there is no pill or technology that can easily be substituted with a placebo. Laboratory studies can use different interventions to compare respondent reaction, but typically the researcher knows who gets the intervention.

CONTAMINATION

Contamination is the unplanned deterioration of a study design when people in the control group are exposed to the program. This exposure can occur when the program is accidentally disseminated to the control group or when another similar program is disseminated simultaneously. The amount of contamination is the percent of the control group subjects exposed to the intervention.

Contamination has two primary forms: control group contamination and treatment contamination. Both types undermine the experimental design. *Control group contamination* occurs when individuals in the control group are exposed to the program. This is difficult to prevent because it is hard to prevent message diffusion. It can occur in three ways: *(1)* directly, *(2)* indirectly, and *(3)* from different sources.

Direct control group contamination occurs when people who should be in the control group are exposed to the program. This exposure can occur when people in the control group travel to the region that received the program or when a campaign is accidently broadcast to a control group. In some cases, new technologies such as VCRs have enabled people from one region to see shows and advertisements that normally would not be broadcast in their region.

Indirect control group contamination occurs when people spread program messages via word of mouth (Freedman and Takeshita, 1968). As people travel and move between control and intervention communities, they can relay messages received in the program. Also, people may show program flyers or brochures to their friends.

Finally, control group contamination occurs when people in the control region receive a program similar to the one being used in the intervention. For example, a campaign to promote better eating habits may have as a secondary message the benefits of daily exercise. If the control region received an exercise promotion campaign, their scores would change and hence the original campaign would not be effective relative to the control.

Treatment contamination occurs when the treatment is not delivered as intended. Treatment contamination in communication campaigns occurs, for example, when the broadcast schedule is not followed because of financial constraints. Treatment contamination weakens the likelihood of a program effectiveness because the intervention group does not get the program at the appropriate rate.

Hawthorne Effect

The Hawthorne effect is named for the Chicago Western Electric plant where a worker productivity study was conducted by researchers at the Harvard Business School. The researchers discovered that reducing the lighting in the factory actually brought about an increase in productivity. Upon investigating the reason for this bizarre conclusion, it was discovered that the "cause" for the increased productivity was that the workers knew they were being studied and they improved their performance because they were receiving attention, not because of the study interventions. The *Hawthorne effect* is the tendency for subjects to react positively to experimental conditions (Roethlisberger and Dickson, 1939; Homans, 1950).

For health promotion researchers who study message effects in artificial settings, there is concern that respondents will react to messages in a favorable manner simply because they know they are being studied. Work site and other institutional interventions may also suffer from the Hawthorne effect. The best remedy is to enlist control groups that resemble the experimental conditions as closely as possible.

SUMMARY

This chapter described the terminology and logic of study designs. It began with an explanation of the conditions needed to demonstrate causality, then described study validity. The distinctions between panel and cross-sectional data and individual versus community-level analysis were discussed. Six study designs with variations in intervention and control groups and in the number and type of pre- and posttests were presented. The relative advantages and disadvantages of these study designs as well as their strengths and weaknesses were discussed.

A table of hypothetical scores was presented to explain how to interpret study results and how the various study groups control for threats to validity. Finally, some guidelines for selecting a study design were presented that stressed the importance of establishing program objectives and bearing in mind practical limitations. Once a design is selected, the evaluator typically needs to select a sample and determine sample size.

Chapter Seven

Sampling and Sample Size

One of the first questions asked of the evaluator is: "What size sample is needed for the evaluation?" It is assumed that sample size will be the primary determinant of cost of the evaluation, but this may not the case, since questionnaire construction and data analysis are often just as costly. Furthermore, it is the procedures of sample selection, not the size, that matter both in terms of cost and interpreting the results. Evaluators need to understand how to develop strategies for sample selection and determine the sample size needed to conduct a valid evaluation.

Virtually all research uses procedures for selecting a sample from the universe of possible units (Babbie, 2001). In health promotion program evaluation, a sample is selected to represent a population. Calculations are made on the sample to make inferences regarding the population. This chapter covers procedures used to determine the type and size of sample to select for the evaluation. Sample types are presented first, then the techniques for sample size determination, and then sample selection. Techniques (and computer programs) for sample size calculations should be used before a program is implemented and after the follow-up data are collected to conduct a valid evaluation. Once a study design has been selected, the sample type and size are determined. Sample type is the selection procedure used to gather the sample.

SAMPLE TYPES

Probability Sampling

There are two basic sample types: probability and non-probability. In a *proba-bility sample*, each element of the population has a known probability of being selected. In most probability samples, each element has an equal opportunity to be selected. The key element, however, is that the probability of being selected is known. There are six types of probability samples, presented below.

Simple random sampling. Each element is assigned a unique number and a series of random numbers are generated to select cases. For example, all students in a school system could be assigned a unique number; a sample would then be selected on the basis of a specified selection of those numbers. If there were 400 students, they would be assigned numbers from 1 to 400 (Table 7–1). To select a simple random sample of 100, a series of 100 random numbers would be generated and those students interviewed. If each person were to be interviewed only once, numbers would be discarded after being selected (sampling without replacement). A simple random sample with equal probabilities of being selected is referred to as the equal probability for selection method (EPSEM).

Systematic sampling. The sample size is determined and a sampling interval created to select every k^{th} case. Like simple random sampling, every case is assigned a number, but the sampling interval is used to select cases. To calculate the sampling interval, the universe size is divided by the desired sample size to get k.

In the school example, the selection interval, k, is calculated by dividing 400 by 100 to get 4. Every fourth case is then selected to be interviewed. If the fourth person is not available, the fifth can be substituted. In practice, since the sample is drawn at one point in time, missing cases are substituted but the remainder of the original sample is still selected. In other words, if person 8 is missing and person 9 is substituted, the researcher does not interview person 13, but instead continues with the original selection strategy and interviews person 12. Systematic sampling is probably the most common sampling strategy.

Stratified sampling. Sample selection is proportionate within distributions on some variable (in conjunction with simple and systematic sampling, ensuring adequate representation of groups). Stratified sampling guarantees over- or underselecting respondents from certain groups. Typically, samples are stratified according to basic demographic characteristics such as gender, age, residential location, and socioeconomic status.

For example, suppose a study was designed to compare career plans of students with different high school grades and samples of 25 students from each

TABLE 7-1. Sample Selection Numbers for a Hypothetical School Population of 400 and Desired Sample Size of 100

	SIZE	SAMPLE TYPE		
		SYSTEMATIC	STRATIFIED	MULTISTAGE
Freshman		*Every 4th*	*Every 5th*	*20 from every 3rd class*
English	30			
Math	30			
Science	30			20 (skip each 3rd)
Physical exercise	30			
Grade total	120	30	25	
Sophomore		*Every 4th*	*Every 4th*	
English	25			
Math	25			20
Science	25			
Physical exercise	25			
Grade total	100	25	25	
Junior		*Every 4th*	*Every 4th*	
English	25			20
Math	25			
Science	25			
Physical exercise	25			20
Grade total	100	25	25	
Senior		*Every 4th*	*Every 3rd*	
English	20			
Math	20			
Science	20			20
Physical exercise	20			
Grade total	80	25	25	
Total	400	100	100	100

grade were needed. The researcher would need to compute separate selection intervals for each grade: freshman, 4.8; sophomore, 4.0; junior, 4.0; and senior, 3.2. Consequently, the researcher would select every fifth freshman student; every fourth sophomore and junior and every third senior.[1]

[1] The final sample would actually have too many seniors and not enough freshmen given the rounding error associated with the selection interval. The researcher could vary the interval to compensate for the rounding such that every fifth freshman selected would be the fourth. A second and usually more advisable option is to round down the interval to oversample all groups.

Census sampling. All elements in the population are interviewed. Census sampling requires the researcher to define the boundary a priori and then enumerate all elements inside the boundary. Census sampling is used in organizations, schools, and rural communities where the boundaries may be defined and the size not too big (<1000). It may be used in conjunction with other sampling strategies. For example, suppose a random sample of organizations is selected and then a census of employees in each organization interviewed. Although statistical inference of data collected from the census may not seem appropriate, it is done to test the strength of associations.

Once the boundary is defined, it can be difficult to get complete response rates, and researchers often settle for less than 100% response rate. Those people who don't respond may be bridges to other groups or to those otherwise on the periphery of the boundary. One major advantage of census sampling is that connections among group members can be measured and studied as a network. Network analysis is an intellectually exciting paradigm of research (see Wasserman and Faust, 1994; Valente, 1995; Scott, 2000).

Multistage sampling. The population is divided into clusters (or strata) and then a sample of clusters is selected from which samples are selected. Multiple stages can be used in the sampling design, depending on study needs. Sampling within each cluster level can be random, systematic, or stratified.

Returning to the hypothetical school example, to avoid having to visit every class, a sample of classes would be selected and then a sample of students from within each class selected. From the population of 16 classes, every third class would be selected, yielding 5 classes, and within each, 20 students interviewed.

Probability proportional to size sampling. This is multistage technique in which the probability of selection is directly related to its cluster size. In (PPS) sampling, the population is divided into clusters and their sizes determined. The sample is selected within clusters randomly or systematically, so that the sample sizes have the same proportions as the population clusters.

A random or systematic sample will be a PPS sample. This sampling is used when a researcher selects a sample from different groups (locations) and has a target sample size for one group (e.g., a required sample size of 500 in one city). Sampling from other groups is performed proportionately so that the sample size for each group is proportionate to the reference group.

Returning to the hypothetical school example, suppose we have data from a sample of 20 randomly selected seniors on their career aspirations and we want to compare them to data from other grades. A PPS sample would need 30 freshman, 25 sophomores, and 25 juniors.

Non-probability Sampling

The second kind of sampling is known as non-probability sampling; each element of the population has an unknown probability of being selected (sometimes referred to as convenience sampling). Non-probability sampling is usually not a wise strategy, as inferences drawn from the data can be misleading. If a non-probability or convenience sample is necessary, then two procedures can be followed to improve its representativeness.

First, a purposive selection of specific cases can be selected. Such quota sampling strategies are used to select respondents that have certain characteristics. For example, the researcher may wish to interview married women with a college education, and although a convenience sample is being selected, the sample is a well-defined one. A second strategy is to interview key informants purposively selected on the basis of their role. For example, a campaign study might interview TV producers to learn how shows are developed. Further discussion of sampling issues can be found in Kish (1965), Sudman (1976), Henry (1990), and Scheaffer et al. (1990).

The most important consideration for constructing a sample is that it represent the population from which it is drawn. Sample bias can be introduced in a number of places: *(1)* when the list is created, *(2)* when a sample is drawn from the list, *(3)* when potential respondents are contacted, *(4)* when respondents decide whether or not to participate, and *(5)* when respondents choose to answer some questions and not others. Biases at any point in this chain distort the data and make them less representative of the population.

The researcher has direct control over all of these sources of bias and therefore should devote considerable energy to attempting to minimize them. The population list should be representative of the population. Appropriate solicitation and questionnaire construction should be used to contact and solicit interviews. A minimally biased sample will be representative of the population and data gathered will accurately reflect the population's characteristics. The central limit theorem, derived from mathematics, has shown that a representative and large enough sample provides an accurate estimate of a population characteristic.

SAMPLE SIZE

There are four alternative methods used to determine the sample size needed for a study. These methods depend partly on the study's analysis plan and partly on expected associations between key variables (i.e., program impact). The four methods are *(1)* the tabulation method, *(2)* the proportions method, *(3)* the differences method, and *(4)* power analysis. This section describes the first three

TABLE 7-2. Hypothetical Cross-tabulation of Program Exposure and Contraceptive Practice

CONTRACEPTIVE PRACTICE	PROGRAM EXPOSURE			
	NONE (10%)	LOW (20%)	MEDIUM (35%)	HIGH (>35%)
Current user (50%)				
Past user (20%)				
Never user (30%)				

methods and introduces two correction factors. The next section discusses power analysis, which relates sample size to confidence in the statistical test.

Tabulation Method

The tabulation method sets a minimum number of cases for the categories of key variables (Fisher et al., 1991). The tabulation method requires that each category of the independent variables contain at least 50 cases. Suppose program exposure is a key variable of interest and is classified in four categories as none, low, medium, and high (Table 7–2). The required sample size would be 500, because 500 interviews would have to be conducted to get 50 people who were not exposed.

The tabulation method also stipulates that the expected number of cases in each cell of a two-variable cross-tabulation is at least 5 (Fisher et al., 1991). To determine this number, the researcher divides the product of the proportions in the smallest categories of the two variables into 5. In the present example, the two least frequent categories are "not exposed" with 10% and "past users" with 20%. A minimum sample size of 250 ($5/((0.10)(0.20)) = 250$) is required. The sample size required for the analysis is the larger of the two conditions, 500.

In practice, the cross-tabulation method is rarely used, as distributions of variables may be unknown. In health promotion program evaluations, it is difficult to predict the reach of a given program a priori. Thus, researchers often use the proportions method to estimate sample size requirements.

Proportions Method

The proportions method is quick and easy to use, and it is often used in meetings to discuss evaluation costs and sample size requirements. It provides a reasonably good estimate of the desired sample size in most situations. The proportions method is used in survey polls that measure public opinion on an issue or voting preference. For example, sample of 1067 respondents provides an estimate that is 95% accurate to within ±3 percentage points.

The proportions method is used to determine the sample size needed for an accurate estimate of a variable such as knowledge, attitude, or practice. To obtain accurate estimates in a population >10,000, Equation 7–1 is used. The researcher specifies three things: *(1)* an estimate of the proportion to have a particular characteristic (*p*); *(2)* the degree of accuracy desired (*d*); and *(3)* the confidence interval around the estimate (*z*). In practice, all three of these parameters can take *customary values*—those that are used in most surveys. The proportions formula is:

$$n = \frac{(z^2)pq}{d^2} \tag{7-1}$$

where *n* is the sample size required, *z* is the standard score for the corresponding confidence intervals, *p* is the estimated proportion of the variable, *q* is $1 - p$, and *d* is the degree of accuracy. The customary values are: $z = 1.96$ (often rounded to 2); $p = 50\%$; $q = 50\%$; and $d = 0.05$. These values correspond to a belief that 50% of the population holds an opinion or engages in a behavior, there will be a 95% confidence interval around the estimate obtained from the sample, and it will be accurate 95 times out of 100 estimations. Using these values, the required sample size is:

$$\frac{1.96^2(0.5)(0.5)}{0.05^2} = 372.4 \tag{7-2}$$

This formula is quite convenient and can be simplified still further to $1/d^2$, since $2^2(0.50)(0.50) = 1$. Therefore, estimating a proportion with 5% accuracy ($d = 0.05$) requires a sample size of 400. Lower or higher estimates of *p*, the population opinion, yield smaller sample sizes, whereas more confident and more accurate restrictions on *z* and *d*, respectively, yield larger sample size requirements.

The proportions method provides a simple formula for calculating sample sizes. Although this method works well in many situations, two correction factors should be considered: *(1)* the design effect and *(2)* the population size.

Design effect. Samples are often selected in a multistage process, clusters (e.g., counties) are sampled, and then households are sampled within clusters. The distortion from simple random sampling introduced by the clusters is known as a *design effect* (Aday, 1989), or the degree of distortion from simple random sampling created by the sampling design. The design effect should be considered when computing sample sizes because it alters the appropriateness of the sample size. A sample drawn from 5 clusters will usually be more biased than one drawn from 20 clusters since the latter covers more of the country's population. The sample drawn from five clusters may be more representative of the five clusters, since there will be larger samples within each one. To account for the design effect, a design effect parameter is included in the numerator of the sample size calculation.

The design effect is the ratio of variances between and within clusters on the variable of interest. If the variance between clusters is greater than that within clusters, the ratio will be >1 and a larger sample will be needed. For example, in an evaluation of a national campaign designed to reduce smoking, urban and rural communities would be compared with regard to smoking. A multistage clustering sample would select rural and urban communities and estimate variance to estimate the design effect. A typical design effect value would be 1.7 so that a sample size of 400 would then be 400 × 1.7, or 680.

Sampling fraction. A second sample size correction factor is used when selecting a sample from a relatively small population such that the desired sample size may be a sizeable proportion of the population (Monette et al., 1998). A *sampling fraction* is the proportion of the population represented by a sample. For example, given a required sample size of 500 in a population of 5000, the sampling fraction is 10% (500/5000). When the sampling fraction exceeds 5%, the required sample size should be adjusted with the following equation (Monette et al., 1998):

$$n' = \frac{n}{\left(1 + \left(\frac{n}{N}\right)\right)} \tag{7–3}$$

where n' = the new sample size, n = the original sample size, and N is the population size. Applying this equation to the hypothetical example yields an adjusted sample size of 454.5.

The tabulation and proportion methods provide techniques to estimate sample size requirements based on simple rules regarding expected variable distributions and customary values. These techniques do not, however, take into account expectations about a program's effectiveness. Expectation regarding program effectiveness is directly related to required sample size. Logically, demonstrating the impact for an effective program (changed many people's behavior) would require fewer interviews than for one that is not effective. The differences method provides an equation to calculate the needed sample size on the basis of expected program impact.

Differences Method

Many evaluations are designed to determine whether a program changed or created a difference between baseline and follow-up (or exposed and unexposed).

The needed sample size is calculated with the same equation as in the proportions method, with a minor modification of multiplying the numerator by 2:

$$n = \frac{2(z^2)pq}{d^2} \qquad (7\text{-}4)$$

where n is the sample size required, z is the standard score corresponding to the desired confidence intervals size, p is the estimate proportion, q is $(1 - p)$, and d is the estimate of the expected difference. For example, suppose a program is expected to increase a behavior by 8%. The sample size needed to conduct this test is:

$$\frac{2(2^2)(0.50)(0.50)}{0.08^2} = 312 \qquad (7\text{-}5)$$

A simple way to use this equation is to reduce the numerator to 2 (2 = 2 × 4 × 0.5 × 0.5), insert the expected effect size as a difference in the denominator, and square it.

In addition to effect sizes, researchers may be interested in comparing results between groups, such as men and women, or between different cities. In such cases, the sample size needs to increase according to the number of groups. Consequently, sample sizes are often at least 500 and are routinely in the 2000–3000 range. Researchers should use the expertise of qualified statisticians whenever possible to compute sample size requirements.

In the evaluation of the Bolivian health communication campaign to be discussed later, the campaign was expected to increase the proportion of individuals who sought information on contraception or started to use it by 7%. To get an accurate estimate with 95% confidence intervals ($z = 2$) and with a current prevalence of 30% ($p = 0.3$; $q = 0.7$), 171 interviews were required. Thus, a minimum of 171 interviews per city were conducted, and the remainder of the sample was then selected according to the population proportions. If the campaign was expected to change behavior by 5 percentage points, d would have equaled 5 and the necessary sample size calculated. Sample size calculations can be complex, thus qualified statisticians and survey methodologists are a great help in this endeavor. It is important, however, that evaluators know the basis for sample size calculations. For additional references, consult Cohen (1977), Lachin (1981), Kraemer and Theimann (1987), Lipsey (1990), and Fisher et al. (1991).

POWER

Calculations of sample size are needed to validly assess impact as well as to assess the robustness of a given statistical test. This line of research is known as *power analysis* (Cohen, 1977; Kraemer and Thiemann, 1987; Borenstein et al., 1997). *Power* is the ability of a statistical test to detect a significant association when such an association actually exists. "The power of a statistical test of a null hypothesis is the probability that it will lead to the rejection of the null hypothesis, i.e., the probability that it will result in the conclusion that the phenomenon exists" (Cohen, 1977, p. 4). In other words, the power of a test is a measure of its ability to detect a true effect.

The most common way to determine the required sample size is to first determine the expected effect size, then use power equations to determine the sample size needed for that effect to be statistically significant. Power analysis is also used to determine the effect size needed to have a significant result given a predetermined sample size. Since sample size is often restricted by the available resources, researchers may have limited sample sizes or may conduct secondary analysis and need to know the power.

Thus, power analysis works two ways: to determine the needed sample size for a given effect size and the needed effect size for a given sample size. In other words, power analysis determines *(1)* a priori the sample size needed for a study to detect impact, and *(2)* a posteriori the power of a test (how often an effect size would be considered statistically significant). Power equations relate four components of an evaluation:

1. Effect size (magnitude of difference, correlation coefficient, etc., also known as Δ)
2. Significance level (type I error or alpha level—usually 0.05 or 0.01)
3. Sample size (number of subjects needed or number already interviewed)
4. Power (the confidence the researcher can have in the test result).

Because these four components are related, if any three are known, the fourth can be computed. Thus a researcher can determine the desired sample size by specifying *(1)* the expected effect size, *(2)* the significance level, and *(3)* power. The basic power equation is:

$$n = \frac{[z_{\alpha/2} + z_\beta]^2 2(p)(q)}{\Delta^2} \tag{7-6}$$

where $z_{\alpha/2}$ is the two-tailed critical value; z_β is the critical value for β (type II error); p is the estimate of sample proportion (can be estimated at 0.5); q is $1 - p$; and Δ is the effect size (e.g., difference in proportions). Note that this formula is quite similar to the one above with the exception that we have a included a term for the power of the test, z_β, in addition to α. The sample size needed to detect a 15 percentage point difference (Δ), at an α of 0.05 ($Z_{\alpha/2} = 1.96$), and 90% power ($z_\beta = 1.28$) is 233 per group:

$$\frac{[1.96 + 1.28]^2 2(0.50)(0.50)}{0.15^2} = 233 \tag{7-7}$$

Similar equations are used for power analysis with different test statistics such as a correlation coefficient, analysis of variance (ANOVA), or t-test. These test statistics are divided by their variances to get Δ, the standardized effect size. There are numerous computer programs available for power analysis, such as Precision (Borenstein et al., 1997), Nquery (Statistical Solutions), and EpiInfo (CDC/WHO).

As an example of power analysis, suppose a study finds that participants improved their knowledge by 10% and reports this as being statistically significant. The power of this result can be specified. Power is the proportion of times the statistical test would have the result if repeated in different settings. If power is 80%, it indicates that out of 100 tests conducted among this population and with this effect size, 80 of them would be considered significant.

Thus far, the effect size has been presented as a percent point difference. Effect sizes are calculated in a variety of ways, and are usually standardized by dividing the measure by its variance. Estimating an anticipated effect size to determine the needed sample size is an important step in the evaluation process, and will be addressed further in the Meta-analysis section of Chapter 13.

It is easy to confuse power with the critical value (also referred to as the alpha level), the probability of rejecting the null hypothesis. The distinction is that power is set before a statistical test is conducted to indicate how likely the researcher will find a statistically significant result and afterwards to indicate how confident one should feel about it. In other words, given a specific statistical result (significant or non-significant), power indicates how likely that result was, given the study parameters of sample size, effect size, and the significance level chosen for the test, α.

The critical value of the statistical test (α) and power are directly related, but represent two different viewpoints of the test. The critical value is the probability that a statistic would have occurred by chance. It is set by the researcher and probabilities lower than it are considered statistically significant. Power, on the other hand, is a characteristic of the test that is dependent on the critical value as well as the test statistic (effect size) and sample size. Both statistical significance and power are derived by calculating the probability of rejecting the null hypothesis if the same test were repeated numerous times. "To obtain the significance level, these hypothetical reruns are done when the null hypothesis is taken to be true. To obtain power, these hypothetical reruns are done when the researchers' theory is true" (Kraemer and Thiemann, 1987, p. 23).

SAMPLE SELECTION

Once the sample type and size have been determined, the sample selection strategy is specified. Typically, a multistage sampling strategy is used, the universe is defined by clusters or strata, and a systematic sample of them is selected. For example, a statewide interview of people at their homes would stratify urban versus rural counties, select every third county, and select every thousandth household to be interviewed.

Clustering saves money spent on data collection. These costs would increase substantially for a random sample of households since the households selected would, in all likelihood, be far from one another, thus increasing the expense of visiting them. To reduce the cost, households are organized and selected by clusters so that interviewers can visit selected households within the same clusters more easily. These multistage sampling designs, however, result in non-random samples.

People in the same group or community will tend to be more like one another, and less varied than people from different groups. Households within the same census track, for example, are likely to be more similar in terms of household education, income, and ethnicity than those in other tracks. Thus, clustering creates bias in sample selection that should be corrected with statistical clustering correction techniques such as the intraclass correlation. These correction procedures are usually referred to as survey design procedures and should be used whenever researchers have a multistage sampling strategy or clustered data.

Figure 7–1 is a schematic representation of a multistage sample selection. The universe of eligible units (e.g., households in a county, students in a school, employees in an organization) is enumerated, then collapsed into clusters (blocks, classrooms, divisions) and a random selection of these clusters is selected. Figure 7–1 depicts households clustered within blocks, clustered within counties. Households are the primary sampling units and would be the unit of analysis.

Selection within Households

A further issue in sample selection is the selection of a person within the household to interview. For example, in telephone surveys, women answer the phone more frequently than men and hence random digit-dial telephone surveys may be biased unless a strategy to select men is used. For example, the interviewer could request to interview the oldest adult male with every second or third call.

Household surveys may require more complex selection strategies. For example, to study parenting, household finances, and health outcomes among moth-

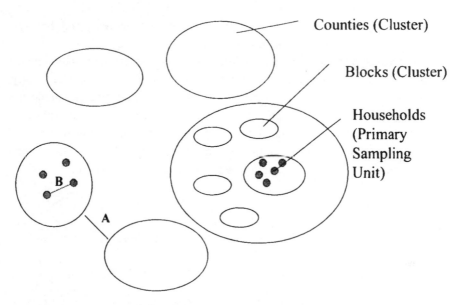

Counties (Cluster)

Blocks (Cluster)

Households (Primary Sampling Unit)

FIGURE 7–1. Schematic of multistage sample selection. Variance for A (between groups) is often greater than B (within group).

ers, researchers may wish to visit respondents in their homes to conduct observations and avoid bias introduced by other methods (phone access, for example). Since some households have several families or several parents, respondent selection procedures need to be developed rather than relying solely on interviewing the person who answers the door. These procedures could include interviewing the person whose birthday is nearest the date of the interview or whose first name begins a with a randomly selected letter of the alphabet. The important point is to develop procedures that create random selection procedures to reduce the bias introduced by interviewing whomever answers the door or the telephone.

SUMMARY

This chapter has outlined issues and procedures to be addressed when designing and selecting a sample. Sampling types were divided into probability and non-probability samples. Probability samples are those in which the likelihood that a particular respondent is included in the sample is known, whereas with non-probability ones, the likelihood is unknown. Probability samples are usually preferred. The most common type of probability sample is the systematic sample, in which every k^{th} element is selected. Usually, systematic samples are selected in a multistage approach in which clusters are selected randomly and then systematic samples selected within clusters.

Sample size considerations and power analysis help researchers determine the appropriate sample size, based on estimates of program effectiveness. Conversely, researchers can determine how much power they have with a given a sample size and program effect. The chapter closed with a discussion of sample selection. Statistical procedures for conducting survey design have been created to control for the biases introduced in multistage sample selection. The next chapter presents techniques for constructing a questionnaire and collecting data.

Chapter Eight

Data Collection and Management

This chapter describes techniques for collecting and managing evaluation data. Faulty collection and management of data can be a significant barrier to successful evaluation; valid and reliable data are needed to make valid and reliable estimates of program effects. This chapter presents procedures for data collection, coding, entry, and management.

Guidelines for proper data management include proper labeling and cleaning of data and variable construction. Data collection is the construction of a questionnaire or other instrument and its administration to a sample. Data coding and entry are used to convert responses to numbers and enter them into a database. Data management is a general term for the storage, labeling, cleaning, and processing of data. Although this chapter addresses these issues primarily in the context of phone and in-person interview methods, the Internet is increasingly being used as a data collection medium. Response rates and their calculation are then discussed. The chapter closes with a discussion of how to combine datasets.

CONSTRUCTION OF QUESTIONNAIRE OR INSTRUMENT

This section presents prescriptions for designing and writing survey questions. Rules for how to compose questions are presented, along with a strong recommendation to pretest questionnaires. A typology of questionnaire items with examples is provided, followed by a review of various interview techniques such as mail, phone, and in-person interviews.

Developing questionnaires can be difficult, yet it is one of the more important aspects of any research project, as the questionnaire determines the type and quality of data. Poorly constructed questionnaires provide misleading data and uninterpretable results, leading to a poor evaluation. Consequently, a well-constructed questionnaire aids in data analysis and interpretation. A number of prescriptions exist for the construction of a good questionnaire. This subsection is based on the advice compiled by Converse and Presser (1986).

The first principle is simplicity. Questionnaires should be simple to administer and easy to understand. The more complex the questionnaire and questions, the more difficult it is for respondents to complete. Short questions should be asked, as they are easier for the respondent to understand. Also, everyday language with simple terms and sentence structure should be used. Interviewers should be taught to speak in clear, common, simple language.

Double-barreled questions should be avoided, as the respondent may be answering one or both parts of the question. An example of a double-barreled questions is: "Do you get health information from the mass media and your friends?" A "yes" response could mean that the respondent gets health information from the media *and* their friends, or one but not the other. A better question for determining where people get health information is: "Where do you get your health information?" The following categories should be provided: friends, my/a doctor, another health professional, newspapers, radio, television, other, don't know, don't get health information. Look for the word "and" in survey questions as a signal that it may be double-barreled.

Double negatives should also be avoided, as they can be confusing. Double negatives, either explicitly or implicitly have two negatives. For example, for the question, "Do you disagree with the following statement: I will not vote in the next election?", a "yes" response indicates that the person will vote in the next election. Double negatives often yield poor data.

Response options should be placed at the end of the question so they are fresh in the respondents' mind. For example, a question about contraceptive attitudes could be phrased as follows: "If your partner was opposed to contraception, would you use it anyway, think about using it or not using it, or definitely not use it?" The three answer options finish the question, facilitating the response.

Whenever possible, closed-ended questions with precoded response categories should be used. Open-ended questions requiring written responses are time consuming both for the respondent and the researcher. It takes a considerable amount of time to read the open-ended responses, develop coding schemes, and enter the data. Open-ended questions should be used only as a last resort. Respondents should be provided with a limited number of response categories that are exhaustive and mutually exclusive.

Few response categories should be used so that respondents are presented with manageable tasks. If respondents get frustrated with the interview, they will terminate it or provide meaningless responses. It is easier to answer questions about facts than opinions.

Also definitions for any terms included in the survey should be provided. For example, when studying immunizations the immunization being asking about should always be defined. Definitions and other instructions should be included on the survey so that anyone reading it knows exactly what the interviewers read and hence to what respondents answered.

Finally, there are a few useful guidelines to asking respondents to recall some event or behavior. Whenever possible, a specific time period should be used, such as, "Have you listened to the radio in the past week?" Typical behavior should be checked against more specific reports. For example, "In a typical day, how many hours do you spend watching TV?" Then the same question should be asked more specifically: "Yesterday, how many hours did you spend watching TV?" Landmarks and cues should be provided to remove guesswork: "Have you visited a health center in the past month, such as the one located on Sixth Street and Lincoln Avenue?"

There is disagreement about whether a middle category should be included on scaled responses. For example, in an attitude question such as, "Please tell me whether you agree or disagree with the following statement: It is OK to advertise contraceptives on television," some researchers argue that there should be four options: strongly agree, agree, disagree, or strongly disagree, with no middle (neutral) category. This technique forces respondents to reply with one of the four options. Others argue that a middle category should be offered, since many respondents may have no opinion on the topic. The best advice is that there should be a "no opinion" or "neutral" category, but the interviewer should not read it (Converse and Presser, 1986).

Intensity should be measured whenever possible—for example, "How many hours per day to you watch TV?" By recording the actual number of hours of TV watched, the researcher can treat the variable as an integer, categorizing it later if desired.

The questionnaire should be organized in blocks so that related topics are asked together. It is helpful to provide a lead-in to a block of questions to give respondents a chance to orient themselves to the new subject and to make the survey conversational. For example, after a block of questions on attitude and before a block of those on media use, there should be a bridge: "Thanks for providing us with your opinions, now I'd like to ask you about your TV viewing habits." The question responses and phrasing should be varied to keep the interview interesting and to help the questionnaire flow logically.

It is usually recommended that questionnaires begin with simple, easy-to-answer, nonintrusive questions. These questions are germane to the research topic designed to get the respondent involved and engaged. The survey should be like a conversation, with the introduction opening the dialogue and creating general impressions. The survey can progress into more detailed and specific questions later, saving the demographic information for the end.

Demographic questions are often asked at the end for a couple of reasons. First, in the beginning, the interviewer has persuaded the respondent to participate on the basis of the importance of the study. If the interview then begins with a series of demographic questions, respondents are likely to feel that this is not what they bargained for. Second, when the interview reaches the demographic section, respondents will know that they are near the end of the survey and are more willing to complete it. Third, the respondent should be more comfortable with the interviewer at the end of the survey and may be more willing to answer sensitive questions.

There are also advantages to asking the demographic questions *early* in the survey. First, it enables the respondent to answer a few questions without thinking and thus can help establish the rhythm of the survey. Second, if the interview is terminated early, the researcher has data to compare respondents who completed the survey with those who did not. There is no absolute rule on whether demographic questions should come first or last, but most researchers prefer to ask them at the end (although in the Bolivia questionnaire included in Appendix B, they are at the beginning).

Questions should progress from the general to the specific. Going from general to specific helps the respondent focus and makes for a more enjoyable interview. Whenever possible, multiple questions on each topic of interest should be asked. This is particularly important for the dependent variable. *A study's significance should never depend on one variable measured with only on question, since it is possible that respondents may misinterpret that question.*

There are several ways to improve a questionnaire. First, have colleagues and noted experts in the field review drafts of the questionnaire. Second, conduct focus group and in-depth interviews with members of the intended audience to develop culturally appropriate language and pilot-test concepts. Third, borrow freely from standard questionnaires and other studies conducted in the same or related area. Standard and previously used questionnaires must still be pretested, because language changes and questions are affected by other questions in the questionnaire. Fourth, conduct declared and undeclared pretests. Declared pretests are conducted with respondents who know they are pretesting a questionnaire and can be interrupted during the interview to determine if they understand the questions. Undeclared pretests are conducted with respondents as if they were enrolled in the study.

Pretest, Pretest, Pretest!

Questionnaires should be pretested extensively. Respondents should be asked how they interpreted the questions, and whether they thought the interview was easy to do and kept their attention. Respondents should be able to follow skip patterns and not get lost during the interview.

The pretest should also be timed, and interviews conducted as quickly as possible. Phone interviews should be shorter than those conducted face-to-face; volunteer interviews should be shorter than paid ones; and commercial interviews should be shorter than pro-social ones. More questions can always be added to a survey. The litmus test for whether a question should be included is whether it is needed to test a hypothesis or is an important control variable. Every question should be submitted to these criteria. Longer interviews create fatigue on the part of the respondent, resulting in lower response rates and poorer data quality. Mailed surveys should take about 20 minutes, but no more than 30 minutes for any respondent. Phone interviews should take about 10 to 15 minutes, in-person ones can take up to 30 minutes. Researchers are obligated to minimize respondent burden by carefully designing their surveys.

When pretesting a questionnaire, ensure that the responses vary. If all pretest respondents answer a question identically, it may not be very useful. A two-response category question (e.g., yes/no) should have 50% to 90% of the response in one category. If more than 90% respond to one category, then the question should be checked. This rule, of course, does not apply to questions that must be asked to test hypotheses.

Question Typology

Questions are open or closed ended. *Close-ended questions* have predetermined and numerically coded response options. Respondents are asked to make a check or circle their answer. *Open-ended questions* do not have predetermined responses, leaving a space for the answer to be written in the space provided.

Open-ended questions should be avoided because there is considerable cost to using them. They are used *(1)* if response options are unknown; *(2)* as part of a closed-ended question for unanticipated responses (the "other" response); and *(3)* if few respondents will answer it and inspection and coding will be easy. Often the final question on a survey is open ended, asking respondents about their impressions of the survey and to comment on the topic. This question can provide rich and useful information, often used for quotes; it is not necessarily coded and entered into the dataset.

There are three types of closed-ended questions: *(1)* dichotomous, *(2)* scaled response, and *(3)* fill in the blank (GAO/PEMD, 1991b) (See Box 8–1). *Dichotomous questions* have two response options (e.g., yes/no, agree/disagree). The yes/no responses may be coded numerically—for example, 1 = yes and 2 = no; or 1 = yes and 0 = no. Many researchers prefer to use the 1 = yes, 2 = no coding to avoid using 0 as a code. The advantages to coding with 1 = yes, 0 = no are *(1)* the variable does not have to be recoded to act as a dependent variable in logistic regression (Chapter 10), *(2)* interpretation is simplified since the

Box 8-1: QUESTION EXAMPLES

DICHOTOMOUS (BINARY CHOICE)

In the past 6 months, have you seen any commercials on TV related to illegal substance abuse?

0. ☐ No
1. ☐ Yes

SCALED RESPONSE, BALANCED (LIKERT)

In the past 6 months, how often have you seen commercials on TV related to illegal substance abuse?

1. ☐ Never   2. ☐ Sometimes   3. ☐ Often   4. ☐ All the time

SCALED RESPONSE, UNBALANCED

How much did you like the last TV commercial that you saw regarding substance abuse? Did you like it very much, somewhat like it, somewhat dislike it, or dislike it very much?

1. ☐ Very much liked it   2. ☐ Somewhat disliked it
3. ☐ Somewhat liked it   4. ☐ Very much disliked it

SCALED RESPONSE, RATING

How entertaining did you think each of the TV commercials was regarding substance abuse? Was [*read name of commercial*] very, somewhat, or not at all entertaining? [*repeat for each commercial.*]

| | ENTERTAINING | | |
	NOT AT ALL	SOMEWHAT	VERY
Commercial A	1	2	3
Commercial B	1	2	3
Commercial C	1	2	3
Commercial D	1	2	3
Commercial E	1	2	3

SCALED RESPONSE, RANKING

Please rank the six TV commercials on substance abuse according to how entertaining each was. Which commercial was most entertaining? Which second most? Third most? Fourth? Fifth? Least entertaining? [*place the rank order next to each commercial.*]

Commercial A _____
Commercial B _____
Commercial C _____
Commercial D _____
Commercial E _____
Commercial F _____

SCALED RESPONSE, SEMANTIC DIFFERENTIAL

For each commercial, I will read two words, and on a scale of 1 to 5, please indicate which word most closely resembles your reaction to the commercial. If the first word reflects your reaction, then respond with a 1, and if the second word reflects your reaction, respond with a 5, and if you feel in between, please provide the number that corresponds to your feeling.

CIRCLE THE NUMBER ON THE SCALE THAT MOST CLOSELY RESEMBLES YOUR REACTION TO [*read for each commercial*]

Entertaining	1	2	3	4	5	Boring
Lively	1	2	3	4	5	Dull
Realistic	1	2	3	4	5	Unbelievable

FILL IN THE BLANK

In the past 6 months, how many different TV commercials related to illegal substance abuse have you seen? _____ (number of unique commercials seen)

---

percentage has meaning, and *(3)* it simplifies summing numerous dichotomous items into a scale (see Chapter 9).

Scaled-response questions provide "a list of alternative responses that increase or decrease in intensity in an ordered fashion" (GAO/PEMD, 1991b, p. 26). Four to seven response alternatives are offered in five ways: *(1)* balanced, *(2)* unbalanced, *(3)* rating, *(4)* ranking, and *(5)* semantic differential. Balanced questions, often referred to as Likert items and scales, use adverbs opposite in meaning to anchor two sides of the scale. For example (Box 8–1), a TV commercial appeal question might be: "How much did you like the TV commercial about substance abuse? Did you like it very much, somewhat like it, somewhat not like it, or very much dislike it?

Unbalanced scaled-response questions have only positive or negative response alternatives. Returning to the TV commercial example, the researcher might ask: "How much did you like the last TV commercial you saw regarding substance abuse? Did you like it a little, somewhat, or a lot?" Unbalanced response options are used when responses are likely to be skewed in one direction, as when respondents are likely to agree to be polite. Use of these questions avoids the problem of all respondents agreeing. The numeric codes assigned to the response categories should increase in value with the response options with the more positive options being assigned higher values. Response codes should consist of evenly incremented whole numbers (i.e., 1, 2, 3, 4, 5 . . .).

Rating scaled-response questions are similar to balanced and unbalanced questions, but are used to compare respondent judgements. For example, to rate six substance abuse commercials on their entertainment value, ratings for each commercial are provided: *(1)* not entertaining, *(2)* somewhat entertaining, or *(3)* very entertaining. Averages for each commercial can be compared to determine which one was the most appealing.

Ranking scaled-response questions ask the respondent to order items according to some criterion. The six hypothetical substance abuse commercials could be ranked from most to least entertaining. Ranking can also be used as a rating, the difference being that ranking forces respondents to chose one commercial as being more entertaining than another and does not allow two commercials to be equally ranked. This may or may not be advantageous, depending on the study's objective. Ranking should not be used when the number of items to be considered is large (i.e., >6).

Semantic differential questions provide a five- or seven-point scale, using words opposite to one another as anchors. To measure TV commercial appeal, respondents are instructed to circle the number on the scale that most corresponds to their opinion of the commercial, such as entertaining/boring; lively/dull; believable/unbelievable; and so on. Obviously, the choice of appropriate anchors is important and determined by study objectives.

These five types of scaled-response questions can be used to avoid respondent and interviewer boredom. Different types of questions in different parts of the questionnaire are used to change the pace and add variety to the interview. However, the researcher should use the same type of scaled-response questions within topics so that individual items can be combined into scales (Chapter 9). Scaled-response questions are generally preferred over dichotomous ones as they allow the researcher to measure the direction and strength of the respondent's response.

One concern in scale construction is the methodological bias that occurs when respondents simply state agreement to all of the statements. To guard against and measure this behavior, some statements are reversed so that they point in the opposite direction of the other statements on the scale. For example, to measure positive attitudes toward family planning, some negative statements about family planning are also used (e.g., women who use contraceptives cheat on their husbands). The analysis should show that this item is negatively correlated with positive-attitude statements.

Fill-in-the-blank questions ask the respondent to report a number that corresponds to some count or frequency of behavior. They are usually used to measure easily enumerated concepts such as age, hours/week watched TV, and so on. For example, a measure of campaign recall might be: "How many TV commercials related to substance abuse did you see in the past 6 months?" The number is simply recorded. Fill-in-the-blank questions are easy to use in statistical analysis.

INTERVIEW METHODS

There are four types of interview methods: *(1)* mailed, *(2)* computer based, *(3)* phone interview, and *(4)* in-person. Mailed surveys are less expensive than phone interviews, which are less expensive than in-person interviews. The lower cost is also associated with less rich information. To some extent, survey method influences the way questions are asked and answered. Mailed questionnaires are the most rigid interview method, providing little opportunity for interviewer and respondent interaction. The survey is received in the mail and completed at the respondent's convenience; confusion or problems with the survey cannot be clarified. A toll-free phone number to answer such questions should be created. Unfortunately, most respondents will not call, and either skip the question or answer it on the basis of their interpretation. Too many ambiguities or difficulties will simply lead respondents to discontinue the survey. Mailed surveys are good for asking sensitive questions because the respondent does not have to verbalize the response or provide it to another person. Importantly, mailed surveys are inexpensive to administer.

Phone interviews are interactive and so respondents can clarify ambiguities during the interview. Also, the interviewer can prompt the respondent for clarification or more information during the interview. Phone surveys are cost-effective and easy to administer. The primary disadvantages are that they provide less rich contextual information and lower response rates than in-person interviews. Phone surveys have been conducted extensively in the U.S., as telephone ownership in the U.S. is nearly universal. It is possible to generate random samples for phone surveys by using random-digit dialing techniques. Phone surveys may not be feasible in regions or among subgroups where phone ownership is lower than 80%. Recent changes in phone technology, such as caller ID and answering machines, are making them less feasible since people can screen calls.

Most survey firms use computer-aided telephone interviewing (CATI) to collect phone survey data. In CATI systems, the questions are displayed on a screen for the interviewer to read, then the interviewer inputs the response directly into the computer. These systems automatically follow skip patterns in the survey, thus reducing human error. For example, CATI systems skip questions about age and gender of children for respondents who are childless.

In-person interviews are the most flexible because the interviewer can observe the respondent and the respondent's surroundings during the interview (GAO, 1991b). In-person interviews often have more trust associated with them because respondents can see and identify with the interviewer. During the in-person interview, respondents can ask for clarification if they are confused. Furthermore, the interviewer can record information that may be pertinent about the environment of the interview, such as whether others were present, what the person was wearing, and so on.

One disadvantage of in-person interviewing is the cost; it is expensive to get interviewers to households or other locations. In-person interviews can and should be longer than other types of interviews. If the survey is short, the cost associated with getting the interviewers to households may be high in relation to the quantity of data, and hence alternative survey techniques should be considered. On the other hand, response rates for in-person interviews are often much higher than for other interview methods.

Increasingly, many organizations use computer-assisted survey interviewing (CASI) for in-person interviews. For CASI, a laptop computer is used to conduct the in-person interview. The survey questions are read from the computer screen and responses are entered directly into the computer (as in CATI). In many situations, respondents complete the survey on the computer with no assistance from the interviewer.

There are numerous advantages to CASI. First, the respondent does not have to interact with an interviewer, increasing confidentiality. Second, advanced audio video, and/or graphics can be incorporated into the survey to prompt respondent recall of a TV spot. Third, the data are entered directly into the computer, thus reducing keypunch errors (although some errors still happen when the wrong keys or options are selected accidentally).

The in-person survey may be conducted in households and at shopping malls, schools, organizations, and other places. When surveys are conducted in schools or organizations, they are often done in a group setting with someone there to answer questions. A group survey has the advantage of being personal while avoiding the cost of getting interviewers to households. The disadvantage is that the interviewer does not interact directly with the respondent and so cannot monitor the quality of each respondent's data or prompt an individual for clarification of a response.

In some instances, researchers combine interview methods, such as mailing a questionnaire in advance and then phoning the respondents to conduct the interview on the phone. It is useful to think of the interview as a conversation between the researcher and the respondent.

Omnibus Surveys

Researchers may not have the resources or desire to conduct their own survey. This is especially true for evaluating smaller campaigns addressed to a specific product or idea. In such cases, researchers can participate in an omnibus surveys, which is conducted on a regular basis among the general population or a subset thereof to monitor attitudes and behavior for a particular industry. For example, there may be an omnibus survey conducted every year to determine the American population's perception and use of household computer technologies.

Omnibus surveys are fielded by large market research firms and used to monitor trends in attitudes, preferences, and purchasing behavior. Individuals and companies can pay to have questions included in an omnibus survey and are typically charged on a per-question basis. The cost depends on the quality and size of the sample and the nature of the questions. Researchers are provided the data on their questions and the demographic characteristics of the sample, but not the data on other questions (paid for by other researchers). Omnibus surveys provide a convenient way to get data on a few items of interest without having to field an entire survey.

RESPONSE RATES

A major variable affecting data quality and the validity of findings is the response rate. Typical response rates depend partly on the interview method used (i.e., phone versus mail) and partly on the type of sample. Also, some respondents might not answer some questions, resulting in missing data for those questions. This section discusses survey response rates, and Chapter 9 explains how to handle missing data.

The *response rate* is the percentage of respondents who complete the survey and is the complement of the *refusal rate*, the percentage who did not. The response rate is computed by keeping a tally of the number of persons or subjects solicited to participate and recording those who refused. For example, in a phone survey, each time a person is contacted and asked to participate, the interviewer records the outcome. If there are eligibility criteria for the survey, such as being married or a homeowner, that information should also be recorded so that the response rate can be calculated relative to the eligible population. For mailed surveys, the response rate is calculated by recording the number of surveys sent and returned. Dillman (1978) provides the following formula for the response rate:

$$\text{RR} = \frac{\text{No. completed}}{N - (\text{Non-eligibles} + \text{Non-reachables})} \times 100 \qquad (8\text{--}1)$$

where RR is the response rate, N is the sample size, non-eligibles are those who did not qualify to be in the sample, and non-reachables, those who could not be contacted.

Suffice it to say that researchers want to achieve the highest response rate possible, and many grants require specifying how a high response rate will be obtained. For example, the U.S. Office of Management and Budget (OMB) requires that government contract research obtain a response rate of 70%.

Dillman (1978) argues that response rates for mail surveys are biased downward, since every survey sent is counted and included in the denominator. In contrast, response rates for phone surveys are biased upward since every number called but not reached is counted as "non-reachable" and subtracted from the denominator. While typical response rates in the past were 30%–50% for mailed surveys of randomly selected households and 40%–60% for mailed surveys from professional lists, these percentages are now considered to be low, given recent developments using the total design method.

The *total design method* (TDM) is the term used to describe the techniques developed by Dillman to improve response rates for mailed surveys. The TDM attempts to "minimize the costs for responding, maximize the rewards for doing so, and establish trust that those rewards will be delivered" (Dillman, 1978, p. 12). The TDM provides specific information on how to achieve maximum response rates for all types of interview methods. For example, in a mailed survey there are three mailings that occur after the original survey is sent: *(1)* a 1-week postcard thank you and reminder; *(2)* a 3-week letter and replacement questionnaire to those who have not responded, and a *(3)* a 7-week letter and replacement questionnaire to those who have not responded.

Dillman (1978) reports an average response rate of 74% in 48 surveys conducted using the TDM either completely or in part. Those studies that followed the TDM completely had an average response rate of 77%, and those surveys that followed the TDM completely and selected respondents from a professional list had an average response rate of 81%. Such high response rates are encouraging, and while there is additional expense associated with achieving high response rates, there is also considerable payoff.

The type of interview method used affects the response rate. For example, in-person interviews have higher response rates than telephone interviews, which are usually higher than mailed ones. Response rates can be increased by following appropriate guidelines and attending to the details of respondent solicitation, question format, and so on.

The response rate is directly affected by seven factors: *(1)* salience of the survey to the respondents, *(2)* quality of the survey, *(3)* reputation of the surveyor, *(4)* persistence and determination of the researchers (for mailed surveys in particular), *(5)* the degree and type of incentives offered, *(6)* notification and cover letters, and *(7)* type of postage outgoing and returning. Salience affects response rates. For example, opinion polls are regularly conducted to determine American attitudes on public affairs. Most people find this activity salient and enjoy expressing their opinion to the pollsters. In a recent survey of clinical supervisors at substance abuse treatment clinics, respondents were asked about their use of guidelines for substance abuse treatment (JBS, 1998). A high response rate was achieved in that survey partly because respondents felt that these guidelines were relevant to their profession.

The quality of the survey instrument, including its format, phrasing, and wording of questions, the survey's length, and any other characteristic pertaining to its administration influence the response rate. The better the quality, the higher the response rate. A good-quality survey can be achieved by following the advice received on question construction, especially to pretest the instrument. In addition, researchers should put considerable effort into the graphical presentation of the survey so that it is easy to read and instructions are easy to follow.

The reputation of the surveyor also influences response rates. More prestigious and well-known surveyors often get higher response rates because potential respondents trust that the firm is legitimate. For example, Gallup is a well-known public opinion polling firm that potential respondents recognize and are more likely agree to be surveyed by than unknown firms.

In a meta-analysis of factors that affect response rates, Fox and associates (1988) found that university sponsorship and stamped return postage had the strongest association with increasing the response rate. Other positive factors included prenotification by letter, follow-up by postcard, outgoing postage as first class, and color of the questionnaire. Notification of a cut-off date and writing a postscript asking for cooperation did not improve the response rate.

Whether to provide an incentive is a difficult decision to make. Whenever possible, an incentive should be included to reward the respondent for completing the survey. Monetary incentives are effective—even small amounts such as $1 or $5 cash gifts. Many researchers have had success enrolling respondents in a raffle.

High response rates substantially increase confidence in survey results because the data accurately reflect the sample and hence the population. With a low response rate, there is always a nagging fear that factors that affected the low response rate also affected survey results.

DATA MANAGEMENT

Data management is the inputting, cleaning, and preparation of data for analysis. Once the questionnaire is designed, pretested, and fielded, the data need to be entered into a computer for processing (Box 8–1). A variety of terms are used to describe data that are important for researchers to know. In most datasets, cases are referred to as *observations,* sometimes as *records* or *respondents.* These observations make up the rows of the data file while the variables are the columns. Sometimes one question may translate into multiple variables, such as when respondents are asked to "check all that apply."

A dataset created from a questionnaire is a "flat file" since it is a two-dimensional array of rows and columns. The datasets are usually rectangular, because the number of cases is usually greater than the number of variables. More complex data structures are possible when respondents or variables are linked to other datasets.

The first variable in a dataset should be the identification (ID) number of each respondent, which should be unique. In some studies, ID numbers are unique within cluster (city, school, etc.), and so each respondent's data can be uniquely identified by combining the cluster and ID variables. Unique identification of observations is necessary to merge datasets (see below) and make subsets of the data.

Variable labels are the textual descriptions that describe each variable and the values are the numeric responses to each question. Each value has a label that is a textual description of the value's meaning. Values should be stored numerically if they are numbers and as strings if they are characters, since computers cannot analyze character data well.

Data Entry

There are numerous computer packages designed to convert questionnaires into databases. For example, EpiInfo, designed by the Centers for Disease Control and Prevention (CDC), can convert an ASCII file of the questionnaire into a data entry template (IMS, designed by the United Nations, operates similarly). Most statistical software can be used to create data entry templates (see Box 8–2).

Accessing Data

Most researchers have data stored in SPSS, SAS, or STATA, the three most widely used statistical analysis programs in the social sciences. Although each program has its strengths and weaknesses, they all provide statistical tools for evaluators. To conduct statistical analysis for measuring impact, covered in Chapters 9 and 10, the data must first be "cleaned" and labeled.

Data Cleaning

Data cleaning entails checking that the values are valid and consistent; i.e., all values correspond to valid question responses. For example, if a question has yes/no response options, then all values should be yes or no. Variable labels and

---

Box 8-2. DATA COLLECTION AND MANAGEMENT

Data from field surveys are input into a computer for storage and processing. These data may be entered with a text editor, spreadsheet, or specially designed data entry program. It is advisable to use a data entry program because it provides the capability to *(1)* enter the data as it appears in the questionnaire, *(2)* establish parameters for checking data entry so that only valid data are entered for each question, and *(3)* build in automatic skipping of non-relevant questions. Epi Info, freeware distributed by the CDC, is useful for this task, as is DataEntry or Survey, produced by SPSS.

Once the data are entered, the researcher writes a program in the statistical package being used to read the data and assigns variable labels (the description of each variable) and value labels (the descriptions of the options for each variable. For example, the variable gender might have values 1 for males and 2 for females, as follows:

NAME	VALUES	LABEL
Gender	1 = male	Gender of respondent
	2 = female	

The researcher then produces a codebook that lists all of the variables, their values, and labels. Then a univariate frequency distribution, the values for all variables, is created so that the data can be inspected. Once these steps are completed, the data are ready for analysis.

For some researchers, the data will be collected by a marketing research or public opinion firm and are provided cleaned and labeled. In such instances, the data may need to be converted to the preferred dataset by statistical programs or with format copiers such as DBMSCOPY. Data that are already entered sometimes need to have variables renamed with new variable and value labels.

---

values are then written. It is not necessary to label values for continuous variables such as years of education since the values are the labels.

Particular attention should be paid to defining missing values as missing values. Often the "don't know" response is coded 8 and "missing" is coded 9. These values need to be defined as such in the computer so that it treats them as "don't know" and "missing," rather than as a valid response.

Consistency checks are then conducted to be sure respondents answered the correct questions (e.g., those who said that they had children provided ages for them). Consistency checks can be extensive with panel data, as certain variables should be consistent between surveys (e.g., being male at baseline and follow-up).

Missing Data

Some respondents will not answer some survey questions. Missing data can be a headache because the number of observations for different variables then varies. For example, a sensitive question such as whether a condom was used at last intercourse may be skipped by a number of respondents. Decisions on how to treat missing data need to be made and documented.

There are at least four options for dealing with missing data. First, cases that have missing data on key variables can be dropped entirely. The number and characteristics of those observations dropped should be documented. If there is a significant number, >5%, analysis should be conducted to determine if the dropped cases are different from the rest of the sample. The remaining data are referred to as the *analytical sample*.

Second, cases with missing values can be recoded to the modal or average value. First a copy of the original variable should be made, followed by recoding of the copied variable, then analysis on both the recoded and original variable conducted to check that recoding the variable conducted did not significantly alter the statistical results. For example, suppose 10 cases have missing values for the variable age and the average is 25. The 10 cases are recoded to 25 and then all cases are included in the analysis. The model is re-analyzed using both variables to ensure that the results are the same. Again, the procedures should be documented.

The third way of treating missing data is to leave them unchanged and cope with varying sample sizes throughout the analysis. Although this option is the most appropriate one statistically, it presents considerable difficulties with interpretation. Different cases are included in different statistical tests, biasing interpretation. In the example for age above, not recoding it would result in different sample sizes for analysis with and without age. Interpretation of the results would be biased because the analysis would consist of different observations in different tests.

The fourth option is to impute values for missing ones, which is done by using other information to make a best guess for the missing values. For example, if data are missing on the variable income, but data exist on age, gender, education, and ethnicity, a regression equation can be computed using these data to determine income values that correspond to the age, gender, education, and ethnicity of the completed cases. These best-guess values are then substituted for the missing ones. Imputation provides the best method for eliminating missing data and retaining the most information in the dataset.

Data cleaning activities can be expected to take at least a month for a moderate-sized dataset of 1000 observations and 500 variables. Once the data are cleaned and missing values accounted for, a univariate or frequency distribution is printed and stored in a notebook for future reference. *The researcher should make a copy of this dataset on a floppy diskette and store it in a safe place.* During the course of the analysis, periodic copies (perhaps every month or every 2 weeks) should be made and stored safely.

Variable Construction

A major component of data management and analysis, the construction of new variables, is done by combining values from different variables. Some variables such as gender will be used as originally collected. Other variables, however, will have to be manipulated and new variables constructed to perform statistical analysis. For example, a variable specifying city of residence may be collapsed to create a new variable with fewer categories, through classifying cities as small, medium, and large.

Box 8–3 describes the importance and use of logic in variable construction and data management. Logical operators are the building blocks of statistical analysis, thus familiarity with logical operators is strongly recommended. Logical operators are used with "compute," "generate," "replace," and other commands to construct new variables.

There are at least three reasons to construct a new variable: *(1)* to collapse or reorder values, *(2)* to combine one or more other variables, or *(3)* to represent a summation of a number of scale items to get a more accurate measure of a concept. If some categories have too few responses, a new variable is created to combine values. Suppose, for example, that respondents were asked how often they watched TV, with categories of 1, never; 2, 1–4 hours/day; 3, 5–8 hours/day; and 4, 9+ hours/day, and further suppose that only 1% of our sample said 9+ hours/day. Because there are so few responses in this category, a new variable would be created to merge those respondents into the two highest categories. A new variable equal to the original one would be created, with 4's being recoded as 3's.

New variables are often created to combine two or more variables. For example, a new variable called "marwom", signifying married women, could be set to 0 for everyone and then replaced with a value of 1 for respondents who are married and female.

The third type of variable construction is scale construction, which consists of adding up the values to a set of scaled response questions to get a summary score. The advantage of using scale construction is that it uses multiple questions to measure one concept. The numerous steps and statistical techniques used in scale construction are explained at length in Chapter 9.

Program Files

After working interactively with a dataset, it is helpful to create program files (also known as batch files or do files) that allow researchers to process commands repeatedly without rekeying them. Program files can be created in the sta-

Box 8–3. LOGIC

The construction of variables, data management, and data manipulation often require the use of logic, a set of operators and rules for these activities. The study of logic was greatly advanced by ancient Greeks and consisted primarily of developing forms of reason. Today, logic forms the basis for computer systems and provides the building blocks for data manipulation and variable construction. The first thing to know about logic is that it consists of the following set of operators:

WORD	SYMBOL	MEANING
And	&	Both things together
Or	|	One thing or the other
Equals	=	Is the same as
Not	^	Is not
Greater than	>	Greater than
Less than	<	Less than

Typically, variables are constructed by using these logical operators to combine values of other variables, thus generating a new variable that is equal (or not equal) to certain values. For example, a new variable that indicates men older than 35 would be created by initializing a new variable set to 0 for all cases. The variable *oldmen* would be set to 1 for each case that has the gender variable equal to men, and the marital status variable equal to single, and the age value greater than 35. The logical operators used are *equal to, and,* and *greater than.*

Importantly, the computer understands parentheses to signify operations that go together. Parentheses are used to instruct the computer when and how to perform operations. For example, if a researcher wanted to add two variables, *attitude1* and *attitude2*, and then divide by the maximum possible on that sum, say 10, the correct syntax would be newattit = (attitude1 + attitude2)/10. If the researcher omitted the parentheses, resulting in newattit = attitude1 + attitude2/10, the statement would provide a completely, and in this case incorrect, result in which attitude1 was added to attitude2/10.

tistical package or with a word processor but saved in ASCII format (since the statistical programs may not understand other program formats). Some text editors such as NotePad or WordPad automatically store files as ASCII.

Learning how to create program files and perform statistical computer programming is a valuable skill that saves considerable time. Program files are usually created to tabulate a list of variables or for a series of statistical analyses. At first programming may seem like a lot of work, and for simpler tasks it may seem easier to type commands interactively than to create a program file. For more complicated work, however, program files are essential and save a lot of time, as data can be added to it and the file can be changed or parts of it deleted. Anything can go into a program file. Researchers can create program files to clean data, to manage data, and to perform statistical analysis.[1]

Saving Data

The data should be saved and backup copies made as frequently as possible. Data should be saved every 15 minutes and always just before trying a command or running a batch file that may not function properly. To retain new variables in a dataset, it must be saved prior to exiting the program.

Coding Open-ended Responses

Typically, a survey questionnaire will have questions with a response category for "other." The "other" category lets respondents write unanticipated responses. For example, a question that asks where respondents get information about reproductive health (question 40 in the questionnaire in Appendix B) may provide the responses "health center," "pharmacy," "doctor," and "other." Many respondents will write in responses that need to be coded.

There are three ways to handle these data: (1) ignore them, (2) back-code them into existing variables, or (3) recode them as new variables. Ignoring these open-ended responses is justified when there are few of them (<10%) or when they are widely scattered among too many different categories. Back-coding consist of inspecting each open-ended response and assigning it a value that corresponds to a preexisting closed-ended response, if possible.

If there is a sufficient number of open-ended responses representing relevant information, the data can be coded as new variables. There are two ways to code open-ended responses into new variables, depending on the type of question. If it asks for one response, the open-ended response is given an unused numeric code. For example, if someone wrote "on the street" to the question "Where did you get that information?", their response would be given a code of 4. The change is made either through search-and-replace in the database or with a recode command.

If the questions asks for multiple responses (e.g., "mark all that apply"), in which multiple variables are generated from one question, a new variable is cre-

---

[1]Researchers will usually write a program file to generate the univariate distribution for all variables in the dataset by getting a tabulation for each categorical variable and the mean, standard deviation, and range for each continuous variable. This program file should generate the variable distributions in the order they appear in the questionnaire.

TABLE 8–1. Univariate Distribution of Education Level for Urban Bolivians Sampled in the National Reproductive Health Program Evaluation*

EDUCATION	FREQUENCY	%	CUMULATIVE
None	76	3.35	3.35
Primary	371	16.37	19.73
Middle	355	15.67	35.39
Secondary	890	39.28	74.67
Post-secondary	574	25.33	100
Total	2266	100	

*Data from baseline respondents ($N = 2266$).

ated to correspond to "on the street." The new variable would be initially set at 0, and then all respondents who checked "other" and wrote "on the street" would be coded as 1.

Labeling Data

Labels are used for tabulations and analyses. There are two kinds of labels (see Box 8–2): (1) variable labels and (2) value labels. *Variable labels* describe the variable and *value labels* describe the response categories for the variable. For example, the variable education, named *educ*, has a variable label of *level of education* and value labels of *none, primary, middle, secondary,* and two kinds of post-secondary. Once the education variable and its values have been labeled, they are tabulated, as in Table 8–1.

A timesaver in the labeling process is the fact that value labels may apply to more than one variable. For example, if variables quest1, quest2, and quest3 all refer to questions with "yes" or "no" answers, the same value label definition is used for all three. Once a value label is created, it can be attached to any variable it corresponds to. If the codes or labels are reversed, i.e., 1 = yes and 2 = no, another value label must be created. (In SPSS, value labels are attached to variables via a template in the data menu.)

Tabulation of Data

Once data are cleaned and labeled, variables are both tabulated singularly and with other variables to begin the process of understanding the data. For example, tabulating the variable for contraceptive method use gives the results shown in Table 8–2. The third column provides the cumulative percentage. It is useful to go through the data by tabulating the important variables to visually inspect that each variable contains valid responses.

TABLE 8–2. Univariate Distribution of Current Users of Modern Contraceptive Methods*

CURRENTLY USE MODERN METHOD	FREQUENCY	%	CUMULATIVE %
No	1565	69.06	69.06
Yes	701	30.94	100
Total	2266	100	

*Data from baseline respondents ($N = 2266$).

Researchers should familiarize themselves with the data by determining whether expected relationships exist in the data. For example, in fertility surveys in developing countries, it is expected that education will be associated with using modern methods of contraception. Table 8–3 presents the cross-tabulation between education and current use of a modern method in the Bolivia study discussed in Chapter 11.

To read this data table, first look at the column and row totals, which show 76 people with no education, 371 with primary, 355 with middle school, 890 with secondary, and 574 with some post-secondary education. For use of contraceptive method, there were 1565 non-users and 701 users. Of the 76 people with no education, 58 (76.3%) were non-users, while 18 (23.7%) were users. For the 371 people with primary education, 312 (82.1%) were not users, while 59 (15.9%) were. Skipping to post-secondary education, 312 (61.2%) were non-users and 223 (38.8%) were users. To interpret this table, read down the column, comparing row percentages. Reading down the second column shows that as educa-

TABLE 8–3. Cross-tabulation of Education with Use of Modern Contraceptive Methods*

EDUCATION	MODERN METHOD USER		TOTAL
	NO	YES	
None	58	18	76
	76.3	23.7	100.00
Primary	312	59	371
	82.1	15.9	100.00
Middle	242	113	355
	68.2	31.8	100.00
Secondary	602	288	890
	67.6	32.4	100.00
Post-secondary	351	223	574
	61.2	38.8	100.00
Total	1565	701	2266
	69.1	30.9	100.00

*Data from baseline respondents ($N = 2266$).

tion increases, the percentage of users of modern family planning increases (indicating that education is associated with method use). It is also possible to get column percentages by reading across the rows and comparing column percentages. The column option can be used instead of the row option, with the same results but a different setup, by switching the positions of the two variables (more discussion of independent and dependent variables is provided in Chapter 10).

COMBINING (APPENDING AND MERGING) TWO DATASETS

To combine two datasets, they can either be appended or merged (see Box 8–4). To append two datasets (e.g., pre- and post-campaign cross-sectional datasets combined into one), it is essential that each contain the same variable names for the same variables (i.e., the variable name *educ* in dataset 1 must also be *educ* in dataset 2). If the same two variables have different names, the combined dataset will contain two variables that cannot be directly compared.

Here are the steps to append two datasets:

Read *data1*
Generate a variable *wave* = *1*
Save the dataset
Drop it
Read *data2*
Generate a variable *wave* = *2*
Save the dataset
Drop it
Read *data1*
Append *data2* to *data1*
Create a value label for wave = 1, *wave1*, and for wave = 2, *wave2*
save the appended dataset, giving it a new name.

The datasets will have different names than these. The combined dataset name should be different from the individual dataset names. Datasets are appended when the survey is administered to different people at different times or different locations. Cross-sectional data are almost always appended.

Panel or cohort datasets are usually merged because they represent surveys of the same individuals at different points in time. Each person (case) should have a unique ID number. (It may consists of a location and interviewer number in addition to the ID, since the data collection group may have assigned the same numbers to different cities or different interviewers.) The two datasets are sorted

Box 8-4. APPENDING VERSUS MERGING DATASETS

The key distinction between panel and cross-sectional studies concerns the way in which they are combined. In panel studies, the datasets are merged and in cross-sectional studies, the datasets are appended.

Since panel studies consist of interviews with the same individuals, the pre-program dataset constitutes the original sample. The ID numbers created for the pre-program sample must be retained and used for the post-program interviews. After the post-program data are collected, they can be merged with the pre-program data, using this ID number. Many questions in the two questionnaires will be identical, since the study objective was to compare changes on these variables. The researcher should then assign similar names to those variables that are identical in both pre- and post-program measures. The two variable names should be identical, with the exception that the post-program survey variable names should have a 2 or something that indicates follow-up survey. For example, the pre-program survey variable *how long*, which measures the number of months a contraceptive was used, should be *howlong2* in the post-program survey.

Cross-sectional studies are conducted with different individuals and so the datasets cannot be merged. A variable is created to indicate whether the data are baseline or follow-up. By appending the data, variable values can be compared between the two waves. For cross-sectional studies, variables that are the same should have the same names.

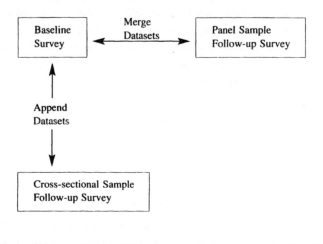

on this (or these) unique identifier(s) and then matched on it (them). Respondents not matched in one or the other dataset will have their values set to "missing." Also, the datasets should have different variable names to distinguish variables collected at different times. For example, education in the first survey should be called *educ* while education in the second survey should be called *educ2*.

Here are the steps to merge:

Read *data1*
Sort the dataset on the ID variable
Save the dataset
Drop it
Read *data2*
Sort the dataset on the ID variable
Save the dataset
Drop it
Read *data1*
Merge *data1* with *data2* using the ID variable
Check that you have the same number of observations in the new dataset that
     you had in the *data1*; if there are more observations, some may exist only
     in *data2*.
Save the merged dataset, giving it a new name.

The number of observations in the new dataset should be equal to the original number of cases that were in *data1*. It may be that some cases appear only in *data2* and hence did not merge with the *data1* cases. Typically, some respondents are lost to follow-up. These will appear only in *data1* and not in *data2* and so have missing values for all the variables in the second dataset.

Successful data appending and merging is required to manage data properly (see Box). Once the data are labeled and cleaned, the process of statistical analysis to determine impact can begin. The next few chapters cover the steps and procedures of data analysis using statistical methods.

SUMMARY

This chapter covered the language and procedures for the collection, inputting, and management of data. Guidelines were presented for survey construction and administration as well as data entry and management. Common survey interview methods and expected response rates were presented, as well as advice on how to secure high response rates. Guidelines for cleaning and handling missing data were also discussed.

The basic language and procedures for managing data were introduced. These include cleaning and labeling data, variable construction, and reading data tabulations. Managing data is a hard task that takes considerable time and attention to detail. Proper data management saves time in the long run since analysis procedures do not have to be repeated to account for variations in missing data and incorrect data coding. The following chapter introduces the next step in the evaluation process: reading univariate distributions and constructing scales.

Chapter Nine
_____

Univariate Analysis and Scale Construction

Chapters 7 and 8 discussed the steps and techniques for selecting a sample, constructing a survey, and collecting and managing data. The data are now ready for statistical analysis to test the theoretical model for the evaluation. Before conducting those tests, however, the data need to be described statistically and collapsed into scales to construct valid and reliable measures.

The first section of this chapter explains the procedures and statistics used to describe variables. These statistics describe a variable's central tendency, the most likely or frequent value, and its variance, or how much values deviate from that central tendency. The second section explains scale creation techniques used to measure, and improve, the validity and reliability of concepts.

UNIVARIATE STATISTICS

Univariate statistics refer to measures that describe a single variable's distribution. The first statistic describes the variable's central tendency or expected value and the second one describes the amount of variation from that expected value. Univariate statistics exist for both categorical variables such as gender and for continuous ones such as age (measured in years).

There are three measures of central tendency: mode, median, and mean. The *mode* is the value that occurs most frequently. The *median* is the value in which half the cases are below and half above it. The *mean* is the average of all of the values. For categorical variables, central tendency is measured using the mode, the percentage of respondents that fall into the most frequent category. For continuous variables (age, distance, etc.), central tendency is measured by the mode, median, and mean, but the mean is used most frequently.

There are three measures of variation or dispersion from the central tendency: index of qualitative variation (IQV), range, and standard deviation (SD). Variation in the variable's distribution for a categorical variable is described by reporting the IQV (Healy, 2001), which is computed with the following formula (Healy, 2001):

$$\text{IQV} = \frac{k(N^2 - \Sigma f^2)}{N^2(k - 1)} \tag{9-1}$$

where k = number of categories, N = number of cases, and Σf^2 is the sum of the squared frequencies. The IQV indicates a variable's variation compared to a standard of all categories being equally likely. If all categories are equally represented (have the same percentages), there is maximum variation. If, however, the distribution is skewed such that one category predominates, then there is little variation.

Variation for a continuous variable is described by reporting the *standard deviation,* which measures the degree to which values vary from the mean. A large standard deviation indicates that values are spread far apart from the mean (deviate from it). The standard deviation is always positive and can range from zero (no variation) to infinity (complete variation). In a normal distribution, 68% of the values fall within 1 standard deviation above *and* below the mean. For example, if the average number of years of education is 12 years with a standard deviation of 2 years, then 68% of the sample has between 10 and 14 years of education (12 ± 2 years). Also, in a normal distribution, 95% of the values fall within 2 standard deviations of the mean. For the years of education example, 95% of the sample has between 8 and 16 years of education. An age variable with a mean of 35 and a standard deviation of 20 indicates that most of the values are very low and very high. In this case, 68% of the sample is 15–55 years old. That same variable with a mean of 35 and a standard deviation of 2 indicates that 68% were 33–37 years old.

Variable description is done, in part, to determine whether variables are normally distributed. A *normally distributed* variable has 68% of cases within 1 standard deviation above and below the mean, and 95% within 2. A *standard* normal curve is a normal distribution in which the mean has been set to 0 and the standard deviation set to 1. A rule of thumb is that approximately normally distributed variables have means that are two times their standard deviations.

Continuous variables are further characterized by two other statistics (also referred to as *moments of the distribution*)—skewness and kurtosis. *Skewness* is the degree of symmetry around the mean. Skewness scores range from -3.0 to $+3.0$, with a negative skew indicating that there are more extreme values less than the mean than there are extreme values greater than it. Positive skew, conversely, indicates that there are more extreme values greater than the mean than less than it. Negative skew is referred to as *skewed left* since the extreme values pull the mean to the left of the peak in the distribution and positive skew is often referred to as *skewed right* since the extreme values pull the mean to the right of the peak in the distribution.

Skewness is also be measured by inspecting the relationship between the mean, median, and mode. If the mean is greater than the median and mode, the distribution is skewed higher by a few extreme scores and thus has a positive skew. For example, income distribution in the U.S. is positively skewed because there are some very high scores in the population. Similarly, if the mean is below the median or mode, then the distribution has a negative skew. If the mean is significantly different than the median or mode, the median may be better indicator of the variable's central tendency.

Kurtosis indicates the degree of "peakiness" in the distribution. Low kurtosis scores indicate a flat distribution and are called *platykurtic,* and high kurtosis scores indicate a sharp peak in the distribution and are called *leptokurtic.*

These four statistics are used to describe variables and estimate the degree of normality in their distribution. For categorical variables, the mode and IQV are reported, for continuous ones, the mean and standard deviation are reported. Variables not normally distributed can be transformed, since most statistical procedures assume normally distributed variables. Deviations from normality affect interpretation of statistical tests and so data transformations that make variables closer to normal can aid statistical analysis and interpretation.

Probably one of the most important concepts in statistics is *variance,* or the amount of dispersion or spread of a variable's measurement. For example, in the measurement of family planning method awareness in Bolivia, respondents knew an average of 6.31 of 11 possible methods. If the variance or standard deviation associated with that average was small, for example, the standard deviation was 1.5, then we would know that most people knew close to the average number. In fact, we would know that 95% of the respondents knew at least 3.31 methods and <9.31 (6.31 $\pm$ 3.0 or 2 standard deviations). If the standard deviation was 3, then we would know that only 68% of the respondents knew at least 3.31 methods and <9.31 (6.31 $\pm$ 3.0, or 2 standard deviations). So the variance measure provides important information about a variable.

Figure 9–1 shows three hypothetical variable distributions with the same mean (average) and different variances (standard deviations). As the variance increases, the distribution of values away from the mean increases, indicating more values

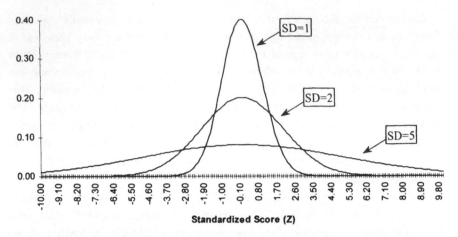

FIGURE 9–1. Three distributions with the same mean and different variances. SD, standard deviation.

further away from the sample's average. Larger variation from the mean indicates that the mean is not necessarily an accurate reflection of the sample's score on that variable, rather it is better characterized as having considerable heterogeneity. Social and behavioral research uses measures of variation to determine if values deviate significantly from expected values and then determine if that variation is associated with variation in another variable.

Most statistical tests were created assuming normally distributed variables. Most variables, however, are not normally distributed. Researchers should check the distribution of their variables. Continuous variables should approximate a normal curve and can be tested for normality using a statistical test (e.g., Shapiro and Wilk, 1965; Shapiro and Francia, 1972). Violations from normality do not invalidate statistical tests, rather they provide additional information to consider when interpreting them.

Variables not normally distributed can be transformed by recoding values or using a mathematical function. For example, suppose age had a high standard deviation, indicating considerable variation from the mean. It could be recoded at naturally occurring intervals to young, middle-aged, and old with roughly equivalent categories.

Mathematical functions are sometimes used to transform variables. The variety and scope of mathematical functions that can be used to transform variables is extensive, and there are an infinite number of ways a variable can be transformed. If a variable has a few values much larger than the average, the logarithm of the variable can be used so that the high values no longer pull the distribution up.

By inspecting variable distributions and transforming those that violate assumptions of normality, data can be more confidently analyzed. It may be that an important variable is not normally distributed, making it difficult to analyze and masking the true relationship between variables. For example, suppose family planning method awareness at baseline is highly skewed to the left so that some individuals have much higher awareness than the rest, but at follow-up the distribution is normal. There may be no change in means between baseline and follow-up, but the distribution has changed, indicating a need to control for those cases that already had high awareness.

Once the univariate properties of the sample have been described and any appropriate transformation made, scale creation can begin. Scale creation is used to assess the validity and reliability of measures, to improve them, and to reduce the number of variables needed to test the impact model.

SCALE CREATION

Scale creation is the set of techniques and procedures used to collapse multiple questions into one or a set of variables whose validity and reliability are measured. These scales are then used in subsequent analysis. A *scale* is a combination of multiple indicators (questionnaire items) combined to measure a concept or set of concepts. For example, attitudes are often measured with a series of agree/disagree statements and an attitude scale created by summing or averaging the responses for the questions. For example, question 16 in Appendix B has a series of 11 agree/disagree statements about family planning. Scores on these items can be added together into a scale ranging from 16 to 48, where 16 represents a negative and 48 a positive attitude toward family planning. The degree to which a respondent agrees with all of these statements represents a measure of a positive attitude toward family planning.

A *scale* is the variable constructed by summing or averaging a set of items, whereas an *index* is a scale constructed by counting the number of conditions or events (such as the number of correct answers to a knowledge test, as in question 29 in Appendix B). Measuring concepts with scales increases confidence that they are measured accurately, since there are multiple questionnaire items rather than just one.

In addition to creating scales by summing items, scales also have dimensions. For example, the 11 items in question 16 may represent one general construct labeled "positive family planning (FP) attitude," or it may measure different subcomponents of it. For example, some respondents may have a positive attitude toward family planning because of its positive impact on children, while others may value family planning because of its positive impact on couples and marital relations.

In this example, people who feel that family planning is good for children may indicate agreement with questions 16a, 16b, 16e, and 16f, whereas people who feel that family planning is good for couples may agree with questions 16c, 16e, and 16g (see Appendix B). Factor analysis is used to determine which of these two patterns describe the data by indicating which items vary together. If all items vary together, the scale has one dimension measuring positive attitude to family planning; if the ones related to children covary and those relating to couples covary, then the scale has two dimensions and measures the two different attitudes.

Factor Analysis

There are numerous texts on factor analysis and many different ways to do it. The most common method is *principle components analysis,* which consists of finding the factors that account for the most variance in the scale items. Moreover, there are various ways to extract factors from the scale items (orthogonal, oblique) and various ways to construct scales once the factor analysis is completed. Factor analysis provides the building blocks for scale construction and measurement theory often referred to as *psychometrics.*

Factor analysis is a statistical technique to measure the validity, dimensionality, and structure of a set of related questionnaire items. It is used to reduce a set of questionnaire items into one or a few concepts. The various procedures and steps for factor analysis make concept measurement more valid. Factor analysis is usually conducted by a method called *principle components* (other methods can be found in Nunnally [1978] and most statistical software guides). In principle components, an imaginary variable is created and each item in the scale is correlated with this imaginary variable, called a *factor,* and the correlation between the factor and each variable is a *factor loading.* The magnitude of the correlation for all variables and the factor is measured as the eigenvalue.

Next, a second imaginary variable called *factor 2* is created and it is correlated with all the variables while simultaneously partialling out (controlling for) the correlations with the first factor. In this way, the second factor measures the degree to which the variables covary with this second factor and not the first one. The process is repeated for a third, fourth, and more factors up to the number of variables being analyzed. The number of factors (imaginary variables) produced is equal to the number of variables in the scale.

If there are eight items in the scale (eight questions on the questionnaire), then the factor analysis will produce eight factors. Each factor will have an associated eigenvalue that measures the strength of that factor—the amount of variance in the items accounted for by the factor. The factors are ordered according to their strength, beginning with the strongest. Factor analysis is conducted to combine questionnaire items into an accurate measure of the concept. The next step is to decide which factors to use, since keeping all of the factors would not result in variable reduction.

Eigenvalues. An *eigenvalue* is a score that indicates how much variation in a matrix of numbers can be accounted for, with the first factor being used to define that matrix. One way to think about eigenvalues is that an eigenvalue of 1 is roughly equal to one questionnaire item. So factors with eigenvalues >1 represent more of the variance in the scale items than a single item. Only factors with eigenvalues >1 should be used, since those <1 are no better than single items. (Usually researchers have to specify this option and can change it if they desire.)

After the initial factor extraction—the process of computing eigenvalues for each factor—the program reports the factor scores (also known as *factor loadings*) for each variable (item) on the factors. The factor scores can range from −1 to +1, indicating how well each item correlates with the factors. For example, a factor score of 0.62 indicates that the item "loads well," or is correlated with that factor. Factor scores for all items on each of factor (those that were retained) are inspected to determine how the items correlate with the factors. Factor loadings should be at least 0.5 or better; 0.6 is good, and 0.7 and above is very good. If the factor analysis shows that the scale has one dimension, its meaning should be straightforward, but if it shows that the scale has multiple dimensions, then the researcher needs to inspect the pattern of covariation in the items and interpret the factor analysis by labeling each factor.

Interpretation. At this point the art of factor analysis begins. The researcher inspects the pattern of factor scores—which items load on which factors—to interpret and label the factors. The item that loads the highest on a factor indicates the meaning of that factor. Since factor analysis creates imaginary variables that measure covariation of survey items, the researcher interprets the meaning of these imaginary variables based on which questionnaire items covary with which factors. Each factor is interpreted and labeled this way.

For example, suppose attitude toward family planning was measured with a series of Likert-type agree/disagree statements. Some of the items measured attitudes toward child spacing and limiting while others measured attitudes toward contraceptive use as being good for couples. It might be expected that the questionnaire items on child spacing/limiting vary together while those on couples vary together. The factor analysis would show whether this was true by providing two factors with eigenvalues >1, with higher factor scores on the child spacing/limiting items for one factor and low factor scores on the second, and the converse pattern for the couples items. The two factors are labeled and the items corresponding to the two scales reported.

In the Bolivia study, respondents indicated their opinion on a series of statements about family planning attitudes by indicating whether they agreed or disagreed with each (Appendix B, question 16). In Table 9–1 the factor analysis results are reported, which show that the first factor had an eigenvalue of 1.99 and

TABLE 9–1. Factor Loading Results for Family Planning Attitudes in Bolivia

FACTOR	EIGENVALUE	DIFFERENCE	PROPORTION	CUMULATIVE %
1	1.99474	1.42690	0.9499	0.9499
2	0.56783	0.32492	0.2704	1.2203
3	0.24292	0.12418	0.1157	1.3360
4	0.11874	0.01287	0.0565	1.3925
5	0.10587	0.09228	0.0504	1.4430
6	0.01359	0.13177	0.0065	1.4494
7	−0.11818	0.02549	−0.0563	1.3931
8	−0.14368	0.03767	−0.0684	1.3247
9	−0.18134	0.05027	−0.0864	1.2384
10	−0.23161	0.03734	−0.1103	1.1281
11	−0.26895	.	−0.1281	1.0000

FACTOR LOADINGS			ROTATED FACTOR LOADINGS		
VARIABLE	1	UNIQUENESS	VARIABLE	1	UNIQUENESS
q16a	0.33430	0.88825	q16a	0.33430	0.88825
q16b	0.49446	0.75551	q16b	0.49446	0.75551
q16c	0.37567	0.85887	q16c	0.37567	0.85887
q16d	0.48924	0.76065	q16d	0.48924	0.76065
q16e	0.56024	0.68613	q16e	0.56024	0.68613
q16f	0.56732	0.67814	q16f	0.56732	0.67814
q16g	0.40823	0.83335	q16g	0.40823	0.83335
q16h	0.33692	0.88648	q16h	0.33692	0.88648
q16i	0.45267	0.79509	q16i	0.45267	0.79509
q16j	0.35864	0.87137	q16j	0.35864	0.87137
q16k	0.09260	0.99142	q16k	0.09260	0.99142

These results were generated in STATA with the command "factor q16a-q16k, minergen(1)"

no other factors had eigenvalues >1. The minimum acceptable eigenvalue was 1, hence only one factor was retained. The single factor indicates that the scale for this population is unidimensional, representing a positive attitude toward family planning in general, and not two or more separate subconstructs (such as beneficial for children and beneficial for couples).

The factor scores for each item on this first factor are shown in Table 9–1. For example, variable q16a ("People who use methods to avoid having children are in a better economic situation.") has a factor score of 0.3343 on factor 1. This is not a particularly high factor score, and so this variable is probably not indicative of the attitude this factor measures, but the item could still be included in the scale. It is customary to use items for a scale with factor scores of at least 0.5 or 0.6. There is no rule specifying the cutoff values for items to be included in a scale.

Q16e and q16f have the highest factor scores and both of these items measure the positive benefits of family planning that accrue to children. Thus, in these data, the family planning attitude measured is that it is good for the children. Notice that item q16k has a very low factor score. This item measured attitude toward abortion ("Abortion is a form of family planning.") and did not load well on the factor. The attitude scale constructed from these items then should not include q16k because this variable is not indicative of the factor. All other items have similar loading, however, and should be included in the attitude scale.

To illustrate factor analysis with more than one factor, we will use data from a survey on TV viewing habits. These data were collected from a random sample of 100 individuals living in the Baltimore area who were given a list of 14 different types of television shows and asked which they watched. The list included informational, news programming, cable news shows, sports, and other programs (Table 9–2). The factors loadings are graphed on a two-dimensional grid in Figure 9–2 to show the factor structure. Each point on the graph corresponds to one questionnaire item, indicating how much the item covaries with the first and second factors. The X and Y values correspond to the loadings on the first and second factors, respectively.

Rotation. After the initial factor analysis is performed, the factors should be rotated onto the items. *Rotation* is the process by which the factors (imaginary variables) are matched (or "fitted") more succinctly to the specific items. In Figure 9–2, many of the variables (questionnaire items) are above the first factor and to the left of the second factor. The items are clustered in the factor space (the space defined by the two factor axes) but not on the axes.

The axes can be shifted or rotated so that they align themselves more exactly with the questionnaire item factor scores. There are two types of rotation: *(1)* orthogonal (the two factors remain at right angles to one another), and *(2)* oblique (the two factors are not required to remain at right angles to one another). If the factor analysis retains only one factor, then rotation has no affect on the factor scores. If there is more than one factor, rotation will usually result in higher factor scores and a better fit of the items onto the factors. Figure 9–3 shows the rotation for the TV viewing factors resulting in more valid measures of TV viewing behavior. Rotation should always be done before trying to interpret factor results.

Table 9–2 shows that the first programming type, informational/documentary, has a low negative loading on factor 1 and a high negative loading on factor 2. Items 1, 3, and 14 all load together, having high negative scores on factor 2. Item 4, daytime dramas, has an opposite pattern, with a strong positive loading on factor 2. Items 6, 8, 11, 12, and 13 (dramas, movies, tabloid TV, daytime talk shows, and night-time talk shows) all load together on factor 1. These 14 TV show types can now be reduced to two variables: factor 1, entertainment TV; and factor 2, news and sports.

TABLE 9–2. Factor Loading Results for Baltimore TV Viewership

I am going to read a list of types of television shows; please tell me which if any you watch on a regular basis. [*Pause after each for "yes" or "no"*]

[ ] 1 Informational/documentary (i.e., Discovery Channel, Learning Channel, PBS)
.[ ] 2 News programs (i.e., *Nightly News, 60 Minutes*)
[ ] 3 Cable news channels (i.e., CNN, CNBC)
[ ] 4 Daytime dramas (i.e., *One Life to Live*)
[ ] 5 Sitcoms (i.e., *Seinfeld, Friends*)
[ ] 6 Dramas (i.e., *ER, Homicide*)
[ ] 7 Music videos (i.e., MTV, VH1)
[ ] 8 Network movies (i.e., *Movie of the Week*)
[ ] 9 Cable movie channels (i.e., HBO)
[ ] 10 Video rentals
[ ] 11 Tabloid TV (i.e., *Entertainment Tonight*)
[ ] 12 Daytime talk shows (i.e., *Oprah, Jerry Springer*)
[ ] 13 Late night talk shows (i.e., *Jay Leno, David Letterman*)
[ ] 14 Sports networks (i.e., ESPN)
[ ] 15 Other (please specify):

FACTOR	EIGENVALUE	DIFFERENCE	PROPORTION	CUMULATIVE
1	1.91884	0.70957	0.4928	0.4928
2	1.20927	0.26462	0.3105	0.8033
3	0.94465	0.41987	0.2426	1.0459
4	0.52478	0.18775	0.1348	1.1806
5	0.33703	0.13256	0.0865	1.2672
6	0.20447	0.14285	0.0525	1.3197
7	0.06163	0.08062	0.0158	1.3355
8	−0.01900	0.07994	−0.0049	1.3306
9	−0.09894	0.00525	−0.0254	1.3052
10	−0.10419	0.09064	−0.0268	1.2785
11	−0.19483	0.04537	−0.0500	1.2284
12	−0.24020	0.06138	−0.0617	1.1668
13	−0.30158	0.04624	−0.0774	1.0893
14	−0.34782	.	−0.0893	1.0000

	FACTOR LOADINGS				ROTATED FACTOR LOADINGS		
VARIABLE	1	2	UNIQUENESS	VARIABLE	1	2	UNIQUENESS
tv1	−0.16382	0.53456	0.68741	tv1	−0.18613	−0.52721	0.68741
tv2	−0.03327	0.38332	0.85196	tv2	−0.20116	−0.32798	0.85196
tv3	−0.04656	0.49068	0.75707	tv3	−0.25431	−0.42220	0.75707
tv4	0.43664	−0.27055	0.73615	tv4	−0.19021	0.47715	0.73615
tv5	0.44677	0.05105	0.79779	tv5	−0.38957	0.22460	0.79779
tv6	0.61520	−0.05341	0.61868	tv6	−0.46289	0.40873	0.61868
tv7	0.26854	0.27159	0.85412	tv7	−0.37740	−0.05870	0.85412
tv8	0.46794	0.19087	0.74460	tv8	−0.48973	0.12477	0.74460
tv9	0.28997	0.15035	0.89331	tv9	−0.32254	0.05152	0.89331
tv10	−0.02470	0.14130	0.97942	tv10	−0.06416	− 0.12830	0.97942
tv11	0.50992	0.04037	0.73835	tv11	−0.43400	0.27074	0.73835
tv12	0.56561	0.08840	0.67227	tv12	−0.50733	0.26522	0.67227
tv13	0.34182	0.24554	0.82287	tv13	−0.42083	0.00582	0.82287
tv14	−0.21783	0.48442	0.71789	tv14	−0.11288	−0.51901	0.71789

These results were generated in STATA with the commands factor tv1-tv14, mineigen (1) and rotate.

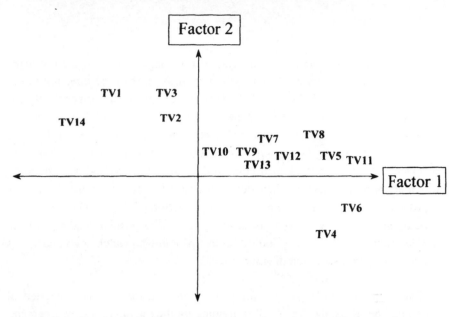

FIGURE 9–2. Graph of initial factors for first two dimensions of TV viewing items.

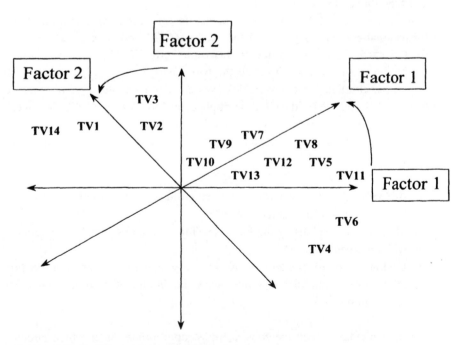

FIGURE 9–3. Factors are rotated to match items.

Negative items. Often factor analysis returns negative loadings on a factor while others load positively. It is very important to consider the direction of the factor loading since it indicates whether the item is positively or negatively associated with the factor. When most items have positive factor loadings and one or some others have negative ones, the negative items need to be recoded so that they "point" in the same direction as the positive ones. Once negative scores are reversed, the factor loadings will point in the same direction and both the positive and previously negative items can be summed to create a scale. In the TV viewership example, three items loaded negatively on factor 2 while one, daytime dramas, loaded positively. Both the negative and positive loadings inform the description of the factors, indicating that people who watch news and sports are not likely to also watch daytime dramas.

Using factor loadings. To this point, scale construction has consisted of summing the items and (optionally) dividing by the maximum to get a percentage. In an alternative approach *factor scoring,* the factor loadings are multiplied by the original item scores to create the scale. In factor scoring, information from the factor analysis is used to construct the scale because each item contributes proportionally to its association with the factor. One drawback to this approach is that it is one more step removed from the original data. Another drawback is that all items are used to create the scale, not just those whose factor loadings exceed the threshold.

For example, in Table 9–2, the rotated factor scores for the first item, informational/documentary, are -0.1861 and -0.5272, and these scores are multiplied by each respondent's value on that variable (0 or 1) to get the first item's contribution to the scales. To create the two scales, factor loadings for all 14 items are multiplied by the variable's values. For example, if a respondent watched PBS and CNN, then 1 is multiplied by -0.53 and -0.42, the factor loadings, to get this person's score on the information variable.

Thus, there are at least three techniques for using factor analysis to create scales:

1. Add items that load well (exceed loading threshold of 0.4 or 0.5 and so on) on each factor with an eigenvalue >1
2. Multiply item values by the factor loadings and add scores for each factor with an eigenvalue >1
3. Explore alternative factor structures by varying the eigenvalue threshold or the factor rotation method, or the factor extraction method (other than principle components).

No rule dictates which methods are most appropriate under which circumstances. The advantage to summing the original values is that the scale is "closer" to the data provided by the respondents. The advantage to using factor loadings is that the scale reflects the weight each item contributes to the concept. Both approaches, as well as others, have their merits and shortcomings. As in much of evaluation research, the choice depends largely on the aims and goals of the study and the conceptual model being tested. Factor analysis and scale construction take time and experimentation to master, but it is worth the effort to obtain valid and reliable measures. Most scales can be constructed following the techniques outlined in this chapter; one exception, however, is when items are hierarchical.

Guttman scaling is used to create hierarchical scales. For example, measuring wealth is usually hierarchical since people buy less expensive things before buying more expensive ones. If they own a house, they are also likely to own a car, and if they own a car, they are more likely to own a household computer. Guttman scaling techniques will indicate the degree to which ownership of items is hierarchical, such that ownership of a house implies ownership of a car which in turn implies ownership of a household computer.

Reliability and Validity

Although often treated as boring sidebars to research projects and nuisances to proper evaluation, reliability and validity provide guides for improving evaluation results. Reliable measures can be interpreted more readily than unreliable ones, which can mask program impacts. Reliability is relatively easy to test and measure, whereas validity is more difficult to assess and often depends more on subjective interpretations. Reliability and validity are related, as an instrument cannot be valid unless it is also reliable (Rossi and Freeman, 1993). Therefore, reliability is tested first.

Reliability is the degree of consistency in measurement. For example, a weight scale may be set to read higher than the person's actual weight, but if it does so consistently, it is reliable (but not valid). A reliable evaluation design yields consistent measurement of a campaign's effect. Reliable survey instruments return consistent responses. Reliability can be assessed by measuring whether the same questionnaire items administered repeatedly yield the same results. Reliability can be measured a number of ways; the literature on reliability and test theory is extensive. In this section four reliability measures are reviewed, with focus on their importance and use, rather than their computation (Cohen, 1960, 1968; Carmines and Zeller, 1979).

Test–retest reliability, the most direct manner to conduct a reliability test, measures the correlation between the same test given to the same individuals at two points in time. Some random fluctuation in responses will occur between the two time points, but a reliable measure will have a strong correlation between the two measures. Although test–retest reliability is important and provides a good measure of reliability, there are few opportunities to conduct it.

Another reliability measure is the *alternative-form method*, which consists of administering an alternative form of the original instrument at a second testing time. The correlation between the original measure and the alternative one indicates the degree of reliability. Although superior to test–retest reliability, it still requires administering two tests.

The *split-halves method* overcomes this difficulty by dividing the scale in half and correlating the two halves; this correlation measures reliability. Specific formulas exist to correct for the number of items in the scales (Carmines and Zeller, 1979). The limitation of the split-halves method is that the correlation may depend on the way the scale is split.

The *internal consistency method* overcomes this problem by averaging the correlations among all scale items. Cronbach's α is the most common internal consistency method, formed by measuring the average correlation of the items in the scale. Cronbach's α is computed by

$$\alpha = N^* \; \frac{r}{1 + r(N - 1)} \tag{9-1}$$

where N is the number of questionnaire items, and r is the average inter-item correlation. Alpha (α) varies from 0 to 1, with higher values indicating more reliability.

When constructing scales and indices, it is important to conduct reliability analysis and calculate α. Some scales may have low reliability, indicating that some items should be dropped from the scale. When constructing indices, or summations of binary variables such as true/false scales, a specific version of Cronbach's α, called *Kuder-Richardson 20* (KR20), is used. In the KR20 method (the 20 refers to equation #20 in their paper), the reliability of a scale constructed of binary items is measured (Kuder and Richardson, 1937). Examples of indices include the number of correct responses on a knowledge test, and the number of agreements to a series of statements. The formula for KR20 is (Carmines and Zeller, 1979, p. 48):

$$KR20 = \frac{N}{(N - 1)} \left[1 - \frac{\sum p_i q_i}{\sigma^2} \right] \tag{9-2}$$

where N is the number of items, p_i is the proportion responding positively to the ith item, q_i equals $1 - p_i$, and σ^2 equals the variance of the total composite score. KR20 ranges from 0 to 1 and is interpreted the same as α.

Researchers should report Cronbach's α and KR20 for a scale. Reliability, α, should be at least 0.7, but scores above 0.9 can be suspect because it indicates that all items in the scale are almost perfectly correlated and hence do not measure different facets of the concept. Ideally, scales should have a reliability of at least 0.8, but lower reliabilities are important to report so that researchers can compare reliability estimates. Importantly, reliability is used to help interpret results and ensure that the scale constructed from the data is the best one.

Validity is the degree to which an instrument measures what it is intended to measure. There are three types of validity: criterion, content, and construct (see Table 6–4 for a description of study validity). *Criterion validity* is the degree to which an instrument measures what it is purported or expected to measure. A test for criterion validity is the correlation between the instrument and the criterion it is presumed to measure. For example, the criterion validity for an IQ test would be its correlation with actual IQ. In the social sciences, the criterion that is being measured rarely has an objective counterpart that can be assessed independent of the measure, such as actual intelligence, and hence criterion validity is often hard to estimate. Criterion validity is usually estimated by comparing a scale to that reported in a recognized standard.

Content validity is the degree to which an instrument measures all of the domains that constitute a concept. For example, the content validity test for a measure of contraceptive knowledge would require that the instrument assess contraceptive method awareness as well as detailed knowledge about the use and function of such methods. Full specification of the relevant domains for most social science concepts is hard to achieve, hence content validity procedures are rarely used.

Construct validity is the degree to which a measure correlates with other measures it is theoretically expected to correlate with. Construct validity tests the theoretical framework within which the instrument is expected to perform. For example, a measure of contraceptive knowledge should correlate with formal education, since education is a strong predictor of contraceptive knowledge in many settings. The degree of correlation between the two concepts is the degree of construct validity.

Criterion and content validity are useful insofar as they provide ways for researchers to think about the instruments used in the study. Their usefulness, however, is limited by the fact that their measure is dependent on *(1)* the degree of correlation with objective external standards (for criterion validity), or *(2)* the ability to specify all the relevant domains of a concept (for content validity). Thus, these two validity measures are rarely used or reported in the scientific literature.

Construct validity, however, is often used in empirical analysis. Construct validity is the degree to which a variable behaves in ways consistent with theoretical predictions. Thus, researchers should examine their measures for construct validity before proceeding to any impact assessment. For example, a researcher using a knowledge scale should be sure it is positively associated with education and income before using it to assess its relationship with behavior.

Validity and reliability are conceptually distinct, but not unrelated. If a measure is valid it will be reliable. Valid measures provide accurate and reasonably true indications of the concepts they are designed to measure. Measurements that are true will tend to be reliable. Reliability, however, implies nothing about validity. Unfortunately, it is easier to assess reliability than validity. Validity is usually estimated using factor analysis and comparison to outside standards, and reliability is estimated with Cronbach's α.

SUMMARY

This chapter covered two topics that are precursors to the statistical testing of the impact model: univariate statistics and scale creation. Univariate statistics describe a variable's distribution by reporting the central tendency and variance. For categorical variables, central tendency is measured by the mode, the most frequent category. For continuous variables, central tendency is measured with the mode, median, and mean, although the mean is often the most accurate. For categorical variables, variance is measured with IQV. For continuous variables, variance is measured with the standard deviation. Continuous variables are also described by their skewness, the degree to which the distribution spreads higher or lower than the mean, and kurtosis, the degree to which it peaks or flattens around the mean.

Scale construct procedures were also described. Scales improve concept measurement because they measure concepts with multiple questions instead of single items. These multiple questions, or scale items, are then aggregated to form scales. Rather than blindly adding the items, factor analysis measure how well items vary together and provides guides for combining items. Two scale construction techniques using factor analysis were presented. The chapter closed with a discussion of reliability and validity and techniques to measure them. Once researchers are satisfied with their understanding of the variables in the study and have satisfactorily constructed scales for key concepts, they can test the hypotheses and conceptual models created to evaluate the program. Chapter 10 provides an overview of the statistical tests needed to test an impact model.

Chapter Ten

Statistical Analysis

The ability to conduct statistical analysis is perceived to be a significant barrier to evaluation. *Statistics* is an applied branch of mathematics for describing and analyzing data. Some researchers feel that statistical analysis is reductionist, and difficult to learn, yet basic statistical knowledge is valuable and essential to an evaluation. Excellent introductions to statistical analysis in social and behavioral research can be found in Healy (2001), Loether and McTavish (1980), Blalock (1988), Williams (1986), among others, and more advanced treatments can be found in Rosner (2000), Pedhauzer (1982), and Harris (1985).

This book cannot cover the many statistical tests used in evaluation research. Instead, the logic of statistical decision-making is described and five techniques that cover 90% of the situations evaluations face are presented. These measures are relatively easy to learn and can be applied to many research settings. Statistical analysis is conducted by programs such as SPSS, SAS, STATA, BMDP, Statistica, and SYSTAT, all of which resemble one another, so experience with one translates into knowledge and ability to use others. To understand which statistical test to use, researchers need to know the levels of measurement.

LEVELS OF MEASUREMENT

Data are usually numbers representing responses to questions or coded observations on behavior. For example, the respondent's gender is stored in the computer data file as the variable sex with numbers (1 for female and 2 for male) representing the two possible alternatives for each respondent. All variables are either categorical or continuous. *Categorical variables* have few response values, whereas *continuous variables* have many values and the intervals between values are equal. Values for categorical variables can be rank-ordered so that the values represent increasing levels or they can be equal. For example, frequency of television viewing is measured with a rank-ordering of often, sometimes, rarely, or never, since "often" is more frequent than "sometimes," which is more frequent than "rarely," and so on. Gender is a categorical variable without rank-ordering because male and female are equally valued.

Level of measurement is a variable classification system based on whether the variables are categorical and equal, categorical and rank-ordered, or continuous. Categorical variables with equal values are nominal, those with rank-ordered values are ordinal. Continuous variables are interval–ratio. The level of measurement dictates the choice of statistical tests used to understand relationships between variables.

Nominal variables are categorical and have equal values so that no value is considered higher or better than any other. For example, gender and ethnicity are nominal variables because none of the values are greater or higher than any others, and categories of male and female are equal in value (Table 10–1).

Ordinal variables are categorical and have rank-ordered values so that each value is greater than or less than (in some sense) the other categories. The magnitude of the distance between values is unknown. For example, frequency of television viewing is measured as none, sometimes, often, every day. Each category is greater than the previous one, but the magnitude of the intercategory differences is unknown. Attitude questions ask respondents to state their agreement on three-, four-, five-, six-, or seven-point scales that are each individually ordinal measures.

TABLE 10–1. Levels of Measurement

	DEFINITION	EXAMPLES
Nominal	Values are not ordered	Gender; religion; ethnicity
Ordinal	Values are ordered but distances between values are unclear	Education categories, Frequency TV viewership
Interval–ratio	Values are ordered and distances known	Age; hours/week watch TV

Interval–ratio variables are continuous and rank-ordered values with equal distances between them. Statistical texts classify interval and ratio data separately, because *ratio variables* have a true zero and interval variables do not. However, since most statistical procedures are the same for both types of variables, interval and ratio data are often treated the same. The values of interval–ratio variables are rank-ordered, each value is greater or less than each other, and the magnitude of those differences is the same so that one unit is the same anywhere in the distribution. For example, age, income (when measured as dollars earned per year), and number of hours of TV watched per week are interval–ratio variables.

Examples of questions for each level of measurement can be found in the questionnaire in Appendix B. Question 2 ("What is your marital status?") is nominal because values are not greater or less than each other. Question 10 ("What is the monthly income of your family?") is an ordinal variable because the response categories are valued, but the distance between values is not equal. (Note that if responses were not grouped into categories but were actual dollar amounts they would be interval–ratio variables.) Question 1, age, is an interval–ratio variable because the values are ordered and the distance between values is equal. Question 16 is a Likert scale of attitudes, asking whether the respondent agrees with the each statement. Each item is an ordinal variable. Chapter 9 described techniques to combine these items into a scale that can be treated as an interval–ratio variable (even though each individual item is ordinal).

Independent versus Dependent Variables

Levels of measurement guide the choice of statistical test for measuring the association between two variables. To interpret the association usually requires deciding which variable influences the other. Variables are either independent or dependent according to their role in a descriptive or causal model. *Dependent variables* are the knowledge, attitude, and behaviors being influenced by the program. For example, in a program to reduce the level of cigarette smoking, cigarette smoking is the dependent variable. Other examples of dependent variables include contraceptive use, knowledge of HIV protection behaviors, voting behavior, instances of drunk driving, drug use, attendance at health clinics, attitude toward drug treatment, and so on. Dependent variables are influenced by independent variables.

Independent variables influence the dependent variables and are not influenced by any other variables (within the model specified in the study). In a media campaign designed to reduce smoking, the dependent variable is smoking and independent variables include exposure to the program, age, education, gender, occupation, and smoking by friends and family.

An independent variable in one study may be a dependent one in another study and vice versa. The classification of a variable as dependent or independent is for model testing and analysis only and is not an immutable characteristic of a variable. This is also true for levels of measurement since different studies can measure the same variable at different levels of measurement. For example, contraceptive use could be measured by asking respondents whether they ever used a contraceptive (nominal variable); whether they used no method, a traditional one, or a modern one (ordinal); or measured continuously by asking how long they have used it (interval–ratio). Contraceptive use can be a dependent variable in an evaluation of a program to promote it or an independent variable in an evaluation of factors that influence fertility.

A hypothesis specifies a relationship between a dependent and independent variable. For example, program exposure (independent variable) increased contraceptive knowledge (dependent variable). Evaluation research consists of testing hypotheses on the effectiveness of the program.

Mediating and Moderating Variables

In specifying a hypothesis between the independent and dependent variables, often the relationship is not direct but involves mediating and moderating variables (Baron and Kenny, 1986). Figure 10–1 is a diagram of moderating and mediating variables, with examples of each. *Moderator variables* affect the relationship between independent and dependent variables such that it occurs more strongly for some categories of the moderator variable than for others. In Figure 10–1, the positive influence of a campaign on smoking behavior is moderated by gender, being effective for females rather than males, for example. Statistical analysis would consist of conducting separate analysis for each gender or constructing an interaction term (multiplying the two variables) and determining its significance. (Note that to test an interaction term, the two variables are also included in the statistical test.)

Mediating variables intervene in an otherwise direct relationship between the independent and dependent variables. In Figure 10–1, spousal communication mediates the otherwise direct relationship between the program and smoking be-

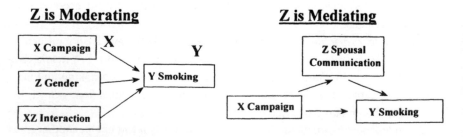

FIGURE 10–1. Diagram of moderating and mediating variables.

havior. There is an association between the program and smoking, but also between the program and spousal communication and between spousal communication and smoking. Mediating variables come between the independent and dependent variable, whereas moderators precede the independent variable. Moderating variables remain unchanged by the intervention, but mediating variables are often changed by it. An excellent discussion of independent, dependent, and mediating variables can be found in Rosenberg (1964).

Conceptual models, such as the one presented in Figure 3–5, specify which variables are independent (gender, age, education, and so on), moderating (gender), mediating (program exposure), and dependent (knowledge, attitudes, and practices). The researcher then sets about the difficult task of measuring these variables validly and reliably, often with scales, and then testing the model with appropriate statistical procedures.

STATISTICAL TESTS

The choice of statistical test to measure the direction and strength of association between two variables is determined by the variables' level of measurement and whether each is independent or dependent. Researchers need to know what statistical test to use, as computer programs will run any test regardless of its appropriateness. There are five statistical tests (Table 10–2) that cover most situations: chi-squared (χ^2), analysis of variance (ANOVA), regression, logistic regression, and t-test. It is recommended that researchers understand these five tests first, then learn about more advanced statistical tests later.

An example of a hypothesis might be, boys smoke more than girls. Gender is hypothesized to influence smoking, so gender is the independent variable and it is nominal, smoking is the dependent variable and it is interval–ratio, so ANOVA (t-test) is the appropriate statistical test.

To understand statistics and their interpretation, evaluators need to be familiar with the following concepts: (1) hypothesis testing, (2) degrees of freedom,

TABLE 10–2. Appropriate Statistical Tests as Determined by Levels of Measurement of Dependent and Independent Variables

INDEPENDENT VARIABLE	DEPENDENT VARIABLE (IMPACT SCORES)		
	NOMINAL	ORDINAL	INTERVAL–RATIO
Nominal	Chi-squared	Chi-squared	ANOVA (t-test)
Ordinal	Chi-squared	Chi-squared	ANOVA (F-test)
Interval–ratio	(Logistic regression)	(Multinomial logistic regression)	Correlation

Box 10–1. HYPOTHESIS TESTING

Hypothesis testing uses logic that can seem odd at first. A *hypothesis* is a statement about an expected relationship between concepts. To test it, the researcher attempts to reject a statement that is its opposite. The research hypothesis is the expected relationship; its opposite is the null hypothesis. Not testing the research hypothesis directly guards against accepting hypotheses that are not true. Hypotheses testing, then, is the specification of the research hypothesis, derivation of the null hypothesis, and performance of a statistical test. If the test shows a relationship that is unlikely (i.e., has a low probability), the null hypothesis is rejected in favor of the research hypothesis.

For example, suppose the research hypothesis is that a media campaign increases knowledge about family planning methods. The research, or alternative, hypothesis is: H_a: Exposure to a family planning media campaign is associated with increased family planning knowledge. The null hypothesis is: H_o: Exposure to a family planning media campaign is not associated with increased family planning knowledge.

In the data from the Bolivia study the correlation between family planning (FP) media campaign exposure and FP method knowledge was 0.21 with a probability of 0.009. Therefore, there is a statistically significant, positive association between FP media campaign exposure and FP method knowledge; the null hypothesis is rejected and there is support for the research hypothesis.

Hypothesis specification and the rules for accepting and rejecting null hypotheses are related to the concept of power. The power of a hypothesis test is derived from the cutoff probability, or critical value, used to decide whether to accpt or reject the null hypothesis, typically set at 0.05 or 0.01. This cutoff, known as α, has a low probability level designed to minimize the likelihood of accepting a false conclusion (type I error). A type II error is the probability of rejecting a true conclusion.

		REALITY	
		DIFFERENCE EXISTS	NO DIFFERENCE EXISTS
Research conclusion	Difference exists	Correct	Type I error Alpha error
	No difference exists	Type II error Beta error	Correct

and *(3)* probability. *Hypothesis testing* consists of stating a relationship between variables in a testable way. The research hypothesis states a relationship between two or more variables that the researcher wants to support. To find support, the researcher attempts to refute a null hypothesis, which is the opposite of the research hypothesis (Box 10–1)—no relationship between two variables. If there

Box 10-2. PROBABILITY

Statistics are based on probability theory, usually measuring the likelihood an association between two variables occurred by chance. Typically a strong relationship (i.e., a high correlation between two variables) is unlikely to have occurred by chance and hence has a low probability associated with it. Conversely, weak relationships are common and hence have high probabilities. For convenience, a probability of 5% is used as the cutoff value for deciding whether a relationship is rare enough to consider it statistically significant, although 1% and lower probabilities are also often used. Probabilities can be put on a number line:

$$0—0.001—0.01—0.05—0.10—0.50—1.0$$

Probability values to the left are less likely, while those to the right are more probable. The lower the probability (the more to the left) the more unlikely it is relative to either random change, or some posited distribution, and hence the more confidence in the strength of the relationship.

is no support for the null hypothesis it is rejected, lending support for the research hypothesis, stating that there is a relationship between the two variables.

The concept *degrees of freedom* provides a measure of the amount of information provided by the data within the context of a specific statistical test. To get an intuitive understanding of this concept, consider the following hypothetical example. Suppose there are 20 blue poker chips and 20 red poker chips in a bag. If 39 are removed, the color of the one remaining would be known. Thus, there are 39 degrees of freedom before one could predict with certainty the color of a chip in the bag. Degrees of freedom is one component needed to determine the statistical significance of a test. *Probability* is the likelihood that an event will occur. Statistical tests indicate how probable it is that a relationship or association between two variables occurred by chance. If it has a low probability, it likely did not occur by chance, indicating a significant association (Box 10–2).

The logic can seem counterintuitive at first: a low probability indicates a higher chance of the association existing, since the probability (also called the significance level, or the *p*-value) is based on the likelihood that the null hypothesis is true. For example, it might be hypothesized that program exposure was higher for males than females. The research or alternative hypothesis states: H_a: There is a significant difference in program exposure between men and women. The null hypothesis is: H_o: There is no difference in campaign exposure between men and women.

The statistical test and the probability relate to the null hypothesis, not the research hypothesis. A *p*-value of <0.05 indicates a 5% probability that the null hypothesis was true and hence a 95% probability that it is false. When the null hypothesis is false (unlikely to occur by chance), there is support for its opposite, the research hypothesis, to be true.

Evaluation research is the specification and testing of hypotheses that specify program impact. Once hypotheses are stated, the level of measurement is determined and then the appropriate statistical test conducted. The results of the tests are interpreted and theory used to guide further tests and specification of moderating and mediating variables.

The following section provides detailed information on how to interpret statistical tests by focusing on three things. First, the independent and dependent variables need to be determined. Second, the magnitude and direction of the relationship need to be defined. Third, one needs to determine whether the relationship is statistically significant, unlikely to have occurred by chance. The experienced researcher becomes proficient at reading statistical output and quickly interpreting it in these terms: direction, strength, statistical significance. To illustrate these procedures, the hypothesis that exposure to a family planning media campaign is associated with family planning method knowledge is tested.

Chi-square

The chi-squared test (χ^2) measures the association between two nominal and/or ordinal variables. Chi-squared analysis produces a Pearson's χ^2 value, which, along with the degree of freedom, has an associated *p*-value (probability of occurring by chance). The χ^2 value and the degrees of freedom determine the probability that the two (nominal or ordinal) variables depend on (significant probability) or are independent of one another (non-significant probability). The χ^2 test is one of the most commonly used tests in the social sciences. Technically, χ^2 is not a measure of association, but rather indicates whether two variables are independent of one another.

In the Bolivia study, campaign exposure was categorized as low and high, and contraceptive knowledge was also categorized as low and high. Table 10–3 reports the cross-tabulation of the two variables, providing the number of respondents in the four conditions (low/low, low/high, high/low, and high/high). The independent variable, exposure, defines the rows, since they total to 100%. Reading across the rows, we find that among those respondents not exposed to the campaign, 68% had low knowledge. The row percentages should be compared between groups to interpret the table. Among those not exposed, 32% had high knowledge while among those exposed, 53.9% had high knowledge. The Pearson χ^2 value of 46.7, with 1 degree of freedom, has a probability of <0.001 of occurring by chance. The conclusion is that there is a significant association between campaign exposure and knowledge.

TABLE 10-3. Output for Chi-squared (χ^2) Test of Association Between Campaign Exposure and Detailed Knowledge

CAMPAIGN EXPOSURE	CONTRACEPTIVE KNOWLEDGE		
	LOW	HIGH	TOTAL
Not exposed	187	88	275
	68.00	32.00	100.00
Exposed	958	1121	2079
	46.08	53.92	100.00
Total	1145	1209	2354
	48.64	51.36	100.00

Pearson chi2(1) = 46.7142, Pr = 0.000.

Analysis of Variance

Analysis of variance (ANOVA) is the comparison of scores for an interval-ratio–dependent variable by the categories of the independent variable. This results in an *F*-score and its associated *p*-value. Again in the Bolivia study, contraceptive knowledge was measured with a scale of knowledge items, and campaign exposure was categorized as low, medium, and high. The ANOVA test was used to compare knowledge score averages for the three exposure groups, and to find the standard deviations within groups and the probability that the differences could have occurred by chance. Table 10–4 shows that knowledge increased between the three groups: the low-exposure group was 41% correct; the medium-exposure group, 53% correct; and the high-exposure group, 58% correct. The *F*-score is 72.14 with 2 and 2351 degrees of freedom and a probability of <0.001 of occurring by chance. The conclusion is a positive and statistically significant association between campaign exposure and knowledge.

Notice that with this test there is another statistical test reported at the bottom, Bartlett's test for equal variance. The *equality of variance test* determines whether the variances between groups are equal. The variances, measured by the standard deviation, for the three exposure groups are 0.23, 0.19, and 0.18, which the Bartlett test informs us are significantly different from one another. (Recall Fig. 9–1, which displayed three distributions with the same averages but different variances.)

Thus, both the averages and variances for contraceptive knowledge are significantly different between groups (low, medium, and high exposure). The significant differences in variances indicate that the variable distributions are different between the three groups in addition to the differences in averages. When the variances differ significantly, the differences in averages should be interpreted with caution. The ideal situation is to have significantly different means with non-significantly different variances.

TABLE 10-4. Output for ANOVA Test of Association Between Campaign Exposure and Detailed Knowledge

CAMPAIGN EXPOSURE	SUMMARY OF % CORRECT RESPONSE OF 14		
	MEAN	SD	FREQUENCY
None	0.41	0.23	275
Medium	0.53	0.19	1476
High	0.58	0.18	603
Total	0.53	0.20	2354

	ANALYSIS OF VARIANCE				
SOURCE	SS	DF	MS	F	PROB > F
Between groups	5.52845003	2	2.76422501	72.14	0.0000
Within groups	90.0804114	2351	0.038315785		
Total	95.6088614	2353	0.04063275		

Differences between groups and probability if each difference occurred by chance

	EXPOSURE GROUP	
EXPOSURE GROUP	NONE	MEDIUM
Medium	0.12 ($p < 0.001$)	
High	0.17 ($p < 0.001$)	0.05 ($p < 0.001$)

The Fisher F-value of 72.14 with 2 and 2351 degrees of freedom was statistically significant at $p < 0.001$.

The Bartlett test for equal variances had a chi-square value of 21.1 with 2 degrees of freedom was statistically significant at $p < 0.001$.

Some investigators argue that differences in variances are a natural outcome of group changes and that an intervention designed to increase knowledge will, in all likelihood, change the variance as well. Others argue that differences in variances indicate an underlying difference in the groups being studied and that this invalidates comparison of the averages. When the variances between groups are significantly different, this should be noted, but there are few options to correct it. One strategy is to transform the variable with a mathematical function that can eliminate differences in variances. This strategy is rarely used, however, since it may not be appropriate to transform the variable being studied. Thus, the best strategy is to note it and interpret the results with caution.

Since the ANOVA statistic determines only that there are differences between groups and not exactly between which groups, it is often wise to determine exactly where the differences are significant and where they are not. This is done using a range test, the Bonferroni test being one example. The *Bonferroni test* provides a table indicating exactly which groups are significantly different from one another. In Table 10–4 there is a significant difference in the average knowledge levels between the no-exposure group and both the medium- and high-exposure levels, and a significant difference between the medium- and high-exposure groups. The range test determines exactly where, and between which groups, any significant differences in group means occur.

Correlation

When both the independent and dependent variables are interval–ratio, the *Pearson correlation coefficient* measures the direction and strength of the association between them. The correlation coefficient can be unstandardized, indicating the amount of change in the dependent variable for each unit change in the independent one. The standardized version, also known as *beta* (β), ranges between -1.0 and 1.0, indicating the direction and strength of the relationship. Again, a probability is given that indicates the likelihood that a correlation of this magnitude with these data occurred by chance.

Returning to the example above, campaign exposure was measured as the number of campaign images recognized by the respondent (covered in Chapter 11), an exposure index of 0 to 8. Detailed knowledge was measured as the proportion of correct responses to 14 true/false questions. Table 10–5 shows that the correlation (also known as regression when there are more than two variables) is 0.21 with a probability of <0.001. The conclusion is that there is a significant association between campaign exposure and knowledge. The magnitude of the correlation, 0.21, indicates a weak positive association between these two variables. Some researchers argue that correlations between 0.1 and 0.3 are weak, between 0.3 and 0.5 are moderate, and 0.5 or greater are strong.

Interpreting the strength of the associations depends on what is measured and the intention and plan of the study. A weak correlation in one context may be strong in another. A weak association between campaign exposure and behavior may seem trivial until one considers that the study may be generalizable to a large population, resulting in a large absolute impact.

Logistic Regression

When the dependent variable is dichotomous (two values), the appropriate statistical test is logistic regression (Aldrich and Nelson, 1984; Hosmer and Lemeshow, 1989). *Logistic regression* computes the probability that the outcome occurred (coded 1 versus 0) for each value of the independent variables. For correlation, a positive association indicates that as values increase on the independent variable, values increase on the dependent variables. For logistic regression, a positive association indicates that as values increase on the independent variables, the probability or the likelihood of the dependent variable occurring in-

TABLE 10–5. Output for Pearson Correlation Test of Association Between Campaign Exposure and Detailed Knowledge (N = 2354)

MODEL: REGRESSION ON KNOWLEDGE

Overall fit statistics

	MODEL	RESIDUAL	TOTAL
Sum of squares	4.97	90.64	90.64
Degrees of freedom	1	2352	2352
Mean square	4.97	0.0385	0.0385

Coefficient estimates

	COEFFICIENT	STANDARD ERROR	T-VALUE	PROBABILITY	BETA
Exposure	0.183	0.016	11.35	0.00	0.23
Constant y-intercept	0.456	0.008	59.90	0.00	—

Statistical significance

F-value (1, 2352 degrees of freedom)	
Probability	0.000
R-squared	0.052
Adjusted R-squared	0.0516
Root mean square residual	0.196

These results were obtained using the STATA command "reg correct tvassp if wave==2, beta".

creases. Thus, the underlying statistical model is a probability curve, not a straight line.

Table 10–6 shows the logistic regression between knowledge and campaign exposure, this time with knowledge dichotomized high (greater than average) and low (less than average), and campaign exposure as the number of TV commercials recognized. Again, the association between exposure and knowledge is positive and statistically significant. For each one unit increase in campaign exposure, knowledge increases 1.17 times. On average, respondents who recognized two spots had a knowledge score 1.17 times higher than respondents who recognized one spot; those who recognized three spots had knowledge scores 1.17 times higher than those who recognized two; and so on.

Campaign exposure has values between 0 and 8. Logistic regression computes the probability of the outcome for each one unit change on the independent variable. If exposure was recoded from a count to a proportion variable ranging from 0 to 1, the probabilities would change, but the statistical significance would be the same. In this example, the odds ratio became 3.62, indicating that respondents who recognized all eight spots had 3.62 times higher knowledge scores than those who recognized zero.

TABLE 10–6. Output for Logistic Regression Test of Association Between Campaign Exposure and Detailed Knowledge (N = 2354)

MODEL: LOGISTIC REGRESSION ON KNOWLEDGE	
Overall fit statistics	
Log likelihood	−1601.2
Chi-square	59.20

Coefficient estimates

	ODDS RATIO	STANDARD ERROR	Z-VALUE	PROBABILITY	95% CONFIDENCE INTERVAL	
Exposure dichotomized	1.17	0.024	7.571	0.00	1.13	1.22
Exposure scale (1–8)	3.62	0.616	7.571	0.00	2.59	5.04

Statistical significance

Probability chi-square	0.000
Pseudo R-squared	0.018

These results were obtained using the STATA commands "logit cordich tvasspd if wave==2, or" and "logit cordich tvassp if wave==2, or".

Multinomial Logistic

Multinomial logistic regression is used when the dependent variable has three to five categories. For example, contraceptive use could be divided into three categories: no use, traditional method, and modern method. A multinomial logistic regression would then be conducted by using no use as the reference category and creating two "dummy variables" (see below)—one to indicate use of a traditional method and one to indicate use of a modern one. Each dummy variable would be set to 0 for all non-users and the traditional-use variable set to 1 for traditional users and the modern method–use variable set to 1 for modern users. Then two logistic regressions would be run to determine the strength and significance of the associations between the independent variables and traditional and modern method use.

T-test

The statistical tests introduced thus far are used primarily to determine whether two variables are significantly associated with one another. There are many instances, however, when a researcher wants to know if two variables are significantly different from one another. For example, suppose an intervention is designed to improve knowledge by testing whether knowledge increased significantly between baseline and follow-up. The t-test indicates whether the average is significantly different between two groups. It is most often used to determine whether a variable changed significantly between baseline and follow-up. It can also be used to determine whether different variables, measured on the same scale, are significantly different from one another.

Table 10–7 reports the t-test results between baseline and follow-up scores for the cross-sectional and panel data from the Bolivia study. The table shows that average knowledge at follow-up (correct2) was 0.518, compared to the baseline of 0.497, a difference of 0.021 (2.1 percentage points). The bottom of Table 10–7 reports whether the difference of 2.1 percentage points is considered statistically significant under three different conditions: significantly *(1)* less than zero, *(2)* different from zero, and *(3)* greater than zero. The t-value is computed by dividing the mean difference by the standard error of the difference. The statistical significance of this t-value is determined using the degrees of freedom. Table 10–7 shows that the difference was significantly different from zero and greater than zero at the 0.05 level, indicating a significant increase in knowledge between baseline and follow-up.

Since some respondents in the Bolivia study were lost to follow-up, the sample sizes were different at the two survey times: there were 797 at baseline and 545 at follow-up. The top of Table 10–7 shows the unpaired results that include respondents without matched interviews. The bottom panel shows the paired results that include matched respondents only. The difference score for matched respondents was 0.014 (1.4 percentage points), having a t-value of 1.60 ($=0.0144/0.009$). The probability that this t-value is significantly greater than zero is 0.0549, which is >0.05, indicating that it is not statistically significant. (Note that for the paired t-test the number of observations is the same at both time points.) These results indicate a significant increase in knowledge between baseline and follow-up for the entire sample but a non-significant increase for those who responded to both surveys.

To summarize, the association between campaign exposure and detailed knowledge has been measured using the chi-squared (χ^2) test, ANOVA, correlation, and logistic regression, depending on the level of measurement. The statistical results consistently showed a statistically significant positive association measured in terms of percentages, a correlation coefficient, or an odds ratio—each with a corresponding probability. The t-test showed an increase in knowledge for the panel sample, although it was not statistically significant when restricted to matched respondents.

These results, however, do not necessarily indicate that campaign exposure *caused* an increase in knowledge. The analysis has only established an association between the two variables and has not met the criteria necessary to demonstrate causality (Chapter 6). To demonstrate a causal relationship, multivariate analysis techniques are often required.

TABLE 10–7. Output for T-test of Association Between Campaign Exposure and Detailed Knowledge

	OBSERVATIONS	MEAN	STANDARD ERROR	STANDARD DEVIATION	95% CONFIDENCE INTERVAL	
Correct follow-up	545	0.518	0.007	0.171	0.503	0.532
Correct baseline	797	0.497	0.007	0.204	0.482	0.511
Combined	1342	0.505	0.005	0.192	0.495	0.515
Difference		0.021	0.01		0.0002	0.042

	DIFFERENCE LESS THAN ZERO	DIFFERENCE NOT EQUAL ZERO	DIFFERENCE GREATER THAN ZERO
Degrees of freedom	1340	1340	1340
T-value	1.99	1.99	1.99
Probability	0.977	0.047	0.024

Paired t-test

	OBSERVATIONS	MEAN	STANDARD ERROR	STANDARD DEVIATION	95% CONFIDENCE INTERVAL	
Correct follow-up	545	0.518	0.007	0.171	0.503	0.532
Correct baseline	545	0.503	0.008	0.197	0.487	0.520
Difference	545	0.014	0.090	0.21	−0.003	0.032

	DIFFERENCE LESS THAN ZERO	DIFFERENCE NOT EQUAL ZERO	DIFFERENCE GREATER THAN ZERO
Degrees of freedom	545	545	545
T-value	1.60	1.60	1.60
Probability	0.945	0.110	0.0549

These results were obtained using the STATA commands "ttest correct2=correct1 if condit~=., unpaired" and "ttest correct2=correct".

MULTIVARIATE ANALYSIS

The statistical analysis thus far has been bivariate, consisting of a dependent variable, knowledge, and an independent variable, program exposure. Other independent variables may mediate or moderate the relationship between these two variables and should be included as controls. They are also referred to as *covariates* or *confounders*. For example, education is often related to both knowledge and program exposure. It is not a dependent variable because it is not hypothesized to change as a result of the program. Since education can influence the relationship between exposure and knowledge, it should be treated as a control, and there are two different methods to do so: *(1)* analyze the relationship separately for each educational level, or *(2)* include it as a control variable in statistical analysis.

Separate Analysis

Hypothesized relationships can be examined for different levels of a control variable to control for its effects. For example, to control for the effect of education, separate statistical tests can be conducted for each level of education. A finding of consistent results across educational levels suggests that the control variable, education, did not affect the relationship between exposure and knowledge. If, however, the association is significant for some education levels and not others, there is reason to believe that it moderates the relationship between exposure and knowledge.

Suppose, for example, that there was no association between exposure and knowledge for respondents with no or primary education, but they were significantly associated for those with secondary and higher levels of education. We would conclude that program exposure was *not* associated with knowledge for those with little or no education, but was for those with secondary or more education. Education is a moderator of the exposure and knowledge relationship.

One difficulty with performing separate analyses by categories of the control variable is the difficulty of including more than one control variable. Two control variables would require analysis for every combination of the two. For example, if both education and gender were used as controls, eight separate tests would need to be conducted and interpreted. Thus separate analysis is usually too cumbersome. A second and related difficulty with performing separate analyses is that it requires larger sample sizes, since analyses are repeated for each category. Given these difficulties, the preferred analysis strategy is to include the control variable(s) in the test in the multivariate statistical analysis.

Including Control Variables

Control variables can be included as additional independent variables in the hypothesis statistical test using multivariate techniques. Multivariate statistical analysis computes the association between all of the independent variables and the dependent one simultaneously. Multivariate ANOVA and regression analysis with one dependent and multiple independent variables is relatively easy using standard statistical packages.

Multivariate ANOVA is used to determine *F*-scores and probability levels for each independent variable. The sign (positive or negative) indicates the direction of the relationship and the *p*-value indicates its statistical significance. Since the analysis controls for other independent variables, a significant association is reported as significant when controlling for the other variables.

Multiple Regression

When there are numerous independent variables and one dependent variable, multiple regression tests the simultaneous association between these independent variables and the dependent one. For example, there may be numerous control variables, such as age, education, and income, that need to be included in the evaluation of whether a campaign was effective at changing knowledge. With multiple regression, these control variables can be included with campaign exposure in the same statistical test.

Multiple regression is used to calculate unstandardized and standardized coefficients for each independent variable with the dependent one. Unstandardized coefficients indicate change in the dependent variable given change in the independent variable. For example, an unstandardized regression coefficient of 0.06 between education and knowledge would indicate that a one-unit change in education is associated with a 0.06-unit change in knowledge. Standardized coefficients are referred to as beta (β) and are used to compare the magnitude of associations between different independent variables. For example, if knowledge is regressed on both education and campaign exposure, and the β for education is 0.30 and for campaign exposure it is 0.21, we can conclude that education is more strongly associated with knowledge.

For logistic regression, unstandardized coefficients also relate changes in the independent variables with those of the dependent variable, but the change is not a linear increase, but rather an increase in the likelihood of obtaining the positive outcome rather than zero. The standardized coefficients for logistic regression are odds ratios, i.e., the likelihood of obtaining the outcome. Odds ratios vary from zero to positive infinity: those that are <1 indicate an inverse, or negative, relationship, and those >1 represent a positive one.

Multiple regression provides the same results, since education is included as an independent variable; the beta value and probability results can be reported as exposure's effect while controlling for education. Since education is not technically an interval-level variable, it should not be included in the regression analysis as is, but rather can be converted into a series of dummy variables.

Dummy Variables

Dummy variables are created from a nominal or ordinal control variable and used in multivariate regression analysis (Hardy, 1993). They are devised by recoding all but one of the values of the control variable into new variables coded as 0 and 1. For example, the four levels of education become three dummy variables: primary, secondary, and some college, each coded as 0 for those without the attribute and 1 for those with. These three dummy variables are then included as control variables in the regression analysis. The strength and significance of each control variable is then assessed to determine which, if any, levels of education influence the relationship between exposure and knowledge.

SUMMARY

This chapter provided an introduction to statistical data analysis. The chapter introduced levels of measurement and hypothesis testing. Table 10–2 showed how to choose a statistical test on the basis of the level of measurement and specification of independent and dependent variables. The conceptual model guiding the evaluation specifies the independent, dependent, mediating, and/or moderating variables in the study.

In the conceptual model, hypotheses are put forth that are then tested by using the appropriate statistical tests. Five common statistical tests were presented using the same two variables recoded to different levels of measurement. Computer output from the tests were presented and interpreted. The use of multivariate techniques and dummy variables was also explained. Learning how to analyze data is challenging and every dataset will have its unique attributes and problems. One should back up the data regularly and explore the relationships within the data. There is no one correct way to analyze data, and no set of guidelines or prescriptions is foolproof. The analysis will take time, but testing hypotheses is a rewarding activity that will answer evaluation questions once the numbers are crunched.

Part Three

Results

This section explains how to analyze data to determine impact. This material is relevant after the data have been collected and the evaluator needs to determine impact. The last chapter describes dissemination procedures and concludes with a summary of evaluation study designs, the book, and assessment of the future of health promotion program evaluation.

Chapter Eleven

Measuring Program or Campaign Exposure

Health promotion evaluations need to measure program or campaign exposure. *Program exposure* is the degree to which the audience recalls and recognizes the program. Evaluating policy changes requires knowledge about how the policy was implemented and expected to work. Evaluating health promotion programs requires knowledge about how the program was implemented and whether the audience was exposed to it.

Program exposure is measured to determine whether it reached its intended audience and how they interpreted it (Unger et al., 2001). Program messages can be interpreted differently and they might not be understood by everyone. Consequently, evaluators need to develop valid, reliable, and comprehensive measures of program exposure that capture the degree to which the audience recalled the message, whether they understood it, and how they reacted to it.

Exposure can be measured as the number or percent of the audience that might have seen a particular program. For example, all people in a baseball stadium could have been exposed to a billboard advertisement. In practice, however, few will have noticed and even fewer remember the message on that billboard. It is preferable to ask respondents directly with both unassisted and assisted questions about whether they recollect specific program messages. In this chapter, *exposure* is audience recognition and recall of the program.

This chapter describes how to measure program exposure, and reports exposure scores for a particular communication campaign evaluation. The data collected were used to evaluate a national reproductive health program (NRHP) mass media campaign broadcast in the larger cities of Bolivia in 1994 and 1996. The Bolivia campaign represents an excellent example of a strategically planned national health communication campaign by targeting policy changes, improving service delivery, and generating demand.

One component of reproductive health is family planning, which has been neglected in Bolivia in the past. Research showed that family planning practice was low and that other reproductive health services in Bolivia were among the poorest in Latin America. The communication campaign was designed to improve Bolivians' knowledge of family planning and encourage them to seek reproductive health services.

The chapter closes with a discussion of the exposure scores and their association with sociodemographic characteristics. There are at least four reasons for measuring program exposure and its association with other variables: to determine *(1)* whether the program reached its intended audience, *(2)* the frequency of exposure for those reached, *(3)* whether the audience understood the program, and *(4)* whether the program had an impact on the audience it reached.

MEASURING EXPOSURE

Campaign exposure is measured on two dimensions (Table 11–1): the type of prompt used to cue the respondent's memory, and the distinction between awareness of the spot and comprehension of its message. The questions can be asked in two different ways, spontaneously and prompted. *Spontaneous questions* are open ended and measure top-of-mind awareness, which is less biased by interviewer demands. *Prompted questions* provide visual and aural cues to assist recall behavior. Spontaneous campaign exposure measures indicate recall and prompted ones indicate recognition.

Recall is spontaneous identification of a spot or message given minimal cuing (also referred to as *unaided recall*). Respondents who recall a spot or message can voluntarily identify them when presented with simple questions concerning awareness of recent mass media materials. *Recognition* is identification of a spot or message given verbal, pictorial, or aural cues (also referred to as *aided recall*). Recognition relies on memory aids to cue respondents about the content and appearance of the program.

Recall and recognition measures have both advantages and disadvantages. The advantage to recall (spontaneous) measures is that the respondent has to be aware of the topic to provide an affirmative response. Recognition (prompted) measures enable the respondent to provide an affirmative response without actually being

TABLE 11–1. Two Dimensions of Campaign Exposure Measures with Data from the Bolivia National Reproductive Health Program Mass Media Campaign

	SPOT	MESSAGE
Recall (spontaneous)	Unprompted generic question that asks respondents whether they heard or saw anything about the campaign in the past 3 or 6 months. TV: 71.7% Radio: 38.7%	Unprompted generic question that asks respondents what they thought was the message in the spot that they heard or saw. TV: 55.6 % Radio: 27.2%
Recognition (prompted)	Pictorial/video/aural cues taken from the campaign and replayed for the respondents, accompanied by questions concerning whether they remember hearing or seeing them. TV: 3.3 spots, or 41.7% Radio: not measured	Themes from the campaign are read to respondents and they state whether they remember them from the campaign. TV: 5.03 messages Radio: 1.65 messages

aware of the campaign. While prompting may introduce demand bias, it also facilitates exposure measurement by presenting agreed-upon cues and the researcher knows that this cue (image, video clip, sound segment) is the one the respondent saw or heard.

The second dimension of campaign exposure is awareness versus comprehension, or the distinction between simply remembering a commercial and understanding its message. *Spots* are the campaign components (ads) disseminated over various media. A TV spot refers to a TV commercial. Spot awareness indicates that the respondent was aware of that campaign element. *Message elements*, in contrast, refer to the content of the spot in the sense of the information or idea being communicated. The distinction between spot and message recall is akin to the distinction between having awareness of something and detailed knowledge of how it works. Respondents may report spot recall and not message recall or vice versa, although generally the two will be highly correlated, since respondents would need to be aware of the spots before they could know the campaign message.

In sum, campaign exposure can be measured by asking recall (spontaneous) and recognition (prompted) questions for both spots and messages. The wording and formatting of questions should be specific to the campaign, as outlined in Chapter 8. The specific channel or medium used to disseminate the campaign should also be measured. For campaigns using both TV and radio, it is necessary to measure campaign recognition and recall for both TV and radio broadcasts, so that eight variables are produced: spot and message recall and recognition for both TV and radio.

While this discussion may make it seem that campaign exposure measurement is a considerable challenge, new technologies such as computer-assisted interviewing have facilitated measuring campaign exposure. For example, computer-assisted interviews can embed specific video or audio clips from a campaign in the survey to prompt viewer recognition. Even without such technology, researchers can use simple photocopying and skillful questionnaire construction to properly measure campaign exposure. Effort should be devoted to this task because it is one of the most useful functions that an evaluation can perform since it provides data on who was exposed to the campaign and how they interpreted it.[1] Before presenting exposure results, some background on the Bolivia National Reproductive Health Program (NRHP) campaign that will be the focus of the analysis.

THE NATIONAL REPRODUCTIVE HEALTH PROGRAM CAMPAIGN

Reproductive health (RH) is the prevention of unwanted pregnancies and the care and treatment of infants and mothers during and after childbirth. This term may also include sexually transmitted diseases among men and women, HIV/AIDS transmission, and contraceptive use and is often linked to women's education and empowerment. Many Bolivians, and others in developing countries, lack access to basic RH information and services (Schuler et al., 1994).

In the Bolivia NRHP campaign, a logo was created for use by all Bolivian RH agencies to advertise their services. A competition was held to solicit designs and a winner chosen through a balloting process. The final design of the RH logo was an adult cupped hand holding a child's hand reaching up, set on a violet background with the words "Salud Reproductiva" (reproductive health) overlaid. The violet color was chosen for all subsequent RH materials because this color was not being currently used by any political party (Fig. 11–1). The logo was created and incorporated into materials distributed to health agencies beginning in 1992. These included a manual, brochures, flyers, wall charts, and key chains (Fig. 11–1).

Service provider training was conducted with more than 500 counselors in 1992–1993, using the RH materials to improve existing services. It was decided that promotion of these services would not begin until sufficient training was conducted to ensure that RH services were of sufficient quality to warrant their promotion. Thus, the campaign was accompanied by considerable service deliv-

---

[1]Campaign exposure measurement can be considered a manipulation check, verifying that study subjects received the intervention as planned and understood it as intended.

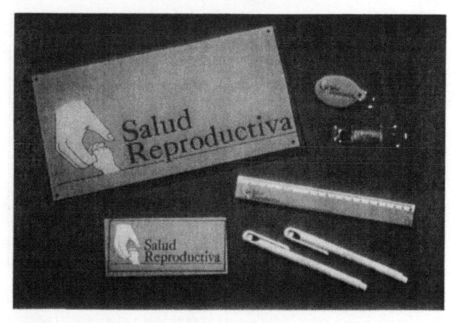

FIGURE 11-1. The National Reproductive Health Program logo and supplemental materials.

ery input that directly affected the supply of family planning and RH services (Lapham and Mauldin, 1985). Box 11–1 lists these other campaign activities and elements produced as part of the NRHP initiative.

To develop message strategy, secondary analysis of existing quantitative data was conducted by studying results from the 1989 Bolivia (DHS, 1989) and from an earlier study of the service provider materials created for the NRHP. In addition, numerous focus groups were conducted among young (15–35 years old) men and women in the major regions of Bolivia. These focus groups revealed that while Bolivians were suspicious of programs designed to promote contraceptives, they were quite concerned about reproductive health and maternal mortality. The initial campaign themes were "Reproductive health is in your hands," "Get information where you see this logo," and "You decide."

The first mass media campaign consisted of 11 different spots broadcast in the major urban cities of Bolivia (La Paz/El Alto, Santa Cruz, Cochabamba, Sucre, Tarija, and Oruro) from May to November 1994 (described in Box 11–2). Each spot had a TV and a radio version. The radio versions were translated and broadcast in "Colla" Spanish, "Camba" Spanish,[2] Quechua, and Aymara (the latter two

---

[2]*Colla Spanish* refers to the language spoken in the Andean region (La Paz; Cochabamba), whereas *Camba Spanish* refers to the language spoken in the Bolivian East Valley (Santa Cruz). The languages are very similar, but there may be a word or phrase used differently in the two regions, and differences in accents.

Box 11-1. OTHER CAMPAIGN ELEMENTS OF THE NATIONAL
REPRODUCTIVE HEALTH PROGRAM

In addition to the mass media campaign, there were other promotional items
produced and disseminated during phase I.

MATERIAL	DESCRIPTION
Counselor training	Over 500 health counselors were trained in interpersonal communication and counseling via a trainer methodology.
Manual	A counselor manual was developed and 400 copies were disseminated.
Clinic poster	One thousand copies of a family planning poster were produced and disseminated.
Flyers	Twelve different flyers on reproductive health were created and 30,000 copies of each were produced and disseminated.
Booklet	A family planning booklet was produced and 127,000 copies were disseminated.
Flipchart	One thousand copies of a family planning flipchart to be used in counselor sessions were produced and disseminated.
Clinic videos	Three different clinic videos were created and 500 copies of each were distributed to health centers.
Advertising	An advertising poster was produced and 6000 copies were disseminated.
Poster	The slogans "Get information and services here" and "Reproductive health is in your hands" were created.
Billboard	An advertising billboard was created and 500 copies were disseminated.

being indigenous languages of the Sierra and Andean regions of South America,
respectively). Box 11–3 shows the broadcast schedule for these 11 spots.

The campaign consisted of the following 11 different spots: *(1)* one of the
Minister of Health stating that reproductive health is beneficial and that contraceptives help women avoid unwanted pregnancies; *(2)* two which introduced the
concept of reproductive health; *(3)* four which covered prenatal care, postnatal
care, breast-feeding, and contraceptives; and *(4)* four testimonials concerning the

Box 11-2. DESCRIPTION OF MASS MEDIA SPOTS FOR
NATIONAL REPRODUCTIVE HEALTH PROGRAM

Eleven mass media spots were created for the Bolivia NRHP campaign. A video-
tape of these spots with English subtitles is available from Johns Hopkins University Center for Community Programs.

SPOT	DESCRIPTION
Ministry of Health	The Bolivian Minister of Health stated the value of of reproductive health and the need to reduce maternal mortality
Introduction	
Reproductive health	Explained the four major components of reproductive health: family planning, prenatal care, childbirth and breastfeeding
Family planning	Presented different contraceptives: calendar, condoms, pills, and IUD.
Prenatal care	Promoted health service attendance during pregnancy
Breast-feeding	Promoted benefits of breast-feeding
Childbirth	Promoted being attended by a provider during delivery
Abortion	Presented family planning as a means to avoid unwanted pregnancy, and being faced with an abortion decision
Family planning testimonial	Presented a satisfied user of family planning
Prenatal care testimonial	Presented a satisfied recipient of prenatal care
Childbirth testimonial	Presented a mother pleased with having a provider attend her childbirth

benefits of reproductive health. These 11 spots were broadcast sequentially over
a 7-month period and totaled approximately 1000 transmissions in each of the
four major cities of Bolivia and about 300 transmissions in each of the three
smaller cities. The television spots were broadcast over local TV channels as well
as the national network; radio spots were broadcast over local radio stations. For
the Aymara and Quechua spots, well-known Aymara and Quechua actors did the

BOX 11-3. BROADCAST SCHEDULE FOR PHASE I OF NATIONAL REPRODUCTIVE HEALTH PROGRAM CAMPAIGN

	MAY	JUNE	JULY	AUG.	SEPT.	OCT.	NOV.	TOTAL WEEKS
Weeks	1 2 3 4	1 2 3 4	1 2 3 4	1 2 3 4	1 2 3 4	1 2 3 4	1 2 3 4	
Minister	X							1
Introduction	X X							2
Reproductive health		X X	X	X	X			7
Family planning		XXXX	X					5
Prenatal care			XXX	X				4
Breast-feeding					XX			2
Childbirth					XXX			3
Abortion					XX	XX		4
Family planning testimonial						X	X	2
Prenatal care testimonial							XX	2
Childbirth testimonial							XX	2
Total								34

voiceovers, thus increasing the popularity of the spots. The target audience was women ages 18–35.

In addition to these Johns Hopkins University–initiated activities, there were other mass media and service delivery activities occurring in Bolivia at this time that were being produced and implemented by other agencies. For example, in 1993, the Bolivian organization Prosalud launched a mass media campaign advertising its reproductive health services. This campaign contained specific references to reproductive health, but did not include the NRHP logo or slogans. Another international public health agency, Mothercare, broadcast a radio and TV campaign in Cochabamba in January through April of 1994.

NRHP CAMPAIGN EXPOSURE

Campaign exposure indicates the degree to which a campaign reached its intended audience. In the NRHP campaign, the baseline survey did not contain campaign recall measures.[3] Because researchers are unsure of a campaign's design and message, it is difficult to measure campaign exposure in baseline surveys. Two storyboard panels were included in the baseline survey in an attempt to measure campaign recognition, but the drawings were so unlike the campaign that a credible comparison was not possible.

It is highly recommended that some measures of campaign recall be included in the baseline instrument, even it is just a phrase such as, "Have you seen anything on TV in the last 6 months concerning health issues?". The researcher can include an open-ended question that allows respondents describe what they were exposed to at baseline and perform an analysis of these data. Unfortunately, to get a credible baseline exposure proxy, one might have to construct the question at the last minute, after the campaign is designed, which creates a logistical challenge.

National Reproductive Health Program Measures

Radio campaign recall was measured by asking, "In the last 6 months, have you heard any commercials on reproductive health, family planning, or maternal health?" (Appendix B, question 60). Those who said "yes" were asked: "Could you please tell me what you heard on radio in those commercials?" After the first campaign, 45.8% of respondents said "yes" ($n = 1077$). A majority of respondents described the spots they heard as promoting prenatal care (12.8%), family planning methods (12.0%), getting services where they saw the *las man-*

---

[3]In the baseline interview for the panel sample we were able to use the follow-up questionnaire and so have an exposure measure at baseline for that subsample.

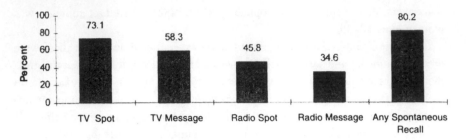

FIGURE 11–2. Spontaneous campaign recall.

itos logo (11.0%), and couples communication (11.0%). Those responses of less than 10% included promotion of reproductive health, breast-feeding, and seeking help from trained providers.

Radio campaign message comprehension was measured by asking, "Thinking about the radio commercials you heard about reproductive health, can you tell me one of the messages in these commercials?" (Appendix B, question 62). Messages were described by 34.67% ($n = 815$) of the respondents, which was 75.7% of those who recalled the campaign. A majority of respondents described messages such as get family planning services (18.3%), get prenatal care (10.9%), and reproductive health (10.9%).

Television recognition and recall were measured with the same format, asking respondents whether they saw anything on TV and then to describe the commercial and the message. TV recall was higher than radio, with 73.1% ($n = 1721$) of the respondents recalling seeing a commercial. Of those, 79.7% recalled a message, and the messages were similar to those reported for radio. There was considerable overlap between those who heard spots on the radio and those who saw them on TV. When combined, 80% of respondents spontaneously recalled the campaign on radio or TV. Campaign exposure in the Bolivia NRHP campaign was thus 80% and constitutes the percentage of the audience that recalled any spot from the campaign. Spontaneous campaign recognition and recall are shown in Figure 11–2.

How Much Exposure Is Enough?

There is no optimal amount of campaign exposure. It is trivial to say "the more the better," as this does not help determine how much time and money should be invested to try and reach various audience segments. A mass media campaign should reach a majority of the intended audience, otherwise it does not capitalize on the economics of scale inherent in mass media. On the other hand, reaching 100% of the population is an unrealistic goal.

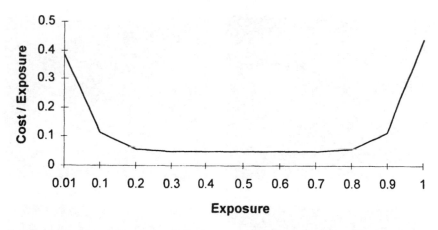

FIGURE 11–3. Campaign cost per exposure by audience reach for levels of theta.

There is a tradeoff between cost and the importance of the message being broadcast. The best metric is cost per exposure, and planners must weigh the cost per exposure according to the importance of the messages. If the message is of extreme urgency, then cost per exposure can be high. If, on the other hand, the messages are of less urgency, then the planner may want to minimize cost per exposure. Most mass media campaigns can expect to reach between 50% and 90% of the target audience and the cost per exposure is likely to rise substantially as the campaign attempts to reach those less accessible. Figure 11–3 presents a graph of cost per exposure, which shows that there is an optimal campaign exposure range. This graph was produced with the equation:

$$C/E = 100((\text{Reach} - 0.5)^\theta) + \rho \qquad (11–1)$$

where C/E is the cost per exposed individual, reach is the audience proportion exposed, and θ and ρ are coefficients to be estimated that determine the shape of the function. For the graph in Figure 11–3, θ was equal to 8 and ρ to 0.05.

Research is clearly needed in a variety of settings to find relevant estimates for θ and ρ. This model posits that reaching the first few audience members in a mass media campaign is comparatively expensive because of production costs. The cost per exposure rapidly drops off as more audience members are reached, but then rises just as dramatically as attempts are made to reach those less accessible via the mass media.

Another topic for future research is whether there are certain efficiencies to reaching certain types of people. Campaign evaluators generally assume that each audience member is equal in terms of the value in reaching them. Some individuals, however, are opinion leaders and often try to change the opinions of others in their community. Consequently, campaigns that reach the more influential people may be more effective than those who do not (Valente, 1995).

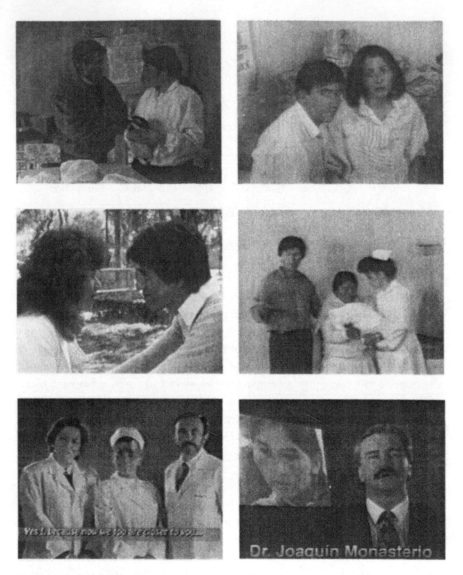

FIGURE 11–4. Images shown to measure TV spot recognition.

Spot and Message Recognition

In the Bolivia study, radio spot recognition was not measured, since that would have entailed recording selected spots or segments on tape and playing them back for the respondent. TV spot recognition was measured by printing selected frames from some of the TV spots and showing them to the respondents (Fig. 11–4). Twelve pictures were shown: eight were from campaign spots, two from in-clinic videos, and two ringers (see below).

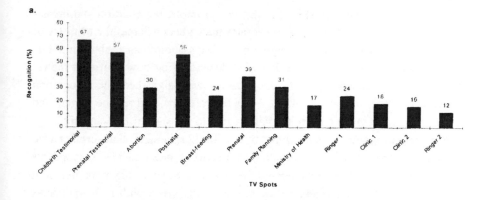

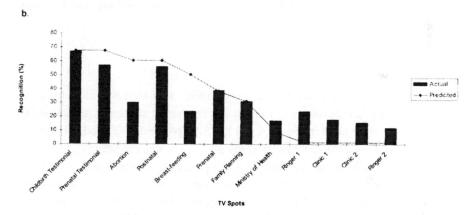

FIGURE 11-5. Assisted spot recall by time of broadcast with predicted recall.

Figure 11–5a shows the level of recognition arrayed by the time since the broadcast of each spot. Spots broadcast more recently had higher recognition levels than those broadcast earlier in the campaign. Respondents were significantly more likely to recall recent commercials than they were to recall older ones. Recognition of the ringers and in-clinic videos was significantly less than that of the campaign spots.

To demonstrate this, we overlaid a graph of the function

$$y = \alpha * \frac{(\text{maxdays} - \text{nodays})}{\text{maxdays}} \tag{11-2}$$

where y is the expected recognition level, α is a discount factor, "maxdays" is the number of days since the beginning of the broadcast and "nodays" is the number of days since each specific spot was broadcast. The distance between predicted and actual recognition indicates which spots were recognized at higher or lower levels than expected (Fig. 11–5b). For example, the abortion and breast-feeding spots were recognized at lower rates than others whereas the Ministry of Health spot was recognized at a higher rate. Two assumptions are built into this model (1) α, the discount factor, is scaled depending on how confident the researcher is that respondents will recognize the campaign (here the recognition value of the most recent spot was used as the referent), and (2) the ringers and clinic spots were given a maxdays value equal to the start of the campaign.

Message recognition was measured by reading 12 statements that corresponded to messages broadcast in the campaign (Appendix B, question 73). Respondents were asked whether they remembered the message, whether they remembered it from TV or radio, and whether they agreed or disagreed with it. Respondents recognized 6.81 out of 12 messages read to them (or 56.8%). There was higher recognition of TV messages, 4.82 (40.2%), than of radio messages, 1.99 (16.6%).

RINGERS

Interviewer demand bias occurs when respondents alter their responses to please the interviewer. Respondents will report that they recall or recognize a campaign even if they were not actually exposed to it. Respondents may confuse another program with the campaign under study and so not intentionally lie, but rather respond truthfully but incorrectly. This is a particular problem when measuring recognition of something as ubiquitous as campaign advertisements. In addition, when individuals feel positively toward some object and if they are asked if they recall an advertisement about it, they will likely say "yes." Demand bias or measurement error can be measured by including *ringers*, or false objects that masquerade as true ones.

The survey in the Bolivia study included two images from campaigns broadcast in other Latin American countries. These spots would not have been seen by Bolivians, but look similar to the Bolivia ones. The degree of positive recognition of these ringers provided an estimate of response bias. As shown in Figure 11–5, ringer recognition was lower than all but one of the campaign images, even though these ringers referred to actual campaign spots. It is estimated, that about 15%–25% of the NRHP campaign exposure is a methodological artifact arising from respondents' desire to answer the recognition questions affirmatively.

Is it possible to include ringer recognition as a correction factor in measures of campaign exposure? Affirmative responses to the ringers are *false positives,* or positive results when negative ones are expected. A variety of techniques can be used to correct campaign recognition by including false positives: (1) divide the scale of true positive by the false ones, (2) subtract the number of false positives from the number of true ones, or (3) include the number of false positives as an independent variable in future analysis. No one method suggests itself over others, and to date the best advice is to use this information as a subjective indication of measurement validity.

Validity and Reliability

Ringers assess measurement validity by showing the degree to which respondents distinguish between ringers and actual campaign images. In the Bolivia study there were 1071 (45.5%) respondents who positively identified at least one campaign image and none of the ringers or clinic videos. The fact that so many respondents identified the campaign and distinguished it from the ringers indicates a high degree of measurement validity.

In addition to being valid, measures should be reliable so that repeated measures return the same results if exposure is the same. In the NRHP campaign, reliability was determined a variety of ways:

1. The same image from a commercial broadcast in both phases of the campaign was included in both surveys. There was a 57% affirmative response to this image in both surveys.
2. The same clinic video image was included in both follow-up surveys, yielding affirmative response rates of 18% and 24% in waves 2 and 3, respectively.[4]
3. Two different images from the same spot were included in the second follow-up survey, yielding affirmative response rates of 63% and 53%.

These three results indicate that this campaign recognition measure was reliable.

The different exposure measures served different purposes. Recall measured top-of-mind awareness and introduced the respondent to that section of the interview. Recognition measured validity and reliability. Message comprehension measures provided more fine-grained analysis of what was understood from the campaign.

The researcher is advised to report all of these, but will usually need to decide on one measure to use for impact analysis. In the Bolivia study, the TV recognition measure was most useful because it varied from 0 to 8, but in each study researchers will have to decide which measure best captures campaign exposure. There are a number of strategies for deciding which exposure measure to use: *(1)* factor analyze the various measures and determine if an exposure scale can be constructed, *(2)* use qualitative methods to debrief selected respondents to determine which exposure measure best captures the concept, *(3)* chose a measure that fits into the mid-range of values provided by the various measures.

---

[4]The 6 percentage point increase could reflect error, increased dissemination of the videos, or increased attendance at clinics.

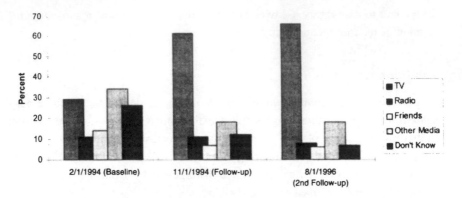

FIGURE 11–6. Reported source of reproductive health information ($N = 7016$).

Source of Reproductive Health Information

One indicator of campaign impact is whether respondents changed their source of information as a result of the campaign. Respondents were asked, "Through what medium did you learn about reproductive health?" The question steered respondents toward eliciting a mass media source; in future studies this question would probably be reworded, such as, "How did you learn about reproductive health?". The proportion of respondents who stated that they learned about reproductive health via TV increased from 29% in the baseline to 61% in first follow-up survey and 66% in the second follow-up survey ($p < 0.01$). Figure 11–6 shows the responses to this question for all three survey waves. In addition to the increase in TV as a reported source of information, there were decreases in other media. Of particular interest is the result that the percentage of respondents saying that they did not have a source of RH information decreased significantly. Thus, the campaign seemed to positively shift expectations about the usefulness of TV to learn about reproductive health.

In sum, in phase I of the Bolivia campaign, 73% of the respondents recalled at least one campaign TV spot, and 80% recalled at least one campaign spot on TV or radio. Most respondents, 78%, recognized at least one TV spot image and the average number recognized was 4.0 (out of 8). In addition, there were message recall and recognition measures.

The seven recognition and recall variables were factor analyzed to create a campaign exposure scale. Results showed that the measure covaried by medium; TV recognition and recall variables covaried and radio recognition and recall variables covaried. This presented somewhat of a dilemma since the results provide two medium-dependent exposure scores instead of one. Factor analysis of the spot and message recall items only yielded one factor with an eigenvalue of 1.70 and each with factor loadings exceeding 0.58. The Cronbach α for the recall scale was 0.71. This spot and message recall exposure scale was used in the impact analysis published in 1998 (Valente and Saba, 1998) but will not be used further in this chapter because, as will be explained below, recall was poorly measured in the second follow-up survey.

The TV spot recognition items were factor analyzed because these included the ringers and provided some measure of reliablity, as discussed above. The TV spot recognition factor analysis had an eigenvalue of 1.83, with no other factors being >1. The Cronbach α for the TV spot recognition scale (eight items) was 0.70. The TV spot recognition index was created by summing the positive responses to the eight spots and dividing by 8. The TV recognition index had an average of 0.40 (SD = 0.25, range = 0–1). For the rest of this chapter, campaign exposure will be measured as TV spot recognition.

CAMPAIGN RECOGNITION BY SOCIODEMOGRAPHIC CHARACTERISTICS (BIVARIATE AND MULTIVARIATE)

It is important to determine whom the campaign reached (recall that the campaign was targeted to young women). For example, among men campaign recognition was 36.6% whereas among women it was 42.4% ($p < 0.001$); among single respondents it was 41.5% whereas among married ones it was 39.3% ($p < 0.05$). Campaign exposure was also higher among those who spoke Spanish, those who resided in the larger cities, and those with more education. In sum, the data show that campaign exposure was higher among younger, single, wealthier, female respondents and lower among Quechua speakers and those who lived in smaller cities.

Exposure by Language

One advantage of developing a national strategy for health promotion is that messages are broadcast on a wider basis and attempts are made to reach all segments of the population. In Bolivia, the radio spots were translated into the indigenous languages of Aymara and Quechua and a conscious decision made to reach these audience segments. The national urban samples analyzed here consisted of 87% Spanish speakers, 9% Aymara, 2% Quechua, and 2% other. The results, shown in Figure 11–7, indicate that Aymara-speaking respondents were much more likely to recall the spots from radio than were respondents speaking Spanish, Quechua, or another language. This is not surprising, given that Aymara speakers are poorer and more likely to not own a television. Thus, translating the spots into Aymara and broadcasting them over radio was an effective strategy for reaching this segment of the population.

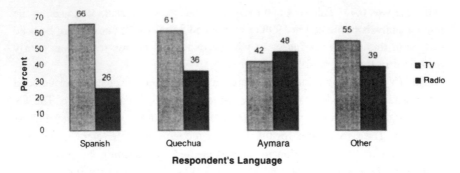

FIGURE 11–7. Message source by language.

To understand who was reached by the campaign, campaign exposure was correlated with sociodemographic characteristics. This analysis can provide a description of the audience that was most highly exposed. For example, if education is significantly positively associated with exposure, this indicates that more educated respondents had higher exposure. Analysis using the standardized multiple regression correlation coefficients of sociodemographic variables on campaign exposure, shown in Table 11–2, indicates that a number of variables are associated with TV spot recognition. Campaign recognition was positively asso-

TABLE 11–2. Multiple Regression Coefficients (β) for Campaign Exposure (TV Ad Recognition) on Sociodemographic Characteristics, the Bolivia NRHP Mass Media Campaigns

	SPONTANEOUS TV AD RECOGNITION				
	URBAN SAMPLES		PANEL SAMPLES		
	NOVEMBER 1994 ($N = 2354$)	AUGUST 1996 ($N = 2396$)	SEPTEMBER 1995 ($N = 798$)	FEBRUARY 1996 ($N = 545$)	AUGUST 1996 ($N = 419$)
Round 2					0.35*
Round 1				0.21*	0.08
Education	0.14*	0.21*	0.07	0.17†	0.14‡
Income	0.03	0.05‡	0.02	0.01	−0.02
Age	−0.04	−0.18*	−0.05	−0.07	−0.08
No. children	−0.03	0.06	−0.04	0.01	−0.01
Female	0.15*	0.13*	0.29*	0.15*	0.03
Married	0.05‡	0.05‡	0.03	−0.04	0.01
City size	0.20*	−0.03	—	—	—
Own TV	0.14†	0.13*	0.12*	0.01	0.01
Spanish	0.05†	0.08†	0.13*	0.03	0.10‡
Adjusted R^2	0.12*	0.12*	0.12*	0.11*	0.22*

*$p < 0.001$; †$p < 0.01$; ‡$p < 0.05$.

ciated with education ($\beta = 0.14, p < 0.001$), being female ($\beta = 0.15, p < 0.001$), living in one of the four major cities (rather than living in the three smaller cities [$\beta = 0.20, p < 0.001$]), and owning a television ($\beta = 0.14, p < 0.01$). There was also a slight tendency for those who are married ($\beta = 0.05, p < 0.05$) and those who speak Spanish ($\beta = 0.05, p < 0.01$) to report higher campaign exposure. These data indicate that the campaign reached more educated women who lived in the larger cities, spoke Spanish, and owned televisions.

While the campaign reached its target audience, there was some concern that the campaign might widen the information gap between more and less educated respondents.[5] (Recall that the sample was drawn from lower- and lower–middle–class neighborhoods and so this widening would occur within an already lower economic group.) The fact that the phase I evaluation showed a strong bias of campaign exposure for the larger cities led us to rebroadcast the phase I campaign over an intensified period to ensure that the smaller cities and the rural audience would have the same information as that provided to the larger cities. In this way, the entire country would be prepared for the phase II NRHP campaign.

EXPOSURE DATA FOR PHASE II OF THE NATIONAL REPRODUCTIVE HEALTH PROGRAM

The phase II campaign was broadcast from March thru July of 1996. Follow-up interviews were conducted in August 1996, with 57.9% recalling a radio spot and 81.7% recalling a TV spot. Radio and TV message comprehension were poorly measured in phase II because of poor interviewer training. In phase II, 87.9% of respondents recalled either a TV or radio spot, and 93.8% recognized at least one campaign image (up from 78.0% in phase I).

The second follow-up survey, like the first, included eight recognition images and two ringers. Factor analysis yielded a first eigenvalue of 2.01 and none other >1, indicating a unidimensional construct. The audience discriminated between campaign spots and ringers: the average recognition level for the eight campaign ads was 56.4%, yet was 22.4% and 22.5% for the ringers (false positives). Recognition of campaign images increased significantly from phase I to phase II (41.7% to 56.4%; $p < .001$) and showed less clustering on recency of broadcast or topic. The reliability coefficient for the second follow-up exposure scale was good, with Cronbach $\alpha = 0.72$.

The multivariate analysis of phase II campaign recognition, also shown in Table 11–2, was more reassuring from a programmatic perspective. Again, more

[5]Part of this bias stems from our method of data collection. More educated Spanish speaking urban women would be more likely to recognize the TV spots whereas less educated Aymara and Quechua speakers are more likely to recall and recognize the radio spots.

educated, Spanish-speaking women who owned a TV reported higher exposure. Note that the negative coefficient between age and TV spot recognition, $\beta = -0.18$ ($p < 0.001$), indicates that younger respondents reported higher exposure. City size was unrelated to campaign exposure in the second follow-up, probably a result of the first campaign's intensive rebroadcast in these smaller cities, priming this audience for the second campaign. The adjusted R^2 for the two equations was relatively low (11%), indicating that sociodemographic characteristics were not strongly associated with exposure and little bias in the audience reached. A high adjusted R^2 with a few variables being strongly correlated with exposure would indicate that the campaign reached specific groups at much higher rates than the general public. It should be acknowledged, however, that education was associated with exposure, which may be a bias of this medium, in this setting, or of this campaign.

The rebroadcast of the phase I campaign provided the opportunity to conduct an additional evaluation consisting of interviews among a sample of residents in one city, Potosí, interviewed before and after the rebroadcast. This panel sample had two advantages not available in the urban cross-sectional data: *(1)* use of the post-campaign questionnaire containing detailed campaign exposure measures at baseline and *(2)* the ability to study change among the same persons interviewed as a panel. Of theoretical and methodological interest then is computation of exposure in this panel sample.

EXPOSURE DATA IN THE PANEL SAMPLE

It is difficult to construct good campaign exposure measures in baseline surveys because the campaign has not yet been developed at the time the survey is fielded. For this baseline panel sample, exposure was measured on the basis of the audience's limited access to the original broadcast of the campaign (Potosí residents could have seen or heard the campaign on some limited national or regional networks and some residents might have traveled to La Paz during the campaign period).

Baseline TV and radio spot recall values for the panel sample, shown in Figure 11–8, indicate that campaign exposure was relatively high before the campaign was broadcast. For example, 54.6% of the Potosí sample interviewed in September 1995 said that they recalled seeing a spot on TV concerning family planning or reproductive or maternal health in the past 6 months. Since the original campaign was finished in November 1994, these high recall values were not expected.

Recall increased over the next year for this sample. For example, TV spot recall increased from 54.6% at baseline to 74.4% after phase I, to 86.6% after phase II. Recall of any spot or message increased from 65.9% to 84.7% to 93.3%. The

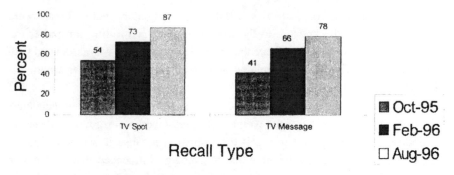

FIGURE 11–8. Recall of campaign for National Reproductive Health Program, for panel data.

Potosí sample was well exposed to the campaign and was undoubtedly sensitized to it by the repeated interviewing. Figure 11–9 reports the spot recognition values for the panel data, which are similar to the exposure values in the cross-sectional data.

Multivariate regression of the recognition scores for the panel sample yielded similar results to those obtained in the cross-sectional samples. Table 11–2 reports the multivariate regression for campaign exposure for each survey wave. At baseline, being a woman, a Spanish speaker,[6] and owning a TV were significantly associated with campaign exposure. For the second and third waves, exposure was significantly associated with being exposed in an earlier survey. Specifically, baseline exposure was associated with follow-up exposure ($\beta = 0.21$, $p < 0.001$), and first campaign exposure was associated with exposure to

[6]Being a Spanish speaker was not associated with other exposure measures. The TV spots were broadcast in Spanish, and so Aymara and Quechua speakers would not recognize these, but as shown earlier, were more likely to recall the radio spots.

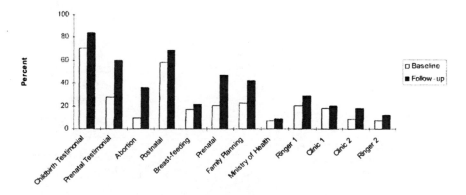

FIGURE 11–9. Recognition of TV spots by time of broadcast for panel sample ($N = 419$).

the second campaign ($\beta = 0.35$, $p < 0.001$). Education and being female were also associated with exposure to the campaign when controlling for earlier exposure. These associations indicate that campaign recognition was associated with subsequent attention to the campaign and that exposure was higher among respondents with more education.

Thus far, campaign recognition has been associated with more educated, Spanish-speaking, and younger women. It is reasonable to argue that these respondents are predisposed to recall the campaign because it was intended for them. Thus, any attempts to infer that a campaign influenced behavior has to contend with the fact that certain types of people will predispose themselves to viewing and recall viewing a particular campaign. This predisposition and its influence on inferring communication impact is selective exposure.

SELECTIVE EXPOSURE

Selective exposure is the degree of bias in campaign exposure that affects measurement and interpretation of communication campaign effects (Sears and Freedman, 1967; Zillman and Bryant, 1985). Selective exposure has been categorized as *(1)* selective attention, *(2)* selective retention, and *(3)* selective recall (also known as *post-hoc rationalization*). These three types of selectivity refer to three stages of health promotion effects: *selective attention* influences who gets the message, *selective retention* influences who remembers the message, and *selective recall* influences who reports that the message influenced their behavior. There are at least seven types of selectivity that occur when trying to measure program impact (Fig. 11–10).

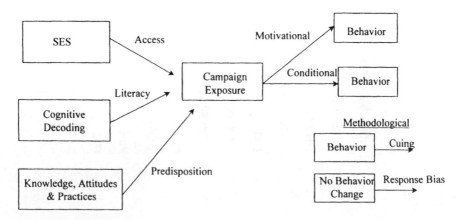

FIGURE 11–10. Conceptual model of selectivity types.

1. Access. *Access selectivity* refers to the ownership and use of specific media and channels within each medium. For a variety of socioeconomic as well as lifestyle reasons, there is considerable variation in the media channels people use and competing outlets within each medium. In a medium-sized U.S. city, most people have access to a number of network and independent TV/radio stations; local, regional, and national print newspapers; and local and national magazines. Increasingly, people use the Internet for news and information. Consequently, a health promotion program over some media and certain channels within each medium will only reach those who have access to and use them.

2. Literacy. *Literacy selectivity* refers to the ability of individuals to understand and process program messages. In any population, there is variability in people's ability to decode the media message and understand it as intended.

3. Predispositional. *Predispositional selectivity* is the effect of existing knowledge, attitudes, and practices (KAP). The KAP levels before the program will influence how ready the population is for it. Generally, populations with higher knowledge and attitudinal levels are more likely to understand the campaign and successfully interpret its message.

4. Motivational. *Motivational selectivity* is the tendency for those already predisposed to change behavior as a result of a campaign. Although related to predispositional selectivity, motivational selectivity is the process set in motion after exposure; predispositional selectivity describes who attends to the campaign, while motivational selectivity describes who will be influenced by it. Motivational selection occurs when individuals change behavior as a result of the program because they were in a ready-to-change state and intended to change their behavior in the near future anyway.

5. Conditional. *Conditional selectivity* occurs when behavior change from a program depends on other factors being present or changed. Conditional selectivity effects indicate that the program is effective under certain conditions but not without them. For example, conditional selectivity would occur if an HIV prevention campaign was effective only among those who reported high levels of perceived susceptibility to contracting HIV.

The following two selectivity categories are methodological, occurring when the researcher does not collect accurate data.

6. Cuing (methodological). *Cuing selectivity* occurs when respondents report an association between exposure and behavior to please the interviewer. Also known as *demand bias*, it occurs when individuals feel that a particular response is expected. Cuing selectivity is a common source of error in survey data because respondents are usually polite and try to please the in-

terviewer. Cuing is particularly problematic when respondents perceive that the interviewer represents the organization sponsoring the survey. For example, in surveys conducted to assess health-care services, respondents will believe that interviewers represent the program being studied and will provide positive answers to avoid insulting the interviewers.

7. Response bias (methodological). *Response bias selectivity* occurs when respondents change behavior independent of a program, but attribute it to the program anyway. Such post-hoc rationalization can occur when the respondents feels no obligation to assign credit to any particular agency.

Understanding these types of selectivity helps researchers determine program effects more clearly. For example, Flay et al. (1993) tested various models of program impact by distinguishing between access and motivational selectivity to determine the portion of behavior change attributable to the program. Results showed that a small but significant program effect was detected when controlling for motivation to quit smoking.

SUMMARY

This chapter presented two dimensions of program exposure: recall versus recognition and awareness versus comprehension. Data on these program exposure measures were reported for the Bolivia study. Choosing among exposure measures is difficult and depends, in part, on the type of program being evaluated. This chapter used an assisted spot recognition measure that captured awareness recognition quite well. Regression analysis showed that more educated, urban, Spanish-speaking women who own televisions had higher exposure. This was due to the type of measurement used, TV rather than radio recognition, and was partly a result of the campaign's focus. Results also showed that residents of the smaller cities were exposed at lower rates than residents of larger cities. This prompted a rebroadcast of the campaign to smaller cities.

The rebroadcast provided the opportunity to gather a panel sample of 798 respondents from one city to supplement the evaluation. Campaign exposure in the panel data showed considerable exposure to the original phase I campaign. Analysis also showed that those who were exposed in early surveys continued to be exposed in later ones. The chapter ended with a discussion of selective exposure and a classification of selective exposure factors.

Measuring program exposure is an important step in the evaluation process, as it informs designers of the degree of message dissemination and among whom. There are a wide variety of ways to measure program exposure and test its validity and reliability. Program exposure measures can be used to revise implementation plans and provide important information for outcome analysis, the topic of the next chapter.

Chapter Twelve

Measuring Outcomes

This chapter explains how to measure program outcomes. Data from the Bolivia National Reproductive Health Program (NRHP) mass media campaigns broadcast in 1994 through 1996 are used to illustrate key points of the analytical procedures. Outcome analysis shows whether the campaign increased *(1)* awareness of family planning methods, *(2)* positive attitudes toward family planning, and *(3)* current use of a modern family planning method. These behavior change variables are often referred to as knowledge, attitude, and practice (KAP).

The Bolivia NRHP campaign evalaution represents a nice case study because it was comprehensive. Many evaluations may not be this comprehensive but would still follow these data analysis procedures so, in that sense, the choice of data is arbitrary. The chapter presents the study design, including the methods and questionnaire used. It then presents the data analysis procedures in some detail to illustrate the process. The analysis is presented in four subsections: preliminary, multivariate, panel, and lagged. The chapter closes with a section on how to report results.

STUDY DESIGN AND METHODS

Encuestas and Estudios (E&E), a Bolivian public opinion firm, was hired through a request for proposals to collect the data. Two urban probability samples were

TABLE 12–1. Study Design for Phase I of Evaluation of the Bolivia National
Reproductive Health Program Campaign

	FEB. 1994	MARCH– OCT. 1994	NOV. 1994	SEPT. 1995	OCT.– JAN. 1996	FEB. 1996	N
Group 1	O_1	X_1			(X_2)		2266
Group 2		X_1	O_2		(X_2)		2354
Group 3		X_1		O_3	X_2	O_4	545*

X_1, Initial broadcast of mass media campaign; X_2, Rebroadcast of mass media campaign.
*Initially 800 respondents were selected at O_3.

selected and interviewed 2 months before and just after the campaign with sample sizes of approximately 2300 proportionately distributed among the seven largest Bolivian cities. The samples were drawn by creating an enumeration of all neighborhoods (manzanas) that met specific socioeconomic criteria (middle and lower–middle income). Every k^{th} neighborhood within each city was randomly selected and every i^{th} household within each neighborhood was randomly selected. Thus, this was a two-stage probability proportional-to-size sample. Interviewers requested an interview with the youngest adult man or woman present in the household (interview times were varied) and then administered the survey face-to-face among same-gender pairs. A deliberate attempt was made to secure an equal distribution of men and women. The study design for phase I is outlined in Table 12–1.

Group 1 is the baseline sample interviewed in February 1994 and then exposed to the campaigns, but not re-interviewed. Group 2 is the follow-up sample interviewed in November 1994 after the campaign was broadcast. Group 3 is the panel sample collected in Potosí interviewed before and after the campaign in September 1995 and January 1996, respectively. The panel sample had 545 respondents interviewed in both waves (out of 798 initially).

Instrument (Questionnaire)

The questionnaire was designed and pilot-tested by a team of researchers, including personnel from Encuestas and Estudios, the Johns Hopkins University Center for Communications Programs (JHU/CCP) Bolivian field office, the Bolivian information, education, and communication (IEC) subcommittee of the NRHP committee, and program and research staff at JHU/CCP–Baltimore. Questions were adapted from the Bolivian demographic and health surveys used in 1989 and 1994 and from the print materials evaluation study conducted in 1990–1993. The questionnaire was extensively pretested. An English translation appears in Appendix B. Since some respondents spoke Quechua and Aymara, the questionnaire was translated into these languages. It consisted of the following eight sections:

1. Demographics (questions 1–15)
2. Attitudes toward family planning and reproductive health (questions 16–18)
3. Family planning awareness and use (questions 19–28)
4. Reproductive health, detailed knowledge (questions 29–31)
5. Reproductive health service access (questions 34–47)
6. Breast-feeding (questions 48–54)
7. Campaign exposure and media use (questions 56–75)
8. Personal networks (questions 76–89).

DATA ANALYSIS

The analysis is presented such that each section tries to provide better evidence for whether the campaign caused a change in outcomes. Data analysis steps are provided in a logical sequence. First, the indicators are created, then their co-variation with campaign exposure is measured, then controls for confounding variables are included.

The data were cleaned, and a new variable called *wave* was created to indicate whether it was baseline ($= 1$) or follow-up ($= 2$). The two datasets were appended, providing a sample of 4620 respondents. Since the intended audience was married women, analysis was restricted to married women, providing an analytical sample of 1929 (915 and 1014).

Constructing Outcome Variables

Knowledge, attitudes, and practices (KAP) were the outcomes used to measure campaign effects. The surveys asked respondents to name the family planning (FP) methods they knew spontaneously and with prompting (Appendix B, question 19). Each FP method awareness variable was coded as 1 for "know" and 0 for "do not know." The FP method awareness scale was created by summing these 11 variables and dividing by the maximum score possible (11) to get a percentage. The percentage is easier to interpret and compare with other variables. Awareness of FP method ranged from 0 to 1, had an average of 0.564, and a standard deviation of 0.26 ($n = 915$) in the baseline survey.

The attitudinal scale was constructed by summing the responses to the first ten attitude questions (question 16 a–j) and then dividing by the maximum possible value, 30 (10×3), to get a percentage. The attitude scale had an average score of 0.870 and a standard deviation of 0.13 ($n = 915$). Both awareness and attitude scales were factor analyzed to make sure they were unidimensional constructs.

Family planning method use, the behavioral measure, was constructed by asking respondents if they had ever used each contraceptive method in the past and then whether they used it currently. Although this measure is not a scale, it is the standard method for measuring contraceptive use (questions 21–23). The variable was set to 0 and recoded to 1 for those who reported current use of any modern method.

In sum, the dependent variables are three commonly used indicators of contraceptive behavior change. Their definitions and reliabilities are as follows:

Knowledge: *Family planning awareness*—percentage of modern and traditional contraceptives (out of 11 possible) recalled by the respondent spontaneously and with prompting (Cronbach's $\alpha = 0.78$).

Attitude: *Reproductive health attitudes*—percentage agreement score on 10 three-point attitude statements (Cronbach's $\alpha = 0.74$).

Practice: *Current use*—whether respondent reported current use of any modern contraceptive technique (yes = 1). These data correspond almost exactly with those collected in the 1994 Bolivia DHS (DHS, 1994).

The next step is to determine whether scores on these three dependent variables increased significantly between baseline and follow-up.

Change in Outcomes

Figure 12–1 shows the change in outcomes between baseline and the two follow-up surveys for female, married respondents. The increase in KAP between baseline and follow-up were as follows: awareness, 56.4% to 60.8% ($p < 0.001$); attitudes, 87.4% to 88.8% ($p < 0.001$); and current modern method use, 30.2% to 35.5% ($p < 0.001$). These modest increases can be attributed to at least the following sources: *(1)* unreliability of measurement, *(2)* historical factors causing change, *(3)* changes in the survey sample characteristics, *(4)* secular trends in the indicators, and *(5)* actual campaign impacts. The outcomes were measured reliably as evidenced by their high Cronbach α scores. There were no historical events occurring over the 9-month period between surveys that could account for changes in the indicator scores. Changes in survey sample and any secular trends will need to be controlled for in subsequent analysis.

To determine if the campaign was associated with these increased outcomes, campaign exposure was correlated with them. Campaign exposure was measured with the TV recognition variable created in Chapter 11. The correlations between campaign recognition and the outcomes were method awareness, $\beta = 0.21$ ($p < 0.001$, $n = 1015$); positive attitude, $\beta = 0.09$ ($p < 0.01$, $n = 1015$); and modern method use, ods ratio (OR) = 2.64 ($p < 0.001$, $n = 1015$). Thus, exposure was associated with outcomes.

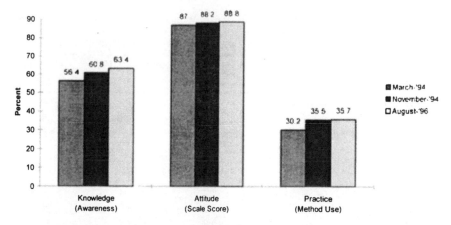

FIGURE 12–1. Knowledge, attitude, and practice scores at baseline, and at 9-month and 28-month follow-up for married women in urban Bolivia ($N = 2818$).

The association between exposure and outcomes does not indicate that the campaign caused these changes, because survey fluctuations and other factors may be responsible for the change or association. The correlation between campaign exposure and outcomes needs to remain after controlling for possible confounding variables, moderators, mediators, selectivity effects, and survey sample fluctuations. Changes in the sample bias the data analysis. For example, if the follow-up sample has more married respondents, then contraceptive use may be higher in the follow-up and it would be inappropriate to attribute this change to the campaign. There are other background variables that influence contraceptive KAP that have to be controlled as well, and this is done using multivariate analysis.

Education, income, age, number of children, contraceptive use in the community, and TV ownership influenced the outcomes and hence should be controlled in multivariate analysis. These variables were measured as follows:

Education: Reported level of education (1 = none, 2 = basic, 3 = middle school, 4 = high school, 5 = technical school, 6 = some college).

Income: Reported monthly income (1 = 0–140 Bs, 2 = 141–500 Bs, 3 = 500–800 Bs, 4 = 501–800 Bs, 5 = 801–1,000 Bs, 6 = 1101 + Bs; at the time of this study, 4 Bs = $1.00). Missing values (5%) were recoded to the modal category 3.

Age: Reported age in years.

Number of children: Reported number of living children (6 cases with more than 10 children were recoded as 10).

City prevalence: Rank ordering from lowest to highest of the percentage of modern contraceptive users in the respondent's city of residence at last survey.

TABLE 12–2. Sample Characteristics for Married Women in Urban Bolivia ($N = 2818$)

FACTOR	CROSS-SECTIONAL SURVEY WAVES		
	MARCH 1994 ($N = 915$)	NOVEMBER 1994 ($N = 1014$)	AUGUST 1996 ($N = 889$)
Family planning awareness (%)	56	61	63
Attitude score (%)	87	88	89
Current modern use (%)	30	36	36
*Education**			
None	5.7	4.4	2.6
Primary	24.9	23.2	20.9
Middle	18.8	17.4	17.2
Secondary	33.8	35.8	38.7
Technical	6.7	8.0	7.4
Some post-secondary	10.2	11.2	13.2
Income‡			
None	0.98	0.7	0.2
80–140 Bs	10.4	5.4	4.3
141–500 Bs	54.2	48.7	40.9
501–800 Bs	19.2	25.4	26.6
801–1100 Bs	8.2	10.6	15.6
1100+ Bs	7.0	9.1	12.4
Age [average (SD)]	31.0 (7.12)	31.4 (7.38)	30.8 (7.41)
No. children [average (SD)]	2.72 (1.82)	2.71 (1.72)	2.65 (1.67)
City prevalence			
El Alto	12	26	14
La Paz	21	35	28
Cochabamba	33	27	32
Sucre	24	25	39
Oruro	31	32	42
Tarija	36	38	49
Santa Cruz	48	46	54
Own TV* [average (SD)]	89.3 (30.9)	92.5 (26.3)	91.1 (28.5)
Speak Spanish‡ [average (SD)]	NA	86.6 (34.1)	81.6 (38.8)
Campaign exposure‡ [average (SD)]	NA	41.7 (26.6)	56.4 (28.7)

*$p < 0.05$; †$p < 0.001$; ‡$p < 0.01$.

Own TV: Whether the respondent owned a television.

Speak Spanish: Whether the respondent spoke Spanish in the home rather than Quechua or Aymara. (Due to an oversight, this question was not asked in the baseline survey, and so all baseline respondents are assumed to speak Spanish.)

Table 12–2 reports the percentages and averages of these control variables. The modal category for education was completion of secondary school. The fluctuation in educational levels was moderately statistically significant between the baseline and the second follow-up survey. Income increased significantly, with the percentage in the modal category of 141–500 Bolivianos decreasing from 54.2% to 40.9% and shifting to higher levels. Age and number of children did not change significantly, while there was some variation in TV ownership and the proportion that spoke Spanish. Multivariate analysis is conducted to control for these changes.

MULTIVARIATE ANALYSIS

Multivariate statistical techniques control for background characteristics. Multiple linear regression and multiple logistic regression calculate the association between campaign exposure and the outcome variables while controlling for these sociodemographic characteristics. The dependent variable level of measurement determines which regression to use: multiple linear regression for continuous variables (awareness and positive attitude) and logistic regression for binary ones (current modern method use).[1] The magnitude of the association between exposure and outcomes after controls is an indicator of campaign effectiveness.

The independent variables can be dichotomous (dummy variables), ordinal, or interval–ratio. The best procedure is to create a regression equation that has the control variables first, followed by substantive ones such as campaign exposure. If interaction terms are included, they follow after the variables entered alone. The same regression model was computed for the three outcome variables and including the same controls. Analysis was restricted to married women to control for these variables. Campaign impact was estimated by using TV spot recognition for campaign exposure.

Table 12–3 reports standardized multiple regression coefficients (β) and adjusted odds ratios (AOR) for the models. The magnitude and direction of the association between the outcomes and the control variables were consistent with past research on reproductive health. For example, education was positively associated with method awareness ($\beta = 0.34, p < 0.001$), reproductive health (RH) attitudes ($\beta = 0.08, p < 0.01$), and modern method use (AOR = 1.27, $p < 0.001$). Income and number of children were also positively associated with the KAP variables indicating that wealthier respondents and those who had more children had higher KAP levels. Age was negatively associated with attitudes, indicating that younger respondents had more positive attitudes to family planning and reproductive health. TV ownership was positively associated with greater method awareness, while speaking Spanish was associated with method

[1] A two-, three-, or four-category dependent variable would use multinomial logistic regression.

TABLE 12–3. Multiple Regression Coefficients for Knowledge, Attitude, and Practices on Sociodemographic Characteristics and Campaign Exposure among Married Women in Urban Bolivia (N = 2818)

	BEHAVIOR INDICATORS		
	MULTIPLE REGRESSION (B)		LOGISTIC REGRESSION (AOR)
	FP METHOD AWARENESS	RH ATTITUDE	CURRENT MODERN FP USE
Education	0.34*	0.08†	1.27*
Income	0.14*	0.06‡	1.26*
Age	−0.02	−0.11*	0.99
No. children	0.07†	0.09†	1.14*
City prevalence	0.03	0.11*	1.16*
Own TV	0.07†	0.06‡	1.55
Speak Spanish	−0.02	−0.07†	2.59†
Campaign exposure	0.10*	0.06‡	1.89*
Adjusted R^2	0.19*	0.04*	0.09*

AOR, adjusted odds ratio; FP, family planning; RH, reproductive health.
*$p < 0.001$; †$p < 0.01$; ‡$p < 0.05$.

use. Interestingly, speaking Spanish was negatively associated with positive attitudes, indicating that non-Spanish speakers had more positive attitudes.

The regression coefficients for campaign exposure show that it was associated with family planning (FP) method awareness, RH attitude, and current modern method use. These associations indicate that the campaign was associated with knowledge and behavior, but less so for attitudes. After controlling for sociodemographic variables there is an association between the campaign and the outcomes it was designed to promote: method awareness ($\beta = 0.10, p < 0.001$), RH attitudes ($\beta = 0.06, p < 0.05$), and modern contraceptive method use (AOR = 1.89, $p < 0.001$).

At the bottom of the results in Table 12–3 are the adjusted R^2 values. The adjusted R^2 reports the amount of variation in the dependent variable explained by the independent variables controlling for the number of variables entered into the model. For method awareness, the R^2 is 0.19, indicating that 19% of the variation in method awareness is accounted for by these variables. The R^2s for attitudes, 0.04, and method use, 0.09, were considerably lower. Although all three R^2s were statistically significant, only the one for method awareness is substantively high.

The Table 12–3 reports both the standardized β coefficient and an asterisk indicating the likelihood that a coefficient of this magnitude would have occurred by chance. Asterisks are used to indicate the probability that the coefficient would occur by chance or to report the confidence intervals (95% or 99%), but not both.

Some researchers prefer confidence intervals because they provide more information about the amount of error or the spread around the estimate, others prefer using asterisks because they are easier to read. The choice of which to report is the researcher's; however, most journals and some academic fields have specific guidelines that dictate that choice.

The analysis thus far has used cross-sectional data, the sample of respondents randomly selected from the seven largest cities. There are numerous reasons, however, for researchers to be wary of conclusions drawn from this analysis. While results from analysis on cross-sectional (or independent) samples may be generalizable to the population, the correlation between campaign exposure and outcomes is still potentially spurious. In spite of the statistical controls employed in the analysis thus far, it is still possible that the association between campaign exposure and the outcomes is due at least in part to spuriousness, selectivity, omitted variables, and other factors. To help control for these factors, panel data were collected using the same questionnaire used in the cross-sectional study.

PANEL DATA

A sample of 798 randomly selected residents in one city, Potosí, was selected in September 1995, almost a year after the follow-up cross-sectional survey. These respondents were re-interviewed in February 1996, after the campaign was rebroadcast. The sampling strategy was identical to that in the first sample described at that the beginning of the chapter. Respondents who completed the follow-up survey in the panel study were generally similar to those who refused, although those who completed the follow-up survey had more children than those who did not (Box 12–1 discusses attrition analysis). In this study, over 50% of the respondents initially interviewed at baseline were retained through wave 3.

Figure 12–2 reports scores for the baseline and follow-up surveys for the panel data. Two of the three variables increased significantly between surveys: FP method awareness (46.8% to 57.3%; $p < 0.001$), and current use of modern contraceptive method (13.5% to 21.0%; $p < 0.001$). Increase in RH attitudes (87.9% to 88.0%; $p =$ NS) was not significant. The panel baseline and follow-up scores were lower than those reported in the urban cross-sectional study, which is a consequence of the fact that Potosí is smaller and less developed than the larger cities sampled above and hence lags behind these cities in RH knowledge and practices. The increased scores can be attributed to one or a combination of the following factors: *(1)* historical factors beyond our control; *(2)* the community increased its scores as a secular trend; *(3)* the baseline interview positively predisposed our respondents to the campaign, which in turn influenced their behavior or their self-reports; or *(4)* the campaign improved these RH indicators.

Table 12–4 reports the standardized multiple regression coefficients for the change in RH variables by subtracting the baseline value from the follow-up

Box 12–1. ATTRITION ANALYSIS

When analyzing data collected on the same respondents over time, some persons included in the initial sample will drop out of the study. This attrition is sometimes referred to as *experimental mortality*. Respondents may be lost to follow-up for at least the following reasons: respondents *(1)* refuse to participate further, *(2)* cannot be found to be re-interviewed, or *(3)* no longer qualify for the study. When analyzing panel data, respondents lost to follow-up should be documented and analysis conducted to determine the nature of any differences between those who remain in the study and those lost to follow-up. This attrition analysis is conducted in part to determine if the remaining sample is biased.

To conduct attrition analysis, the researcher first creates a variable in the baseline dataset that indicates the respondent status at follow-up (refused, not found, not qualified, or re-interviewed). Then the researcher conducts bivariate and multivariate analysis using the follow-up status variable as dependent and any and all sociodemographic characteristics that might bias the results as independent ones. For example, in the baseline panel data, a variable that indicated if the respondent was re-interviewed and the reason that he or she was not re-interviewed was created. Analysis was conducted comparing this variable to contraceptive use and showed that interview status was not significantly associated with contraceptive status (Valente and Saba, 1998).

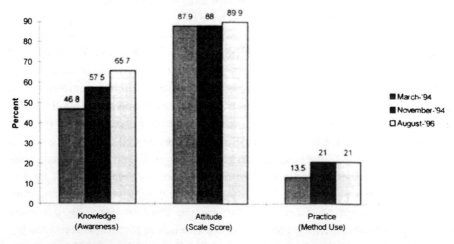

FIGURE 12–2. Knowledge, attitude, and practice scores at baseline and at 6-month and 11-month follow-up for the panel sample of married women in Potosí, Bolivia ($N = 212$).

TABLE 12–4. Multiple Regression Coefficients for Change in Knowledge, Attitude, and Practices on Sociodemographic Characteristics and Campaign Exposure among Married Women in Potosí, Bolivia ($N = 212$)

	CHANGE IN		
	MULTIPLE REGRESSION (B)		LOGISTIC REGRESSION (AOR)
	FP METHOD AWARENESS	RH ATTITUDE	CURRENT MODERN USE
Education	0.39*	0.06	1.39
Income	−0.05	−0.14	1.02
Age	0.26†	0.15	0.98
No. children	−0.11	0.03	1.23
Own TV	−0.04	0.01	0.57
Speak Spanish	−0.43*	−0.22†	1.31
Campaign exposure	0.11	0.07	3.84
Adjusted R^2	0.17*	0.03	0.06*

AOR, adjusted odds ratio; FP, family planning; RH, reproductive health.
$p < 0.001$; †$p < 0.01$; †$p < 0.05$.

value. These difference scores provide a measure of how much each respondent changed between surveys; positive scores indicate an increase while negative scores indicate a decrease. Three variables were significantly associated with change in method awareness; education ($\beta = 0.39$, $p < 0.001$), age ($\beta = 0.26$, $p < 0.01$), and speak Spanish ($\beta = -0.43$, $p < 0.001$). This indicates that respondents who were more educated, older, and did not speak Spanish were more likely to increase their method awareness. Changing to a more positive attitude was slightly associated with not speaking Spanish ($\beta = -0.22$, $p < 0.05$). In sum, a few variables were associated with change in outcomes, indicating a modest ability of the variables to explain changes in outcomes among this sample.

The panel data results deviated significantly from the cross-sectional results in that campaign exposure was not associated with change in outcomes (KAP). In the cross-sectional data, sociodemographic variables such as education, income, age, and so on were associated with variation in KAP, but in the panel data they were less associated with change in KAP. The advantage to using change scores with panel data is that the change variables (difference in scores between baseline and follow-up) are a direct measure of the concepts under study. That is, the campaign aims to increase FP knowledge, attitudes, and practices and the change variables are a direct measure of that increase. A second advantage to using change scores is that the same variable can be used to make comparisons on subgroups (e.g., was change different for men and women, or was change significantly greater in the intervention group than the control). Box 12–2 describes a study that used change scores to compare outcomes between subgroups.

Box 12–2. EVALUATION OF NALAMDANA STREET THEATER
IN MADRAS, INDIA

Nalamdana means "are you well?" in Tamil and is the name of a drama group
started in 1993 by young people of various professional backgrounds but with
a common interest in theater. Nalamdana performs health-related street theater
in India, each performance lasting between 1 and 3 hours. In January of 1996,
an evaluation of Nalamdana was conducted to determine the effectiveness of
three HIV/AIDS dramas created to disseminate HIV/AIDS information. Pre-
and post-performance interviews were conducted with a panel of randomly selected audience members from 10 separate performances in Tamil Nadu state,
India ($N = 93$); and a post-only comparison group ($N = 99$).

Results showed a significant increase in HIV/AIDS–related knowledge as a
result of watching the drama (Valente and Bharath, 1999). Before the drama,
audiences had relatively high levels of accurate knowledge about HIV/AIDS,
but lower knowledge levels of common HIV/AIDS misconceptions. The drama
reduced these misconceptions.

KNOWLEDGE SCALES	PRE-DRAMA ($N = 93$)	POST-DRAMA ($N = 93$)	T
Total (12 items)	71	97[*]	14.0
Accurate subscale (6 items)	89	99[*]	6.8
Misconceptions subscale (6 items)	54	95[*]	14.6

[*]$p < 0.01$.

Change scores provide the opportunity to determine who was most influenced
by the drama. One-way analysis of variance (ANOVA) tests were conducted on
the difference scores by sociodemographic characteristics. Results showed that
men and women had about the same level of knowledge change for both the
accurate and misconceptions subscales. The drama was differentially effective,
however, for less and highly educated respondents, and for low- and high-
income respondents. This table shows that accurate knowledge changed more
for respondents with no education (19 percentage points) than those with some
post-secondary (1 percentage point).

	KNOWLEDGE CHANGE	ACCURATE KNOWLEDGE CHANGE	MISCONCEPTIONS KNOWLEDGE CHANGE
All respondents	26	10	42
Males	25	9	41
Females	29	13	45
Education[*]			
None	37	19	54
Elementary	27	12	42

	KNOWLEDGE CHANGE	ACCURATE KNOWLEDGE CHANGE	MISCONCEPTIONS KNOWLEDGE CHANGE
Education (Continued)			
Middle	25	10	40
Secondary	25	7	43
Some Post-secondary	14	1	26
Income†			
Low	28	13	43
High	24	7	40

*Overall knowledge and accurate knowledge were significantly different by education levels ($p < 0.05$).

†Accurate knowledge was significantly different by income categories ($p < 0.05$).

There are researchers, however, who criticize using change scores as outcome indicators.

Lagged Analysis

At least two major criticisms of change scores have been raised (Cronbach and Furby, 1970). First, often there is an association between the change and baseline scores because of regression to the mean. People who score high on the baseline measure will have a tendency, all other things being equal, to score lower on the follow-up and those who score low on the baseline will have a tendency to score higher on the follow-up. When reporting analysis using change scores it is important to analyze and report the correlation between the baseline score and the difference score to measure regression to the mean. The correlations between difference scores and the baselines ones were as follows: FP method awareness, -0.55 ($p < 0.001$); positive attitude, -0.64 ($p < 0.001$); and current contraceptive method use, 0.34 ($p < 0.001$). The strong negative correlations for awareness and attitudes indicate considerable regression to the mean since those who scored high at baseline had lower change scores.

The second criticism of change scores is that they implicitly assume a perfect correlation between baseline and follow-up scores. To understand this concern it will help to digress a little to present the models used in statistical analysis. When conducting linear regression, researchers attempt to predict the score on the dependent variable, Y, by estimating the Y-intercept, α, and the coefficient of the X independent variable, β. The linear regression equation is some variant of the following:

$$Y = \alpha + \beta X + E \qquad (12\text{--}1)$$

When using the change score, the regression model predicts the difference score, which is Y at follow-up minus Y at baseline, giving the following equation:

$$Y_{t+1} - Y_t = \alpha + \beta X + E \qquad (12\text{--}2)$$

Rearranging these terms by putting the Y_t component on the righthand side of the equation shows that difference analysis assumes a coefficient of 1 for the correlation between Y_t with Y_{t+1} as in the following equation:

$$Y_{t+1} = (1)Y_t + \alpha + \beta X + E \qquad (12\text{--}3)$$

Thus, difference score regression analysis cannot estimate the multivariate correlation coefficient for the association between the outcome variable at baseline (Y_t) with the follow-up (Y_{t+1}). Lagged analysis provides a way to estimate the association between the outcome variable at follow-up with its score at baseline using the following equation:

$$Y_{t+1} = \beta_1 Y_t + \alpha + \beta_2 X E \qquad (12\text{--}4)$$

in which β_1 estimates the association between outcomes at baseline and follow-up.

There are advantages and disadvantages to using change scores or lagged independent variables. There is no absolutely correct way to conduct the analysis and the researcher's choice of analysis method is dependent on the ultimate objectives of the analysis. If the study puts substantial emphasis on understanding how change occurs differently among subgroups (e.g., men versus women), then perhaps the outcome variables should be treated as change scores (e.g., Valente and Bharath, 1999). On the other hand, if there is substantial correlation between baseline and difference scores, then perhaps a lagged analysis is best. If the researcher anticipates multiple time points in the data, then lagged analysis will probably be the most appropriate test for the influence of multiple time lags.

Lagged analysis is the use of one or more prior time period variables to predict later ones. The Bolivia panel data analysis was re-run using lagged dependent variables as the first independent variable to compare the lagged results with the difference score analysis. Table 12–5 reports the multiple regression coefficients with the outcome variable at baseline entered first, followed by the sociodemographic variables (education, income, age, number of children) and then campaign exposure.

The lagged variables for FP awareness, attitudes, and modern FP method use were significantly associated with the outcomes. For example, baseline awareness was associated with follow-up method awareness ($\beta = 0.23$, $p < 0.001$), in-

TABLE 12–5. Multiple Regression Coefficients for Knowledge, Attitude, and Practices on Lagged Dependent Variables, Sociodemographic Characteristics, and Campaign Exposure among Married Women in Potosí, Bolivia ($N = 212$)

	OUTCOME AT FOLLOW-UP		
	MULTIPLE REGRESSION (B)		LOGISTIC REGRESSION (AOR)
	FP AWARENESS	RH ATTITUDE	CURRENT MODERN USE
Baseline score	0.23*	0.25†	6.84*
Education	0.47*	−0.04	1.36
Income	0	−0.03	0.87
Age	0.22†	0.03	0.96
No. children	−0.15	0.11	1.34
Own TV	0.04	−0.02	0.54
Speak Spanish	−0.26*	0.02	1.43
Campaign exposure	0.24*	0.15	1.91
Adjusted R^2	0.38*	0.06	0.13†

AOR, adjusted odds ratio; FP, family planning; RH, reproductive health.
*$p < 0.001$; †$p < 0.01$.

dicating that respondents who knew many FP methods at baseline knew more methods at follow-up. Education was significantly associated with awareness and use, but not attitudes once the prior score was controlled. Campaign exposure was positively associated with FP method awareness, but not positive attitudes or method use. The coefficients for the campaign exposure variable, in general, were stronger than those reported in the previous analysis using difference scores and were also quite strong compared to the sociodemographic variables.

Also, notice that the adjusted R^2, the amount of variance explained in the dependent variable, is much higher for the lagged model than in the others (the cross-sectional or difference models). Lagged variable models generally return higher R^2s because the lagged variable often accounts for a lot of the variance in the dependent variable. In sum, outcome analysis was conducted by creating indicators, measuring their change between baseline and follow-up, and then correlating this change with exposure when controlling for other factors through difference scores and lagged analysis.

REPORTING RESULTS

As mentioned above, there are different preferences for reporting statistical results. Parameter estimates in multiple regression can be unstandardized (b) or standardized coefficient (β). The unstandardized coefficient indicates the degree of change in the dependent variable for each unit change in the independent variable. The standardized coefficient is constrained to vary between −1 and +1.

The unstandardized coefficient is more practical when the researcher wishes to make statements about changes in Y based on changes in X, whereas the standardized ones are useful for comparing the magnitude of the coefficients between variables (e.g., education was more strongly associated with awareness than income).

The researcher can also report the probability value or the confidence interval of the parameter estimate to indicate its degree of statistical significance. The probability value is a quick indication of whether the estimate is likely to have occurred by chance (its statistical significance). Typically, one asterisk is used to signify the 0.05 level, two indicate the 0.01 level, and three, the 0.001, but this can vary and different symbols can be used for different levels. The confidence interval provides an estimate of the spread around the parameter estimate. Confidence intervals provide more information, but they take more room than simply using an asterisk. Some researchers prefer reporting the standard error of the estimate, which also indicates variability and is used to calculate statistical significance. Convention typically dictates which is reported in a particular journal.

Although many of the examples in this book have been from developing countries, many health promotion programs are being implemented and evaluated in the U.S. Box 12–3 describes an evaluation of a media campaign designed to reduce smoking among youth in Massachusetts.

SUMMARY

This chapter presented a series of analyses designed to demonstrate how to conduct statistical analysis appropriate for a health promotion program evaluation. The first section demonstrated how the outcome variables were constructed using the scale development steps discussed in Chapter 9. The outcomes used were knowledge (family planning method awareness), positive attitude, and practices (current modern family planning method use). These are known as KAP variables and data were reported that showed that KAP increased between baseline and follow-up surveys.

The increased KAP values were associated with campaign exposure. These associations are likely a consequence of numerous factors, including sample fluctuations, existing trends historical events, selectivity, or the campaign. Multivariate regression analysis was conducted to determine if the association between exposure and outcomes would persist after controlling for sociodemographic characteristics. Cross-sectional data cannot control for some selectivity threats and so analysis of panel was conducted.

Difference scores were analyzed and the results were not consistent with the cross-sectional analysis. The limitations of difference analysis were described and the procedures for lagged analysis presented. The lagged analysis, prior time

Box 12-3. MASSACHUSETTS ANTI-TOBACCO MEDIA
CAMPAIGN EVALUATION

Many studies have linked tobacco advertising and tobacco use (Tye et al., 1987; Flay, 1989) such that promotional campaigns are associated with increasing tobacco use. Other studies have shown the anti-tobacco campaigns can delay smoking initiation and prevent tobacco use. The advent of the tobacco settlement and other policy innovations has provided the impetus for government-sponsored anti-tobacco campaigns in a number of states (e.g., California, Florida, Massachusetts). Siegel and Biener (2000) conducted an evaluation of the Massachusetts anti-smoking campaign launched statewide in the 1990s.

Siegel and Biener (2000) interviewed 592 randomly selected Massachusetts youths age 12 to 15 years. Two interviews were conducted: a baseline measure after the campaign had been launched and a follow-up 4 years later. The study was designed to determine whether those who reported being exposed to the campaign at baseline would be less likely to become an established smoker (defined as having smoked 100 or more cigarettes) 4 years later. The authors measured campaign exposure as spot recall for each medium: TV, radio, and billboards. Baseline exposure was nearly optimal at 71.3% and was significantly associated with follow-up exposure.

Youths ages 12–13 who recalled anti-smoking TV advertisements were less likely to become established smokers (AOR = 0.49; 95% CI = 0.26–0.93) after controlling for age, gender, race, baseline smoking status, baseline smoking exposure (parents, friends and siblings), television viewing, anti-smoking messages on the radio, and exposure to anti-smoking messages not related to the campaign. The authors speculate that "the effect of the media campaign on smoking initiation may be mediated, in part, by its effects on perceived youth smoking prevalence" (Siegel and Biener, 2000, p. 384). It seems that those respondents who recalled the campaign were more likely to correctly report that less than a majority of the students at their high school were smokers.

Note that the Siegel and Biener (2000) study used an innovative approach to create a pre/post-study design by using an evaluation conducted when the campaign was first launched and re-contacting respondents who had participated in the earlier study. In this way, Siegel and Biener could use statistical controls to show a rather robust correlation between campaign exposure and subsequent behavior.

period outcome variables are entered into the model, had ressults consistent with the cross-sectional ones, with the addition that the campaign was more strongly associated with the outcomes and the explained variance was much higher.

These data indicate that the campaign was somewhat effective at improving reproductive health knowledge, attitudes, and practices among married, female, urban, Bolivians. There are other more advanced analysis used to evaluate programs to be presented in the next chapter.

Chapter Thirteen

Advanced Design and Statistical Topics

This chapter focuses on some advanced design and statistical topics that expand the evaluators toolbox. Eight topics are presented; some require certain types of data while others offer different analysis strategies. The first section provides a description of stepwise regression, followed by a discussion of statistical procedures for three wave data (e.g., baseline, midpoint, and follow-up). The third section introduces path analysis and structural equation modeling, used to analyze multiple dependent variables. The fourth section explains event history analysis, which is used to study time-varying and time-constant covariates and censored data. The next section presents time series analysis used to study count data from multiple time points (usually more than 30). This is followed by a review of meta-analysis procedures and its use in evaluation. Data weighting procedures used for comparing data to an external standard, or to make samples comparable, are then discussed. Finally cost–benefit and cost-effectiveness analysis is explained.

Advanced methodological and statistical techniques are useful tools in the evaluation process, but should not be mistaken for methodological rigor (GAO/PEMD, 1991a, p.16). Advanced statistical techniques cannot compensate for poorly designed studies or poor-quality data. The classic experimental method in which a treatment group is compared to a control group (Chapter 6) can use very simple statistics in the determination of impact (a t-test of the difference of differences for example). In the real world, however, practical limitations and pressures often force researchers to use less than ideal study designs and more complex statistical analysis.

Researchers should be prepared to cope with and take advantage of these different opportunities, some of which can improve inferences made from the data. For example, path analysis allows the researcher to include multiple dependent variables in the analysis. This can be useful when impacts are expected on multiple outcomes. Sometimes the methods complement one another as when time series analysis of clinic statistics are compared to regression results.

STEPWISE REGRESSION

Studies with multiple dependent (outcome) variables and many independent variables present considerable risk of type I error (concluding that an independent variable was significantly associated with the outcome when it was not). On the other hand, there is a need to guard against type II error (concluding that an independent variable was not significantly associated with the outcome when it was). As Cohen and Cohen (1985) state, "the investigator can neither afford to make spurious positive claims (type I) nor fail to find important relationships (type II)" (p. 169). In the analysis presented in the last chapter, it is possible that one or more of the statistical tests will be spurious given the number of variables.

Stepwise regression balances type I and type II error by only including those independent variables in a regression model that contribute significantly in explained variance to the dependent variable. The independent variables can be treated singularly or can be grouped together in blocs in which case it is referred to as hierarchical stepwise regression. The block is entered into a multiple regression model and its significance in explaining variance in the dependent variable measured. If the block adds significant explained variance then it (all variables in the block) is kept in the model, if it does do not, then it is dropped. Stepwise regression can be done forward, blocks are included in the model successively in the order listed, or backward, the blocks are removed from the model successively in the order listed. Blocks are created by grouping conceptually related variables. For example, sociodemographic variables may be grouped, attitude variables grouped, and so on. A typical stepwise regression equation will have some variables grouped in blocks and others entered alone.

The analysis presented in the next section uses backward stepwise regression with sociodemographic variables (education, income, age, and number of children) entered as a block, and other variables (prior behavior and campaign exposure) entered independently. Each variable or block was assessed to determine if it contributed significantly to the explained variance in the dependent variable at the $p < 0.15$ level. If a variable or the block did not contribute significantly (at the $p < 0.15$ level) to the explained variance in the dependent variable it was dropped from the model.

THREE- AND MULTIWAVE DATA

Chapter 12 presented two-wave data from the Bolivia campaign evaluation in which data were collected before and after the mass media campaign was broadcast. Two-wave data are quite common, as many evaluations have one campaign and there is no need to collect additional information. There are circumstances, however, when more than two waves of data are collected. For example, the campaign may be long and a mid-term measure desired, or there are various phases of a campaign and each phase requires a separate evaluation. For the National Reproductive Health Program (NRHP), a second mass media campaign was created to expand and promote other aspects of reproductive health, providing a third wave of data.

Phase II of the campaign was broadcast from March 1996 to July 1996 and the third wave of data were collected in August 1996. The cross-sectional sample was selected as in waves 1 and 2; interviews were conducted with 419 of the 545 panel respondents from Potosí wave 2 (77%). Among married women, 171 of the of 212 respondents who completed wave 2 (81%) were re-interviewed.

Three or more data waves are challenging because it is no longer possible to look specifically at change from baseline to follow-up. There are three change scores to choose from: time 1 to time 2, time 2 to time 3, and time 1 to time 3. Hence, lagged analysis is the appropriate technique with time 3 outcomes as dependent variables and time 2 and time 1 scores on those variables as predictors.

Figure 12–1 presented the time trends for the cross-sectional data. The data show that the outcomes increased over time, reflecting an increase in reproductive health knowledge, attitude, and practice (KAP). For example, awareness of family planning (FP) methods increased from 56.4% to 60.8% to 63.4% ($p <$ 0.001) in the three samples ($N = 2818$) over the $2^1/_2$–year period. This 7 percentage point increase represents a 12% increase in method awareness. Figure 12–2 presented the time trends for the panel data and also showed that KAP increased during the study. For example, FP method awareness increased from 46.8% to 57.5% to 65.7% ($p < 0.001$) among the Potosí married women interviewed in all three waves ($N = 171$). Stepwise multiple regression results for the three KAP variables for the three survey waves are presented in Table 13–1. Note that in this analysis, past modern FP method was added as an additional control variable in the cross-sectional data.

For the cross-sectional data, past modern FP method use is an important and significant variable associated with all three outcomes. For example, past method use was associated with knowledge ($\beta = 0.18, p < 0.001$), positive attitudes ($\beta =$

TABLE 13–1. Stepwise Multiple Regression Analysis for Three-Wave Data[a]

	CROSS-SECTIONAL DATA (N = 2818)			PANEL DATA (N = 171)		
	MULTIPLE REGRESSION		LOGISTIC REGRESSION	MULTIPLE REGRESSION		LOGISTIC REGRESSION
	KNOWLEDGE	ATTITUDE	USE	KNOWLEDGE	ATTITUDE	USE
Outcome at time 1	0.18*	0.13*	1480*	0.32*	0.37*	15.8*
Outcome at time 2				Dropped	Dropped	4.9†
Past modern use	0.32*	0.01	Dropped	0.11*	Dropped	Dropped
Education	0.08*	0.04	Dropped	0.25†	Dropped	Dropped
Income	−0.02	−0.07†	Dropped	−0.01	Dropped	Dropped
Age	0.05‡	0.05‡	Dropped	−0.03	Dropped	Dropped
No. children	−0.01	−0.01	Dropped	0	Dropped	Dropped
City method use rank			Dropped	—	—	—
Campaign recall	0.09*	Dropped	Dropped	Dropped	Dropped	Dropped
Campaign recognition	0.07†	0.05†	2.19†	0.28*	0.15‡	Dropped
Adjusted R^2	0.24*	0.03*	0.51*	0.49*	0.15*	0.32*

[a]Education, income, age and number of children were entered as a block.

*$p < 0.001$; †$p < 0.01$; ‡$p < 0.05$.

0.13, $p < 0.001$), and current use (AOR $= 1480, p < 0.001$). Education, income, and, to a lesser extent, having more children were associated with method awareness. Being younger was slightly associated with more positive attitudes. For current modern method use, the block of sociodemographic variables did not contribute substantively and were dropped. Campaign recall (spontaneous recall of TV and radio spots and messages) was associated with method awareness, but was dropped from the other two models. Campaign recognition was significantly associated with all three outcomes. The explained variances were 24% for awareness, 3% for attitudes, and 51% for use.

For the panel data, past KAP were important and significant variables associated with all three outcomes. For example, past method awareness was associated with wave 3 awareness ($\beta = 0.32$, $p < 0.001$); past positive attitudes was associated with wave 3 positive attitudes ($\beta = 0.37, p < 0.001$); and past method use was associated with wave 3 method use (wave 2, AOR $= 15.8$, $p < 0.001$; wave 1, AOR $= 4.9$, $p < 0.01$). Education and income were associated with method awareness. No other sociodemographic variables were associated with change in outcomes. Note that the sociodemographic characteristics drop out of the model once time 1 and time 2 values on the outcomes were included in the model. Campaign recall was not associated with outcomes in the panel data. Campaign recognition was positively associated with method awareness and, to a lesser extent, positive attitudes in the panel data. The explained variance was relatively high for awareness (49%), weak for attitudes (15%), and moderate for use (32%).

These results show that the campaign was relatively effective in increasing FP method awareness and had a modest impact on behavior. The lack of an association with attitudes is probably because attitudes were high at baseline (approximately 88%). Thus both knowledge and behavior could increase, but attitudes could not. The sociodemographic variables did not explain change in outcomes once prior behavior (past method use) or prior states (wave 2 and wave 1 indicators) were included in the model. The campaign recognition variable was significantly associated with outcomes in both datasets.

To summarize, the multivariate analysis of the cross-sectional data indicate that *(1)* contraceptive knowledge and behavior change in Bolivia occurred among better educated, wealthier, married women of lower socioeconomic status (recall that the sample was selected from this group); *(2)* younger women and those with more children had more positive attitudes to FP; and *(3)* the campaign was significantly but weakly associated with increased knowledge and practice.

The multivariate analyses of the panel data show that *(1)* prior knowledge, attitudes, and behavior were the strongest predictors of current behavior and change was not common; *(2)* few sociodemographic characteristics were associated with change; and *(3)* campaign recognition was associated with change in knowledge and positive attitudes, but not with adoption of a modern method.

PATH ANALYSIS OR STRUCTURAL
EQUATION MODELING

Researchers often wish to understand the simultaneous role of multiple dependent and independent variables. For example, a program may be expected to increase knowledge and that knowledge expected to simultaneously influence behavior. In addition, multiwave data with multiple variables may posit complex
pathways of influence between variables. For example, increased FP method
awareness at time 2 might translate into adoption of a method at time 3. Furthermore, researchers may want to simultaneously model variable measurement
and the interrelationships between those measured variables at the same time.
For example, a scale's reliability can be estimated and its association with the
outcome measured at the same time. To conduct these simultaneous estimations,
a technique referred to as structural equation modeling (SEM) has been developed (Hayduk, 1987; Bollen, 1989; Jöreskog and Sörbom, 1989).

Figure 13–1 shows a path model of campaign impact using multiple outcomes
at multiple points in time. The model posits a set of independent variables predicted to impact dependent variables, some of which mediate relationships between other dependent variables. The actual measurements, questionnaire items,
are known as *manifest variables*. For example, question 16a in Appendix B is a
manifest variable (also known as a *manifest indicator*). The manifest variables
are indicators of concepts referred to as *latent variables*, which are the concepts

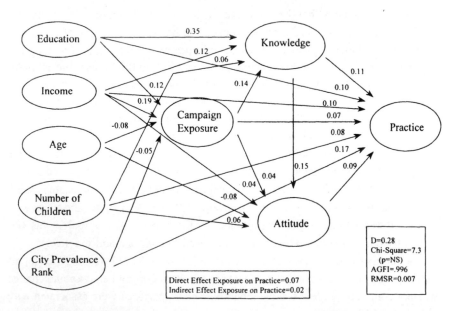

FIGURE 13–1. Conceptual model of health communication campaign impact for the Bolivia National Reproductive Health Program. AGFI, adjusted goodness of fit index; RMSR,
root mean square residual.

enclosed in ovals in this path diagram. The independent and dependent latent variables are referred to as *exogenous* and *endogenous* variables in path analysis, respectively. The *measurement model* in the path diagram assesses how well the manifest variables (indicators) measure the concepts, while the *theoretical model* assesses the relationships between concepts as specified in the conceptual model. Figure 13–1 presents only a theoretical model.

The relationships between concepts specified by the researcher constitute the theoretical test of impact, and most studies use structural equation modeling to test conceptual models without including the measurement components. The theoretical model is compared to the data and the correspondence between them measured with a statistical test. The conceptual model is tested with data from the Bolivia study.

The path analysis was conducted using the LISREL (Linear Structural Relations) computer package (Hayduck, 1987; Jöreskog and Sörbom, 1989), but some researchers prefer EQS (Bentler, 1984; Bollen, 1989). In LISREL and EQS, researchers specify a theoretical path model to test and then they use a correlation or covariance matrix computed among the variables included in the model. The information structure contained in the correlation matrix is compared to the information that would exist if the theoretical model were true. The degree of fit between the theoretical model and data provides a measure of how well the theoretical path model is supported by the data. The fit between the model and data is reported as the coefficient of determination, which is analogous to R^2 in multiple regression. The SEM also provides an adjusted goodness-of-fit index for the overall model and estimates of the strength and significance of all paths in the model.

Figure 13–1 shows the standardized coefficients and goodness-of-fit results for the impact model. Education ($\gamma_{1,1} = 0.12$), income ($\gamma_{1,2} = 0.19$), age ($\gamma_{1,3} = -0.08$), and city prevalence rank ($\gamma_{1,5} = -0.05$) were associated with campaign exposure (TV recognition), indicating the degree of selective exposure to the campaign. Education ($\gamma_{2,1} = 0.35$), income ($\gamma_{2,2} = 0.12$), and number of children ($\gamma_{2,3} = 0.06$) were associated with method awareness. Income ($\gamma_{3,2} = 0.04$), age ($\gamma_{3,3} = -0.08$), and number of children ($\gamma_{3,4} = 0.06$), were associated with positive attitudes. Education ($\gamma_{4,1} = 0.10$), income ($\gamma_{4,2} = 0.10$), number of children ($\gamma_{4,4} = 0.08$), and city prevalence ($\gamma_{4,5} = 0.17$) were associated with current method use. These results are consistent with those multiple regression.

Campaign exposure was associated with FP method awareness ($\beta_{2,1} = 0.14$), positive attitudes ($\beta_{3,1} = 0.04$), and current modern method use ($\beta_{4,1} = 0.07$). Knowledge was associated with attitudes ($\beta_{3,2} = 0.15$), and FP method use ($\beta_{4,2} = 0.11$). Positive attitude was associated with FP method use ($\beta_{4,3} = 0.09$). The goodness-of-fit indicators provide an indication of the overall fit of the theoretical model to the data. The coefficient of determination (D) was 0.28, indicating a moderate amount of explained variance. The chi-squared value was nonsignificant, indicating that the model does not deviate significantly from the data, which is good. The adjusted goodness-of-fit index (AGFI) is quite high (0.996), indicating that the model fits the data well; the root mean square residual (RMSR) is low (0.007), indicating little error. In sum, the model fits the data well and explains a moderate amount of the variance in the dependent variables.

The SEM also provides measures of direct and indirect effects. The direct effect of campaign exposure on method use is shown by the β coefficient linking exposure to practice ($\beta = 0.07$). The indirect effect of exposure on use is derived by tracing the indirect paths that link exposure to practice. The two indirect paths are through knowledge and attitude, which act as mediators of the influence of exposure on use. In this case the indirect effects are computed by multiplying the coefficients for each indirect path: $0.14*0.11 = 0.0190$ and $0.04*0.09 = 0.0036$ and adding them to get an indirect effect of 0.02.

Although these results are consistent with the regression analysis presented above and consistent with prior research, it is possible that the impact model is misspecified because the paths from exposure to the outcomes could be reversed. Specifically, method awareness, positive attitudes, and method use could influence campaign exposure. This model was run and returned similar fit indices, indicating that this selectivity model fits the data well. The cross-sectional data cannot be used to test a bidirectional influence to determine whether exposure influences awareness or awareness influences exposure. The impact model in Figure 13–1 is known as a *non-recursive model* (no feedback loops) that can be tested with cross-sectional data. However, recursive models, those with feedback loops, require panel data, since the time-ordering of variables is known.

Figure 13–2 shows a path diagram of the expected relationships between sociodemographic characteristics, campaign exposure, awareness of FP methods, and use of FP methods from the panel data. Attitude was dropped from the model since it did not change much during the study. The model has five exogenous (independent) variables influencing all three endogenous (dependent) variables at time 1, which in turn influence the same concepts at waves 2 and 3.

Results show that education is an important correlate of all three variables at baseline and the positive association between education and method awareness persists through time periods 2 and 3, even when controlling for prior method awareness. Thus, more educated respondents were more likely to learn about FP methods over time, further exacerbating the knowledge gap (Gaziano, 1983). Note also that education was positively associated with campaign exposure at time 3, even when controlling for exposure at time 2.

The endogenous variables, exposure, awareness, and use were significantly associated with themselves over time. Campaign exposure at time 1 was associated with campaign exposure at time 2 ($\beta = 0.13$; $p < 0.001$), and time 2 was associated with time 3 ($\beta = 0.20$; $p < 0.001$). Note that exposure at time 1 did not influence exposure at time 3, indicating that perhaps selectivity fades over time. Method awareness and use also influence themselves at successive time pe-

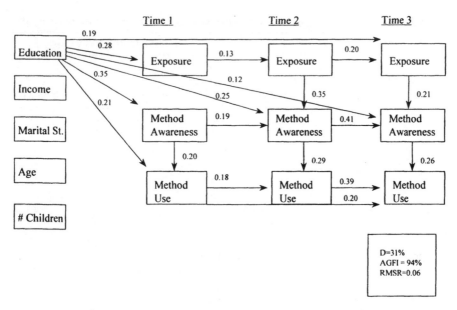

FIGURE 13–2. Path diagram of longitudinal effects for panel data in Potosí, Bolivia. AGFI, adjusted goodness of fit index; RMSR, root mean square residual.

riods with the persistence in the effect of prior states for method use lasting longer than exposure or awareness (method use at time 1 was significantly associated with method use at time 3, controlling for method use at time 2 [$\beta = 0.20$; $p < 0.001$]). The contemporaneous campaign exposure measure was associated with method awareness ($\beta_{6,5} = 0.35$; $p < 0.001$ and $\beta_{8,7} = 0.21$; $p < 0.001$), consistent with the three-wave regression reported above.

In sum, structural equation models provide a linear regression technique used to model multiple dependent variables simultaneously and including certain aspects of the measurement model simultaneously. The results presented in this section were consistent with those presented above and confirm that the campaign created a modest increase in FP method awareness and, to a lesser extent, method use. The next advanced statistical technique, event history analysis, models time more explicitly.

EVENT HISTORY ANALYSIS

Event history analysis (EHA) can be conducted when data are collected over time or contain a time or date indicator. It provides ways to measure the influence of variables that vary over time and those that remain constant over time (Allison, 1984). For example, suppose the data contain the date at which people adopted a new behavior (Valente, 1995) as well as variables that vary over time (e.g.,

TABLE 13–2. Schematic Diagram of Data Reconfiguration for Event History Analysis

ORIGINAL DATA			RECONFIGURED DATA			
OBSERVATION NO.	ID NO.	YEAR OF ADOPTION	NEW OBSERVATION NO.	ID NO.	ADOPTION YEAR	INDICATOR
1	1	6	1	1	1	0
2	2	4	2	1	2	0
3	3	2	3	1	3	0
			4	1	4	0
			5	1	5	0
			6	1	6	1
			7	2	1	0
			8	2	2	0
			9	2	3	0
			10	2	4	1
			11	3	1	0
			12	3	2	1

price) and others that are constant over time (e.g., educational attainment). To conduct event history analysis, the data are reshaped so that each case or row represents a person by time period observation. There are multiple observations for each respondent—one for each year he or she did not adopt the behavior and one for the year he or she did. Table 13–2 depicts a hypothetical dataset of three respondents and their adoption times (6, 4, and 2). The reshaped dataset has 12 cases with new and old ID numbers and a dummy indicator for whether the respondent had adopted by that year.

Statistical analysis is conducted using the adoption indicator as the dependent variable and performing a maximum likelihood estimation with the independent variables. Both the time-varying and time-constant variables are input into the equation and effects are estimated along with standard errors. Event history analysis is also used when data are censored. *Censoring* occurs when data collection is terminated prematurely before all respondents have adopted the behavior (right-censored) or when data collection is begun after behavior change has started and some respondents already adopted the behavior (left-censored).

Snyder (1990) used event history analysis to evaluate the effectiveness of a communication campaign in The Gambia that was designed to promote oral rehydration solution (ORS) use as a treatment for diarrhea. Snyder (1990) collected monthly data for 30 months to determine whether various communication activities were effective at teaching women about ORS, whether they retained that knowledge, when they first used ORS, and whether they continued using it. Event history analysis was used because the respondents had different values of exposure to different media channels over time. Snyder (1990) found that only exposure to the flyer was consistently associated with all four outcomes.

TIME SERIES

Data on behavior over a long period of time are an asset to an evaluation. For example, evaluation of a communication campaign designed to promote product sales is enhanced by having sales data over a long time period before and after the campaign was launched. Time series data are often obtained from management information systems (MIS) established to track data on the following (Keller, 1991):

1. Inputs, the infrastructural components that provide product supply
2. Outputs, counts of product sale or distribution
3. Quality, an assessment of the caliber of the service or product provided
4. Outcomes, an assessment of programmatic effect.

An MIS would ideally contain data collected on all four of these activities, but this is not usually possible given the expense and difficulty of tracking indicators over time.

In health care evaluations, it is desirable to collect data *(1)* tallying the total number of clients who visited service locations on a daily basis, usually aggregated by week or month; *(2)* categorizing those clients as new or continuing clients; *(3)* recording the type of service received (whether the visit was to obtain information or a product); and *(4)* the source of motivation for the visit (i.e., whether it was a mass media program, a friend, or outreach worker). Clearly, these should be collected, whenever possible, from both public and private sector agencies.

All MIS data collection systems should have the following qualities:

1. Periodic. The data are aggregated daily, weekly, monthly, or yearly, depending on the topic of study (monthly is the most common).
2. Accurate. The data should be accurate and the researcher should ask the following questions: Do the data make sense? Do centers that serve fewer people report lower levels of use? Are the data consistent with other data sources?
3. Reliable. The data should be reliable and the researcher should determine if they are relatively consistent over time. Are there any radical shifts that cannot be explained?
4. Consistent. The data should be consistently collected. The instruments (intake forms) and procedures should not vary over time. When significant changes are made, they should be documented.

5. Sufficient. The data should be collected over a substantial period of time, especially prior to and after an intervention. In general, approximately 30 time periods are needed to perform time series statistical analysis.
6. Diverse. The data should come from as many diverse sources as possible. For example, try to get data from *(a)* public and private sectors providers; *(b)* rural and urban centers; *(c)* intervention and control sites; and *(d)* a variety of socioeconomic levels.

Clearly these conditions are difficult to meet in many applied settings, but the advantage of such data is that they often provide an unobtrusive and sometimes unbiased measure of program impact. The Brazilian vasectomy promotion campaign by PRO-PATER (Box 13–1) provides a good example of how clinic statistics collected over an extended period time provided a good way to measure campaign impact (Kincaid et al., 1996).

META-ANALYSIS

Meta-analysis is a statistical technique that combines results from numerous evaluation studies to get a combined estimate of effect. Meta-analysis can be used to determine whether an intervention is effective, based on a population of studies collected by literature searches and compiling the effect sizes into a database. The average across studies, after some statistical adjustment, provides an estimate of the true effect size. Meta-analysis is useful when there are at least 30 or 40 similar studies measuring similar variables. The studies can then be aggregated to determine if an overall generalization can be made about the relationships under study.

When compiling studies, the researcher must decide whether to restrict them to those that have been published in referred journals or to include studies that may exist in the gray literature. (Gray literature studies are reports or conference papers not published in peer-reviewed journals.) Once criteria for inclusion have been determined, studies are located by using computer database searches, literature searchers, making announcements on Internet lists, and at conferences. Studies are then collated and entered into a database.

If the studies are rigorous and comparable enough, meta-analysis is performed by aggregating the direction, magnitude, and variances of the effect sizes to get an estimate of the true effect size (Glass, 1976; Hunter and Schmidt, 1990; Durlak and Lipsey, 1991; Cordray, 1993; Kim and Hunter, 1993). Determining the test statistic to compare studies can be a challenge, but most often, difference scores or correlations are used. The test statistic is averaged with statistical adjustment for the variances and sample sizes of each study to obtain an estimate of the true effect size.

Box 13-1. BRAZIL PRO-PATER VASECTOMY PROMOTION

Kincaid and others (1996) reported that use of modern contraceptives and voluntary female sterilization were fairly high in Brazil, but voluntary male sterilization, vasectomy, was not. PRO-PATER provides information and medical services regarding contraception and sexuality and offers vasectomies in its clinics for a fee. PRO-PATER has been offering vasectomies since 1981 and has launched various campaigns to promote its services. Specifically, it was involved in the following mass media promotions in 1983, 1985, and 1989 (Kincaid et al., 1996):

1. 1983: 3-minute TV and radio broadcast that reached an estimated 40 million people
2. 1985: 10-week print campaign using newspapers and magazines
3. 1989: Multimedia campaign using print, TV, and radio. The 1989 campaign featured a dancing hearts TV spot that won numerous international awards for its appeal. The slogan was, "Vasectomy is an act of love." This campaign generated considerable pre-campaign publicity—70 news stories on TV and radio. The campaign was broadcast three times (5/18/89–6/30/89; 9/19/89–9/29/89, and 1/1/90–3/4/90).

Evaluation of the 1989 campaign showed that the number of telephone calls to clinics increased dramatically during the campaign broadcasts. Additionally, the number of clinic visits and the number of vasectomies performed increased during the campaign (Kincaid et al., 1996).

Time series analysis was conducted using data on the number of vasectomies performed per month from February 1981 to December 1992 in one clinic located in São Paulo. The analysis was performed using Poisson regression, the appropriate statistical technique for analyzing count data. The data and predicted regression lines are shown in Figure 13-3. The number of vasectomies starts out low and climbs steadily until November 1985, when, during the 1985 campaign, there is an increase. The increase was not sustained after the campaign and the number of vasectomies decreases until the 1989 campaign, when there is another significant increase. Again, this increase is not sustained but drops off until the end of data collection.

In statistical analysis, the number of vasectomies performed each month was used as the dependent variable and the independent variables consisted of time (the month), dummy variables for the campaign times. Results showed that the campaigns were associated with creating an increase in the number of vasectomies performed. The data, however, also showed a substantial decrease in the number vasectomies performed during the post-1989 campaign period. Why, if the campaign was successful, did vasectomy use decrease in these data? Kincaid and others (1996) point to at least three reasons for the decrease after the 1989 campaign: (1) the cost of the operation at PRO-PATER increased during this time period, (2) the cost of living in Brazil increased during this time period, and (3) substitution—other private physicians, trained at PRO-PATER, opened clinics in the São Paulo area to offer vasectomies at competing clinics.

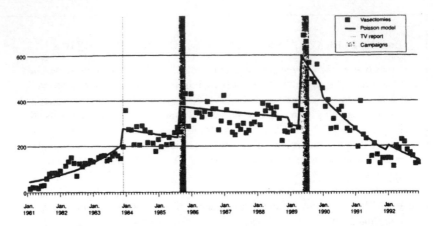

FIGURE 13–3. PRO-PATER vasectomy rates. (From Kincaid et al., 1996, with permission.)

A meta-analysis of 48 health campaigns was conducted by Snyder and colleagues (Snyder, 2001; Snyder and Hamilton, 2001; Snyder et al., 2001). Snyder (2001) showed that the average effect size for mediated health communication campaigns was a correlation of 0.09, which translated into an 8.6 percentage point change. Snyder (2001) was then able to analyze characteristics of the campaigns and studies to determine if certain study types were associated with stronger or weaker campaign effects. For example, campaign topic was associated with effect size such that campaigns that promoted smoking cessation were less effective than those promoting non-addictive behaviors. Snyder and others (2001) found that the baseline behavior rate influenced campaign effectiveness such that campaigns were more successful when between 30% and 50% of the audience already performed the behavior at baseline. They also found that campaigns consisting of enforcement messages, such as seat belt use, were more effective (average correlation of 0.17) than those without an enforcement component (average correlation of 0.05). These results are consistent with those reported by Freimuth and Taylor (1998) and Ratzan (2000).

The series of studies by Snyder and associates provide valuable results for communication campaign evaluators. First, they provide compelling evidence that media campaigns can change behavior, and although the effect size is modest, given the large audience reached by most campaigns, this modest effect size can translate into large absolute effects. Second, they provide an estimate of the expected effect size for sample size calculations (Chapter 7). One major limitation to meta-analysis is the suspicion that the scientific literature favors publication of positive results rather than null ones. It is more likely that an evaluation of a successful campaign will get published rather than an unsuccessful one. Comparisons between published and unpublished studies, however, have not supported this concern (L. B. Snyder, personal communication).

WEIGHTING DATA

There are times when biases in data collection result in a sample that is different from the general population or different from what was desired. For example, the Bolivia sample had more women than men relative to the general population. It is possible to control for this sample bias by weighting data. Data are weighted by creating a new variable that signifies the proportion that each case should represent in the analysis. For example, if a sample was 60% women and 40% men, yet equal representation was desired, a variable would be constructed equal to 0.83 for women and 1.25 for men. Subsequent analysis would multiply corresponding cases by this variable so that men contribute 1.25 more to the analysis whereas women contribute 0.83.

Survey samples can be weighted to each other or to some external standard, and statistical programs have made it easy to do. In SPSS, the researcher indicates that the data are to be weighted in the "data" menu under the "weight cases" option and specifies the variable or variables that contain the weighting information. In STATA, the researcher needs to specify the weighting variables in brackets for each statistical command. If a weighting variable is not already in the data, it can be constructed. To construct a weighting variable based on characteristics in the data, the researcher calculates the multipliers needed for each category of the existing distribution to match the desired one. In the gender example above, the existing distribution for women was 60% and the desired distribution was 50%, so the weight factor would be the solution for $60x = 50$ or $x = 0.83$.

COST–BENEFIT AND COST-EFFECTIVENESS ANALYSIS

Many evaluation studies are conducted to determine whether the benefits of a program are greater than the cost needed to implement it (Nas, 1996). Some studies explicitly use cost data along with outcomes to determine the relative effectiveness of various interventions. For example, suppose an organization wanted to communicate the importance of good dental hygiene to its employees. The designers could compare different geographic sites by comparing the relative effectiveness of various communication strategies such as an employee newsletter, posting messages on physical and electronic bulletin boards, or including inserts in payment envelopes. The costs and impact for each strategy can be compared by conducting cost–benefit or cost effectiveness analysis.

Cost–benefit analysis consists of converting all program inputs and outputs into monetary terms and then determining whether there is a net benefit to the program by subtracting costs from benefits. This cost–benefit determination provides a measure of net value (Thompson, 1980). More commonly, evaluators compute a benefit-to-cost (BC) ratio by dividing the benefit number by the cost number to compute the BC ratio. The BC ratio provides a measure that quantifies the gain provided by the investment. Those BC ratios >1 indicate programs that provide a positive return while those that are <1 do not. One advantage to the BC ratio is that it provides a means to compare the relative return of various interventions.

The major shortcoming to cost–benefit analysis is the difficulty of converting program outputs or impacts into monetary values. For example, many programs are designed to inform the public or change their behavior, but it may be difficult to assign a dollar value to human knowledge. How much money should be equated with accurate knowledge concerning the benefits of breast-feeding? The difficulty inherent in monetary valuation of human knowledge, behavior, and potential life-saving information has given rise to cost-effectiveness research.

Cost-effectiveness analysis consists of recording the dollar costs associated with program inputs, but leaving outputs recorded in their original metric and then dividing program impacts by their costs. Cost-effectiveness (CE) analysis provides a ratio indicating the amount of impact gained per dollar spent. For example, suppose in the hypothetical dental hygiene example, the inserts raised knowledge by 15% while the bulletins raised it 10%. If both interventions cost $2.00 per person reached, the respective CE ratios are 7.5 and 5, indicating that the inserts were more cost-effective.

Typically CE analysis is conducted to summarize the impact of an intervention in an intuitive and easy to understand way. This analysis is also conducted when a researcher or policy-maker is trying to decide between various programmatic alternatives. Cost-effectiveness ratios for strategic or programmatic alternatives can be compared to decide which is the more cost-effective approach (Flay, 1986).

SUMMARY

This chapter has provided some advanced statistical techniques used to measure impact. Stepwise regression procedures for balancing type I and type II errors were presented, and data used to illustrate the technique. Structural equation modeling (SEM) was presented and a communication campaign impact model tested using SEM analysis. Results were presented using both the cross-sectional and panel data. Statistical analyses were consistent and showed that the campaign increased FP method awareness and to a lesser extent, FP method use.

The chapter also discussed some related evaluation issues such as time series, meta-analysis, weighting data, and cost-benefit and cost-effectiveness. Each of these topics was presented briefly and their use in health promotion evaluation discussed. Every program evaluation will present unique challenges and unique statistical requirements. While it is never possible to anticipate all the challenges presented by an evaluation, the evaluator must be prepared to learn new techniques and develop methods to overcome these challenges.

Chapter Fourteen
_____

Dissemination of Evaluation Findings

The evaluation framework presented in Chapter 1 (Fig. 1–1) indicated that dissemination is the last step in the evaluation process. Dissemination (sometimes referred to as *feedback* or *feed-forwarding*) is neglected in many evaluation budgets because before the findings are known, there is little thought as to how best to disseminate them and to whom they should be disseminated. In fact, dissemination is one of the most controversial aspects of the evaluation process; the first section of this chapter discusses why. In the second section, dissemination of findings is explained, including estimates on how long it takes. In the third section, a model of the policy process is presented and the ways in which dissemination affects policy are discussed. The chapter then turns to some ancillary material not yet mentioned but crucial to research–ethics and budgeting. The chapter closes with a summary of the book and an assessment of the future of health promotion program evaluation.

DISSEMINATION CONFLICT

There are at least three reasons why controversy or conflict emerge during dissemination of evaluation findings. First, designers and evaluators may disagree on the appropriate audience or vehicle for dissemination. For example, researchers in academic institutions may need to publish the results in prestigious peer-reviewed journals. This process is time consuming and usually a particular methodology or result is emphasized. In contrast, designers are usually interested in disseminating a report that looks good and is comprehensive and understandable to a professional audience of other designers and policy-makers. These two competing pressures can cause considerable friction. Second, there is usually pressure to report positive results. Designers want the evaluation to stress the successes of the project, since it is partly an evaluation of their performance. The evaluator is interested in accurately reporting on the results, regardless of the positive or negative effects detected. Third, proper dissemination takes considerable time to conduct statistical analysis and money to pay for it. Resources are needed to write the report, and publishing it can be expensive when done professionally.

Despite these potential controversies, the evaluator may be obligated to expend considerable effort in disseminating findings. These findings should be distributed even when, or particularly when, the results show that a specific program did not work. Many researchers acknowledge that evaluations that show a lack of success can be more informative than those that report success.

DISSEMINATION

Evaluation findings can be disseminated in at least four ways. The first is for the researcher to meet with designers to present findings and other results of the evaluation. One reason to meet with designers first is so they can prepare to respond to their stakeholders. If the evaluation shows that the program was successful, the designers can be prepared to answer questions about how they intend to sustain the program or expand it if more resources were available. If the evaluation shows that the program was unsuccessful, the designers may be able to explain why. A second reason to apprize designers is to enlist their help in interpretating the findings. There may be anomalies in the data or findings that are difficult to interpret yet may be understood by those involved in the program's implementation. For example, if a program was not successful in a particular location, the designers may know that dissemination was not well implemented there. Finally, sharing findings with designers provides an opportunity to test presentation of findings.

The second means of dissemination is to present findings at scientific meetings. Health promotion evaluations are routinely presented at conferences of groups such as the American Public Health Association, the Society of Public Health Educators, the American Evaluation Association, the International and National Communication Associations, the American Sociological and Psychological Associations, and the Population Association of America. These conference presentations provide the opportunity to get feedback from colleagues that can improve exposition of the results or provide valuable advice on evaluation theory and methodology.

The third means of disseminating findings is through a key findings or technical report in which the methods, operations, and key findings of the study are summarized. It should be written in clear, concise language, and free of technical jargon. Typically, this report is targeted to the study funders, the designers, the policy-makers, and other interested audiences. The audience is likely to be sophisticated and knowledgeable, but not one that has time to read much about the details concerning the study.

A key findings report should include the following:

1. An executive summary
2. A program description
3. The study design, including sample size, sampling strategy, response rate, and data collection methods and procedures
4. A description of the sociodemographic characteristics of the sample, including scores and values on key variables of interest such as program exposure, knowledge, attitudes, and practices
5. An estimate of the program's effect or the major findings to be communicated
6. A discussion of conclusions, implications, and next steps to be taken.

The key findings report is often written by the evaluator and simply photocopied and distributed. There should be a list of those who should receive it and a strategy for distribution, with some money set aside for using quality graphics (if the project is large enough to warrant printing). The key findings report is a resource for planning future activities and provides lasting documentation of the program.

The fourth option available for disseminating findings is the academic paper submitted to and published in a journal. Most studies do not reach this level of dissemination because the time and effort needed to get research results published are extensive. For researchers working in an academic center such as a university, publishing research results is essential to professional promotion. For many evaluators, however, this type of publishing is not necessary, and the time required for it is generally not deemed worthwhile. Since most research journal articles are directed at academics, not practitioners, they rarely have an impact on program implementation.

Journals are sponsored by professional associations, some have rotating editorships while others have more or less permanent editors. Most academic fields or disciplines have one or a few top-tier journals that accept very few submis-

TABLE 14-1. Refereed Journal Submission and Publication Process

STEP	ACTIVITY	TIME (MONTHS)
1	Data analysis is completed and results/interpretation agreed upon	12
2	Paper is drafted (see Becker 1995)	3
3	Paper is circulated to colleagues for internal review (co-authors, mentors, and colleagues)	1
4	Paper is circulated to colleagues for external review	3
5	Paper is presented at a conference during this time period (allow time to create materials needed for the conference)	1
6	Paper is submitted to academic journal, editors notify author of receipt	1
7	Editors decide whether it is appropriate for the journal and notify author of the estimated review time. Paper is sent to three reviewers; the identity of author and reviewers is known only only to the editor (blind review)	3
8	Editor receives comments from reviewers and decides whether to *(1)* reject the article, *(2)* ask the authors to revise and resubmit the article, based on the reviewers' and editor's comments, *(3)* accept the article pending certain revisions, or *(4)* accept the article without change. The most common result is that the author is asked to revise and resubmit the article. Usually the editor provides guidance for revisions	1
9	Paper is revised and co-authors and possibly one or more of the internal or external reviewers are consulted	6
10	Paper is resubmitted, notice is received from editor, paper is returned to all or some of the original reviewers (note that some journals send the paper to new reviewers)	1
11	Paper is re-reviewed and editor receives comments	3
12	Author receives acceptance notice and editor asks for a final draft on diskette and provides an estimate of when the article will appear in print	1
13	Journal sends author(s) page galleys, which are page proofs of how the article will appear in the journal. Author proofreads the page proofs immediately (and sends copies to co-authors). This activity is expected to occur within 2 days of receiving the galley proofs since the journal is usually on a tight publication schedule. Authors are not permitted (except at great expense) to make modifications to the paper at this time, other than to change small typographic errors.	4-6
14	Paper appears in print	3
	Total time for paper to be published after it is first drafted	28+

sions (perhaps <10%). In addition to general-audience journals, there are specialty journals that target specific subareas of the discipline.

The steps to publishing a journal article are detailed in Table 14-1. Researchers are forewarned that the publication process can easily take 2 to 4 years to complete and that publishing in high-profile journals can be difficult. Briefly, the publication process consists of the following three phases: *(1)* the paper is drafted and reviewed internally and externally by colleagues; *(2)* it is submitted to the appropriate journal and then sent out for review by the editor(s); *(3)* a decision is made regarding the manuscript and, after revision, it is published. Each of these phases has a set of substeps, reviewed in detail in Table 14–1.

Given the difficulties and time costs of journal publication, many researchers opt to publish their results in "working papers" series, and many are increasingly turning to the Internet as a forum for information exchange. Another forum is the publication of selected findings in books or as chapters in edited books. These techniques are usually considered less rigorous scientifically but often provide a more concise and streamlined option for dissemination than peer-reviewed journals.

POLICY PROCESS

The dissemination of research results is further complicated by the variety of terms used to describe the process of sharing results and working in the policy arena. This text has provided detailed information about the challenges to the development, implementation, and evaluation of health promotion programs. The same issues often arise when evaluators attempt to develop, implement, and disseminate their research results to other relevant audiences. Figure 14–1 diagrams the various institutions or stakeholders present in the dissemination process and offers a conceptual clarification to the terms used to describe them.

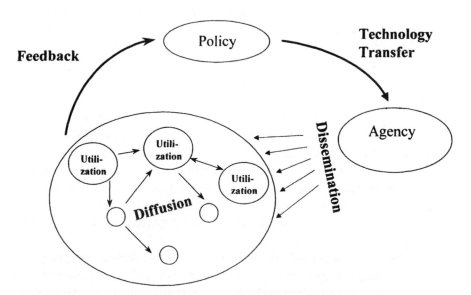

FIGURE 14–1. Research findings inform many stages in the social change process.

Technology transfer is the conversion of research into commercial application or the conversion of a technology from one application to another. Technology transfer is often employed by federally sponsored research laboratories that attempt to turn inventions created for one use into commercial applications. For example, considerable effort is expended to convert inventions created in the space program into commercial products to offset the government's investment in space exploration.

Dissemination is the communication of information to constituent populations by agencies and organizations. Dissemination is akin to public communication or marketing efforts designed to inform and educate the public about available services and new products. Dissemination may or may not accelerate utilization of findings, depending in part on the effectiveness of the dissemination strategy and the diffusion process.

Diffusion is the spread of a new idea or practice within a community (Rogers, 1995). Diffusion of innovations is the process by which new ideas and practices spread through certain channels (see Chapter 2; Rogers, 1995; Valente, 1995). The diffusion process occurs as individuals and agencies interact with one another and share their experiences with the innovation.

Utilization is the study of how individuals, a community, or public use or implement the innovation. Utilization addresses the way individuals or agencies practice the knowledge, information, or persuasion received from dissemination or diffusion activities. Utilization studies are particularly concerned with modification to the practice during its use. Research results are often underutilized.

Figure 14–1 depicts the separate domains encompassed by these different activities. The process starts with research findings being transferred to an agency (often a government agency). The agency is responsible for disseminating this finding to the field. Some organizations or individuals in the field will use the new practice and utilization research conducted to understand how it was implemented. Use of the innovation diffuses through the network of orgnizations or individuals, and research on that is fed back in the form of new research findings.

Clearly the four domains are interrelated, as decisions and processes embedded in each domain affect those other domains. The most successful technology and policy changes occur when all four domains are linked strategically and conceptually and the transfer process is attuned to the forces that drive successful utilization. Health promotion programs are embedded in this process when they are used as part of the dissemination strategy. The evaluation of the program in the context of diffusion and utilization also gets fed back as new research findings.

One frustrating aspect of evaluation research is that findings are rarely used to inform programs and policy as much as desired. Policy and program decisions are often made for reasons other than scientific evidence on the effectiveness of a specific program or campaign (Flay, 1986). For example, a mass me-

TABLE 14–2. Dissemination Activities in the Bolivia Study

ACTIVITY	DATE	MONTHS SINCE FOLLOW-UP DATA
Baseline data collected	March 1994	−7
First follow-up collected	November 1994	0
Presentation made to Bolivian IEC subcommittee and policymakers	July 1995	9
Technical report sent to funders	September 1995	11
Presentation at professional association meeting	November 1995	12
1000 copies of report printed and distribution	February 1996	15
Second follow-up data collected	August 1996	22
Academic paper submitted to journal	January 1997	26
First academic paper appears in press	February 1998	39
Second academic paper submitted to journal and rejected in June 2000	April 1999	52
Resubmitted to different journal	August 2000	68
Paper appears in press	November 2001	81

IEC, information, education, and communication.

dia communication campaign might be launched to inform and influence the public because it is a politically high-profile intervention, not because it is the most appropriate intervention. Consequently, evaluators often find themselves in difficult situations regarding the appropriateness of a specific intervention and the difficulty of communicating research results. There are no clear solutions to such problems and suffice it to say that policy-makers, designers, and evaluators have multiple constituencies and influences. To some extent, resolving issues concerning proper dissemination strategies is dependent on whether the evaluator is external or internal to the organization implementing the program (see Chapter 2).

Table 14–2 provides a list of the dissemination activities that occurred in the Bolivia study. After the follow-up data were collected, it took approximately 9 months to prepare the data for debriefing to relevant policy-makers and designers in Bolivia. Professional association presentations were made and a copy of the technical report printed during the next 2 years. An academic paper suitable for journal publication was produced and appeared in print approximately 39 months after the data were collected. In the interim, a second follow-up survey was fielded and the results from those data were available within a year; a second academic paper was submitted approximately 20 months later.

Data Sharing and Reporting

After data have been collected, it is desirable and sometimes necessary to share it with other researchers and/or the funding agency. For example, data collected with federal money are public data and should be shared with other individuals or groups that qualify for access to them. The evaluator is responsible for ensuring that the data contain no information that could potentially be harmful to any respondents. For example, datasets should not contain information on residential location so that unscrupulous individuals cannot use it for criminal means. Likewise, when reporting findings, the researcher should not print or disseminate information that would permit others to identify specific individuals within a dataset. These "identifiers," if any exist, are typically stripped from a dataset before it is shared with anyone so that location of a specific individual is not possible.

INTERPRETATION

One reason evaluation findings are often underutilized is that researchers neglect to interpret their findings for their constituencies. Evaluators are often deeply involved in the research aspects of their work, making it difficult for them to translate findings, and the nuances of those findings, for lay audiences not well versed in the more arcane aspects of sophisticated data analysis. Furthermore, researchers are often overwhelmed with many other responsibilities, thus they may have little time to translate their work for other audiences.

The most challenging of these tasks is the interpretation of evaluation findings. Although the researcher may be content with reporting that a program had a 10% impact on the immediate outcome of study, for designers and policy-makers this may not be enough information. Designers and policy-makers are likely to want to know the impact on the ultimate outcome of study. For example, if there was a 10% change in contraceptive use, how many births averted would this translate to? How will this affect overall fertility levels or reductions in abortion?

Furthermore, designers and policy-makers are interested in the characteristics of those individuals who were influenced by the campaign. Was the campaign more effective among women or among those less educated? This type of analysis will help determine what types of interventions and messages should be planned next and how they should be carried out. What does the research say about existing barriers to behavior change? Interpretation takes time; the time pressure in most organizations results in an underutilization of research data to explore these issues as deeply as warranted.

GRAPHICS

A picture is worth a thousand words. Evaluation research often consists of communicating complex information. Using graphics and pictorial displays to facilitate this communication is strongly recommended. There are at least three opportunities for using graphics—when presenting *(1)* a logical model to describe program or evaluation components, *(2)* a conceptual framework of the theoretical approach, and *(3)* study results.

Graphics can show the steps in a program or evaluation. For example, a campaign to promote seat belt use may involve formative research among different target audiences, baseline and follow-up surveys, focus group discussions, and police checkpoints. A diagram showing the interrelationship and timing of these activities could help the various teams understand the components of the project. Such a diagram, often referred to as a logic model, is particularly useful during planning meetings.

Graphics can be used to describe the conceptual framework guiding the investigation. Figure 2–6 is a general framework for understanding the influence of communication campaigns on behavior change, providing a more concise and more easily interpretable description of the ways in which a program might influence behavior than a textual description. With Figure 2–6, researchers can discuss the various components of the model, alternative paths of influence between variables, postulate on those variables that have been omitted from the model, and debate methods for testing the model. Researchers often discover that drawing the conceptual framework and/or the specific model to be tested enables them to specify their research goals and interests more clearly.

Graphics can also be used to display study results. Paragraphs of text reporting variable values and study results can be tedious to read. Many studies consist of baseline and follow-up survey results that can more easily be communicated with bar graphs. For example, Figures 12–1 and 12–2 reported baseline and follow-up scores for the evaluation's knowledge, attitude, practice (KAP) variables. These bar graphs communicate the data more clearly and quickly than a textual description of the values. Line graphs are often used to show the relationship between two variables and to show trends over time.

ETHICAL CONSIDERATIONS

There are certain ethical concerns and standards relevant to research on human behavior. Above all else, there is a responsibility to act decently and appropriately while conducting research. In the long run, responsible behavior improves evaluation efforts and reduces the likelihood of harm to the intended beneficiaries of the program. Ethical considerations occur both during data collection and during data sharing and reporting.

Data Collection

Study participation should be voluntary; that is, potential participants should be informed of the study procedures and given the option to agree to participate or agree not to participate at any time. An accurate description of the burden from study participation should be given to the participant. Many institutional review boards (IRBs) now require that participants sign an informed consent form to be kept on file.

Informed consent must clearly state that participation is optional and that participants may refuse to answer any question at any time (Faden and Beauchamp, 1986). Most health promotion evaluations consist of questionnaire surveys that are not likely to be intrusive or harmful to the subjects. Indeed, most respondents will be familiar with survey techniques that ask respondents to answer a series of questions about their knowledge, attitudes, and practices regarding some topic. An example of an informed consent notice is provided in Appendix C.

It is important to give the potential respondent an estimate of how long the interview is expected to take and whether any sensitive questions will be asked. It is also imperative that the researcher be truthful when providing this information. Telling a potential respondent that an interview will take 20 minutes when it will take 40 is unethical, unkind, and inappropriate.

Sensitive questions may be asked on surveys and it is polite to warn the respondent before asking a question that may be considered sensitive. It is also advisable to remind respondents that they may choose not to answer these sensitive questions. It is also polite to provide the respondent with options that allow the respondent to provide vague or non-revealing responses. For example, a question about the frequency of substance abuse should have a response option of "not sure."

Institutional Review Boards

Most universities and many research organizations have an institutional review board (IRB) that is responsible for approving research protocols. These boards (also known as Committee for Human Research or Committee for the Protection of Human Subjects) are responsible for reviewing study procedures to ensure they do not cause harm to study subjects. The federal government has guidelines for study implementation; studies funded directly by the federal government are reviewed by the Office of Management and Budget.

There is a range of strong opinions regarding the jurisdictional boundaries for the IRB. Most researchers, not surprisingly, feel that an IRB should be restricted to ensuring that researchers follow ethical procedures and obtain informed consent. Others feel that the IRB is responsible for minimizing respondent burden, and so it should be able to prohibit research that is of dubious scientific merit because it places an undue burden on the respondents. For example, if a study design does not have appropriate sample size estimates (see the section on power analysis, Chapter 7) should the research be permitted to proceed if it may pose an unnecessary burden on respondents?

The IRB review process typically takes 3 to 6 months. Although getting IRB approval can be time consuming and costly, it is a necessary step in the research process. Evaluators are advised to establish familiarity with the processes of the IRB that oversees their research. Often the IRB has considerable experience with research activities and can be very helpful to the researcher.

Researchers should know the distinction between confidentiality and anonymity. *Anonymity* in data collection indicates that the data will be collected so no information specifically identifying the individuals will be recorded. Examples of identifying information are the respondent's name and address or phone number or Social Security number. *Confidentiality* in data collection indicates the data will not be used or shared with anyone or any agency unless all identifying information is removed from the data.

BUDGETS

Obviously, financial resources play a large role in determining program development and evaluation. Many people argue that resource scarcity prohibits conducting an evaluation, yet evaluations must be conducted to reduce the likelihood of wasting those scarce resources on misdirected and ineffective programs. The question then arises of how much an evaluation should cost and how evaluation expenses are budgeted.

A general rule of thumb has been to allocate 10%–15% of program costs to evaluation. This percentage might be larger if *(1)* the topic of promotion is new or there is little information about it and more baseline research is needed to determine appropriate messages; *(2)* the topic is critical or sensitive, hence it is important to monitor the program's impact closely; and *(3)* the program is the first in a series of activities and so early evaluation data will be important later. The evaluation percentage might be smaller if the program is the later part of a series of activities and hence data are already plentiful and messages and strategies are well developed. In sum, the newer the program the greater the need for research and evaluation while more mature programs may decrease the resources allocated to evaluating it.

The two mass media campaigns for the National Reproductive Health Program in Bolivia cost approximately $560,000 and the evaluation costs for data collection and entry were approximately $68,000, yielding a 12.1% research and evaluation budget. Other expenses included further data analysis and dissemination activities of approximately $60,000, bringing the cost to 20% of the overall budget. The projects were conducted by the Johns Hopkins University Center for Communication Programs and funded by the U.S. Agency for International Development under contract number DPE-3052-A-00-0014.

Appendix D provides a sample program evaluation budget. This sample provides a start and should not be considered comprehensive and not necessarily accurate in all situations. The evaluator is forewarned that budgeting is a complex, political, difficult, and essential component of evaluation.

In most evaluations, the principal investigator (PI) is the person responsible for project administration and overseeing every aspect of the study. Research assistants (RA) are responsible for carrying out many of the activities, and administrative assistants (AA) responsible for coordinating and maintaining many of the logistics. In the Bolivian study, the PI was allocated a total of 33 days (15%), the RA a total of 220 days (100%); and the AA, 55 days (25%). Many evaluation projects will apportion time commitments at roughly these rates.

BOOK SUMMARY

This text has presented the procedures and steps necessary for evaluating health promotion programs. The components of evaluation are discussed in roughly the sequence they occur, with the recognition that a good evaluator will anticipate these steps and plan accordingly. The goal has been to provide the frameworks, theories, tools, and formulas that evaluators use to evaluate programs, and every attempt has been made to be comprehensive so that researchers may find this guide useful to have with them in the field.

It is also anticipated that some researchers may find this material useful for writing evaluation study proposals. Box 14–1 describes the components needed to write a study design proposal. Programs and their evaluations are rarely funded blindly with a blank check. Rather, government agencies, foundations, and other organizations will request a proposal that details the programmatic and research steps for which funding is sought. Funding for the evaluation will only occur after the proposal is reviewed and judged to be appropriate.

Every evaluation will be unique because health programs vary considerably. The components outlined in Box 14–1 provide a guide for what to include in an evaluation proposal. Some proposals may require more emphasis on quantitative measurement and multiple survey waves, while others may emphasize the collection of qualitative data for formative research. Regardless, a good evaluator incorporates the many different elements in the evaluation process to avoid making false conclusions about program outcomes.

The evaluation process consists of the steps outlined in Box 14–2. These steps are a broad summary of the activities diagramed in Figure 1–1. Although every step is crucial, the third one, the study design, is often the most critical because the baseline data provide the benchmark for measuring success, yet are collected before everything about the program is known.

In sum, this text has stressed the importance of setting program objectives and specifying the theoretical basis for the program and its evaluation. In Part I, for-

Box 14-1. STUDY DESIGN

Health promotion program evaluators should get advice from the program designers and other evaluation experts. The designers know the intended scope and goals of the program and may help the evaluator understand how to measure the program's effects. Other evaluation experts can help improve the study design and instruments.

To get this input, others will need to see a study design. In many cases, a proposal to conduct the evaluation study will need to be written. Although it is difficult to anticipate the needs and challenges of a study before a program is launched, it is essential to have the study design planned in as much detail as possible. A study design usually consist of the following components:

1. Goals and objectives. The goals and objectives of the study should be stated precisely and clearly (Chapter 2).
2. Theory. The theoretical rationale for the intervention and how it is expected to achieve the objectives should be described (Chapter 3).
3. Study design. The number of waves of data to be collected and whether the interviews will be conducted among a panel or cross-sectional sample should be detailed (Chapter 6).
4. Sample size and sample selection. The number and types of respondents needed for the study and how they will be selected should be outlined (Chapter 7). An explicit rationale for the sample sizes should be provided.
5. Threats to validity. The potential threats to validity that are controlled and those that are not controlled should be given (Chapter 6).
6. Formative research. Descriptions of the formative research including pilot test and feasibility analysis to be conducted should be provided (Chapter 3).
7. Process research. A plan for monitoring the program and collecting data on its implementation should be detailed (Chapter 5).
8. Analysis plan. Data management and analysis procedures, including the types of statistical tests and their interpretation, should be described (Chapters 9–13).
9. Budget. Information about the projected costs for the study should be included (Chapter 14).
10. Instrument. A draft of the questionnaire or other instruments used to collect the data, such as registration forms, should be provided (Chapter 8, Appendix B).
11. Timeline. The design description should contain estimates of when each phase of the study will be conducted, including instrument (questionnaire) revision and completion, pilot-testing, data collection, data entry, statistical analysis, and dissemination.
12. Dissemination plan. Specific dissemination vehicles and intended audiences should be described and budgeted (Chapter 14). The dissemination plan should also include information on how the data will be used for further health promotion activities.

Box 14-2. STEPS IN EVALUATION PROJECT

Evaluating health promotion programs is a process involving many steps. While not required in all evaluation projects, the following list provides a convenient checklist useful to monitor the steps to an evaluation project.

1. Project is initiated by the need or desire to create a program.
2. Evaluation design proposal developed (see Box 14–1).
3. Pre-program data measurements are collected, literature reviews of current situation conducted, and intervention and evaluation monitoring procedures established. Data and analysis have been feed-forwarded to program designers.
4. Program is monitored.
5. Post-program data (i.e., follow-up or outcome measurement) are collected.
6. Data to measure outcome of program are analyzed.
7. Findings to designers and other stakeholders are presented.
8. Preliminary findings report is written that can be widely distributed to stakeholders and other interested parties. Results are disseminated to interested parties.
9. Analysis is conducted for learning lessons from the evaluation process.
10. Evaluation data are used to make recommendations for future programs.

mative research and monitoring were described and guides for conducting them presented. Part II presented study designs, and rules and guidelines for selecting study subjects, interviewing them, and managing the data they provide, and provided rules for analyzing these data. In Part III, data from the Bolivia National Reproductive Health Program campaign were used to demonstrate basic and advanced statistical analysis techniques for measuring outcomes. It is hoped that the guides, rules, and examples presented will enable evaluators to more easily conduct program evaluations in the future. Evaluation data provide measures of the audience's knowledge, attitude, and practice that are essential for setting goals, determining impact, and planning future activities that are essential to strategic and informed management. I hope this text facilitates that process.

THE FUTURE OF HEALTH PROMOTION PROGRAM EVALUATION

Health promotion program evaluation should be consistent conceptually, operationally, and empirically. Conceptually, does the evaluation make sense by telling a plausible story? Operationally, does it describe how the program and its evaluation were conducted in a way that provides the opportunity for replication? Empirically, are the data presented in an understandable and appropriate way? These three domains can be used to judge the appropriateness and quality of health promotion program evaluations.

There will always be considerable demand for evaluation research because, unfortunately, there is an abundance of social and public health problems to be addressed. Humanity will never be perfect, but we will continue to strive to improve our lot and to do so requires health promotion and communication campaigns (among other things) to inform people of their options so they can make informed choices. The demands for conducting rigorous evaluations will increase and the training necessary to conduct these evaluations will become more challenging.

Statistical and survey sampling tools are getting better, and at the same time getting more complex. Consequently, program evaluators must keep abreast of these developments to implement scientifically valid evaluations. As the computing technology gets more complex, ostensibly to save time, it requires more time to manage.

The future looks bright in terms of challenges. It is hoped that this guide will make facing those challenges a little less daunting and the benefits of these evaluation endeavors more fruitful.

Glossary

Alpha (α): The critical probability value for rejecting the null hypothesis. Typically, α is set at 5% or 1%. α is also used to represent the reliability coefficient.

Attrition: The loss of study subjects during the course of the study which can occur because they drop out, move, or are hard to contact.

Beta (β): The probability of type II error in which the researcher concludes that the null hypothesis is true when in reality it is false. Typically, β is set at 20% (or 0.20). β is also used to signify a standardized regression coefficient.

Between subjects: A study design that uses cross-sectional (or independent) samples and makes comparisons between respondents or subjects.

Bias: A factor associated with study design that distorts measurement from being true.

Blind review: The process by which the identity of the author(s) of submitted journal articles is (are) kept anonymous and the reviewers' identities kept from the author. The blind-review process helps maintain the objectivity of the review process.

Blinded study: A study in which the study subjects (and perhaps the researchers) do not know whether they are in the intervention or control group.

Case study: An in-depth description of the activities, processes, and events that happened during a program.

Case–control study: A study design in which persons with an outcome (cases) are compared to those without it (controls). A matched case–control study is one in which

257

the cases have been identified and controls are selected to match them on as many characteristics as feasible.

Causality: The determination that one event, action, state, or behavior is responsible for another.

Ceiling effect: When the baseline level of a variable is high (>80%) and there is little room for improvement, hence the program may have limited impact.

Cohort study: Following longitudinally a group of people who enter the study at the same time.

Comparison group: Individuals selected to be used like a control group to compare to the intervention group.

Contamination: The unplanned deterioration of a study design either because the control/comparison group was exposed to the intervention or the intervention was not implemented as intended; for example, when information in a media campaign to promote a health behavior is disseminated to the control communities.

Content analysis: The quantitative coding of symbolic or communication material (e.g., coding of political orientation of selected opinion pieces from selected newspapers).

Control group: Individuals not exposed to the treatment or intervention, to be compared to the intervention group.

Cost–benefit analysis: Subtracting program costs from program benefits (both valued in U.S. dollars) to determine net benefits either with a scalar or with a ratio.

Cost-effectiveness analysis: Dividing program impacts (however measured) by program costs to determine an effectiveness ratio.

Critical value: The value of the statistic that must be exceeded for the researcher to conclude that the test results were statistically significant.

Cronbach's α: The measure of scale reliability, which ideally should be >0.70.

Cross-sectional sample: Potential respondents selected independently at each survey time.

Degrees of freedom: The amount of information provided by the data within the context of a specific statistical test.

Dependent variable: A variable hypothesized to depend on other variables and thought to be influenced by independent variables, represented as Y. For example, getting regular exercise might be a dependent variable promoted in a campaign. Knowlege, attitudes, and practices (KAP) regarding reproductive health were the dependent variables in many of the examples in this book.

Design effect: The degree to which sample selection procedures deviate from simple random sampling by sampling clusters. The researcher can adjust the sample size calculation to control for this bias.

Dose: The amount of intervention that the study subjects receive.

Double-blind experiment: When neither the researcher nor the subject knows who gets assigned to the intervention and control conditions (both researcher and subject are blind to the subjects' assignment).

Ecological fallacy: When data collected at one level of analysis are used to make statements about indicators at another level, falsely ascribing group characteristics to individuals. For example, using state-level data to make inferences about individual behavior.

Endogenous variable: A dependent variable in path analysis.

Evaluation: The systematic application of research theories and methods to determine if and how a program achieved its objectives.

Event history analysis: A set of statistical techniques used to study probabilities over time; particularly useful when the researcher has independent variables that vary over time.

Exogenous variable: An independent variable in path analysis.

Experimental design: When subjects are randomly assigned to treatment and control conditions.

External validity: The generalizability of a study's findings—the degree to which the findings are representative of the population's behavior.

Factoral design: A study design. A 2 × 2 factoral design consists of two different conditions crossed with two other conditions. For example, a researcher might have a mass media intervention compared to an interpersonal one in two high- and two low-prevalence communities.

Fidelity: The degree to which a program's implementation matches the intended one.

Focus group discussion (FGD): A semi-structured group interview, typically conducted among 8–12 relatively homogeneous subjects and moderated by a trained researcher.

Formative research: Activities conducted before an intervention to inform program development.

Framework: A conceptual model that guides the steps in an evaluation.

Goal: The general purpose of an intervention.

Hypothesis: The statement of a relationship between variables to be tested in a study. Typically, hypotheses are derived from theory.

Hypothesis testing: The process of determining whether a hypothesis can be supported by the data or study.

Impact: The expected result of an intervention.

Independent sample: A new sample collected at each time point not linked to respondents who were interviewed previously.

Independent variable: A variable not hypothesized to depend on other variables and thought to influence the outcome variable(s) under study. Typically, gender, age, and education are independent variables.

Indicator: A variable that measures a desired programmatic outcome, such as level of contraceptive use.

Information, education, and communication (IEC): An umbrella term that includes many aspects of communication actities.

Informed consent: The process by which subjects (respondents) are informed of the purposes and activities of the research and given the opportunity to participate voluntarily.

Institutional review board (IRB): The committee at an organization responsible for reviewing and approving research to guarantee that it is ethical (also known as the Committee for the Protection of Human Subjects or Committee for Human Research).

Internal validity: The accuracy or truthfulness of the conclusions drawn from a specific study.

Intervention group: Individuals exposed to the treatment who are to be compared to a control group, with the expectation that the treatment will influence them. Sometimes referred to as the experimental group.

Level of measurement: Classification of how variables are measured that is dependent on their value and ordinality. There are three levels: nominal, ordinal, interval–ratio.

Likert scale: Series of questionnaire items rated as strongly agree, agree, neutral, disagree, and strongly disagree, usually summed to create a scale. Likert items typically have three to seven values (or points).

Longitudinal study: Any study in which observations are made over time. Typically used to refer to panel or cross-sectional samples that are collected at multiple points in time.

Manipulation check: Procedures and measurements used to verify that subjects received the intervention the way it was intended.

Meta-analysis: The statistical analysis of similar studies to estimate a parameter from the population of studies.

Monitoring: Research conducted during program implementation to measure how the intervention was delivered.

Mystery or simulated client studies: Studies in which imposters are recruited to pose as clients to determine what happens at services sites.

Needs assessment: The process by which the prevalence and degree of a problem is identified and the existing situational, organizational, and contextual factors that influence the behavior are analyzed.

Nonreactive measures: Data collection techniques in which the respondent/subject is not disturbed and perhaps is unaware that data are being collected (also known as unobtrusive measures).

Normal distribution: Variable distribution in which the mean and standard deviation (SD) are such that 68% of cases fall within 1 SD of the mean and 95% fall within 2 SD of the mean. The mean is two times larger than the SD and the distribution is symmetric (neither skewed left or right).

Null hypothesis: A hypothesis that is the converse of what the researcher wishes to prove. Rejection of the null hypothesis implies support for the research hypothesis.

Omnibus surveys: Surveys conducted on a regular basis among the general population, usually by market research organizations, to monitor attitudes and behavior in a particular industry.

Outcome: Expected result of an intervention.

Panel sample: A study sample in which the same individuals are interviewed repeatedly.

Panel study: A study in which the same respondents are interviewed repeatedly.

Participant observation: The researcher observes study participants in naturalistic settings.

Pilot study: A small study conducted to test the feasibility of a larger study.

Pilot testing or pretesting: The act of testing study instruments to detect errors and improve measurement.

Power: The ability of a study to detect a specified effect, with a specified degree of accuracy and replicability $(1 - \beta)$; the ability to detect a true difference when there is one.

Process evaluation/ research: Research conducted to understand program creation, implementation, dissemination, comprehension, and effects on the audience. Also referred to as monitoring.

Prospective study: A study conducted in such a way that data are collected before the intervention is put into place so that predictions can be made before the intervention occurs.

Qualitative research: Research procedures aimed at providing in-depth analysis ("thick description") of behavior. The emphasis is on understanding the phenomenon and generating theory, not on generalizability.

Quantitative research: Research procedures aimed at collecting data to test theories of behavior. The emphasis is on generalizability, replicability, and theory testing.

Quasi-experimental design: An analogue of experimental or case–control study, but the researcher does not have control over whether subjects receive or do not receive the intervention. In quasi-experiments, the intervention is often available to everyone and so the researcher cannot control who receive it and who does not receive it.

Ratings and coverage data: Data that represent the type, reach, and frequency of media attention to a given issue.

Reliability: The consistency of a measurement.

Response rate: The percentage of respondents who participate in a study.

Retrospective study: A study that collects data after the fact and attempts to look back to see what happened.

Scale: A composite score derived from combining multiple questionnaire items.

Scaled-response question: A question in which response categories vary. Typically, scaled-response questions are referred to as Likert-type question in which the respondent may agree, feel neutral, or disagree.

Secondary analysis: Re-analysis of data originally collected for a different purpose.

Simulations: Systematic hypothetical scenarios extrapolated from existing conditions to process "what-if" scenarios.

Standard deviation: A measure of the degree to which individual scores vary from the average score. A standard normal curve has a standard deviation of 1.

Study validity: Whether a study accurately measures what it is intended to measure.

Summative research: Research conducted to determine the effect or impact of a program.

Theory: A conceptual model that explains the phenomenon under study.

Treatment group: Another term for the intervention group.

Type I error: See Alpha.

Type II error: See Beta.

Variance: The degree of dispersion or spread around the mean. The standard deviation is one measure of variance for individual scores, whereas the standard error is a measure of variance in parameter estimates (such as a correlation coefficient).

Weighting data: The process of assigning probability values to observations to adjust the importance that each case contributes to the analysis.

Within subjects: A study design that uses panel (or cohort) samples and makes comparisons within observations.

References

Aday, L. A. (1989). *Designing and Conducting Health Surveys*. San Francisco: Jossey-Bass.

Ajzen, I. (1988). *Attitudes, Personality, and Behavior*. Chicago, IL: Dorsey Press.

Ajzen, I. (1991). The theory of planned behavior. *Organizational Behavior and Human Decision Processes 50:* 179–211.

Ajzen, I. and Fishbein, M. (1980). *Understanding Attitudes and Predicting Social Behavior*. Englewood Cliffs, NJ: Prentice-Hall.

Aldrich, J. H. and Nelson, F. D. (1984). *Linear Probability, Logit, and Probit Models*. Newbury Park, CA: Sage.

Alexander, C., Piazza, M., Mekos, D., and Valente, T. W. (2001). Peer networks and adolescent cigarette smoking: an analysis of the national longitudinal study of adolescent health. *J. Adolescent 29,* 22–30.

Allison, P. D. (1984). *Event History Analysis: Regression for Longitudinal Event Data*. Newbury Park, CA: Sage.

Anderson, J. G. and Jay, S. J. (1985). The diffusion of medical technology: social network analysis and policy research. *Sociol. Q. 26(1):* 49–64.

Andreasen, A. R. (1995). *Marketing Social Change: Changing Behavior to Promote Health, Social Development, and the Environment*. San Francisco: Jossey-Bass.

Babbie, E. (2001). *The Practice of Social Research* (9th Ed.) Belmont, CA: Wasdworth.

Backer, T. E. and Marston, G. (1993). Parternship for a drug-free America: an experiment in social marketing. In T. E. Backer and E. M. Rogers (eds.) *Organizational Aspects of Health Communication Campaigns: What Works?* Newbury Park, CA: Sage.

263

Backer, T. E., Rogers, E. M., and Sopory, P. (1992). *Designing Health Communication Campaigns: What works?* Newbury Park, CA: Sage.

Bandura, A. (1977). *Social Learning Theory.* Englewood Cliffs, NJ: Prentice-Hall.

Bandura, A. (1986). *Social Foundations of Thought and Action: A Social Cognitive Theory.* Englewood Cliffs, NJ: Prentice-Hall.

Barnett, G. A. and Danowski, J. A. (1992). The structure of communication: a network analysis of the International Communication Association. *Hum. Commun. Res. 19:* 264–285.

Baron, R. M. and Kenny, D. A. (1986). The moderator–mediator variable distinction in social psychological research: conceptual, strategic, and statistical consideration. *J. Pers. Soc. Psychol. 51:* 1173–1182.

Bauman, L. J., Stein, R., and Ireys, H. (1991). A framework for conceptualizing interventions. *Sociol. Practice Rev. 2:* 241–251.

Becker, M. (1974). The health belief model and personal health behavior. *Health Educ. Monogr. 2:* 328–353.

Becker, M. (1995). *Writing for Social Scientists.* Newbury Park, CA: Sage.

Bentler, P. M. (1984). *EQS: Structural Equations Program Manual.* Los Angeles, CA: BMDP Statistical Software.

Berelson, B. (1952). *Content Analysis in Communications Research.* New York: Free Press.

Berelson, B. and Freedman, R. (1964). A study in fertility control. *Sci. Am. 210(5):* 29–37.

Berelson, B., Lazarsfeld, P. F., and McPhee, W. (1954). *Voting: A Study of Opinion Formation in a Presidential Campaign.* Chicago: University of Chicago Press.

Bernard, H. R. (1995). *Research Methods in Anthropology: Qualitative and Quantitative Approaches,* 2nd ed. Newbury Park, CA: Sage.

Bertrand, J. T., Santiso, R., Linder, S. H., and Pineda, M. A. (1987). Evaluation of a communications program to increase adoption of vasectomy in Guatemala. *Stud. Fam. Plan. 18:* 361–370.

Blalock H. (1988). *Social Statistics.* New York: McGraw-Hill.

Bollen, K. A. (1989). *Structural Equations with Latent Variables.* New York: John Wiley and Sons.

Borenstein, M., Rothstein, H., and Cohen, J. (1997). *Power and Precision: A Computer Program for Statistical Power Analysis and Confidence Intervals.* Teaneck, NJ: Biostat.

Broadhead, R. S., Heckathorn, D. D., Weakliem, D. L., Anthony, D. L., Marday, H., Mills, R. J., and Hughs, J. (1998). Harnessing peer networks as an instrument for AIDS prevention: results from a peer-driven intervention. *Public Health Rep. 113(S1):* 42–57.

Bruce, J. (1990). Fundamental elements of the quality of care: a simple framework. *Stud. Fam. Plan. 21(2):* 61–91.

Bruce, J. and Jain, A. (1991). Improving the quality of care through operations research. In M. Seidman and M. Horn (eds.) *Operations Research: Helping Programs Work Better,* pp. 259–282. New York: Wiley-Liss.

Campbell, D. T. and Stanley, J. C. (1963). *Experimental and Quasi-experimental Designs for Research.* Boston: Houghton Mifflin.

Carlson, R. O. (1964). School superintendents and the adoption of modern math: a social structure profile. In M. B. Miles (ed.) *Innovation in Education,* pp. 329–342. New York: Bureau of Publications, Teachers College, Columbia University.

Carmines, E. G. and Zeller, R. A. (1979). *Reliability and Validity Assessment.* Newbury Park, CA: Sage.

Cartwright, D. (1949). Some principles of mass persuasion: selected findings of research on the sale of United States War Bonds. *Hum. Relat. 2:* 253–267.

Cartwright, D. (1954). Achieving change in people: some applications of group dynamics theory. *Hum. Relat. 4:* 381–392.

CDC AIDS Community Demonstration Projects Research Group (1998). Community-level HIV intervention in 5 cities: final outcome data from the CDC AIDS community demonstration projects. *Am. J. Public Health 89:* 336–345.

Chaffee, S. H. and Mutz, D. C. (1988). Comparing mediated and interpersonal communication data. In R. P. Hawkins, J. M. Wiemann, and S. Pingree (eds.) *Advancing Communication Science: Merging Mass and Interpersonal Processes*, pp. 19–43. Newbury Park, CA: Sage Annual Reviews.

Chaffee, S. H. and Roser, C. (1986). Involvement and the consistency of knowledge, attitudes, and behaviors. *Commun. Res. 13:* 373–399.

Chen, H. T. and Rossi, P. H. (1983). Evaluating with sense: the theory-driven approach. *Eval. Rev. 7(3):* 283–302.

Church, C. A. and Geller, J. (1989). Lights! camera! action!: promoting family planning with TV, video, and film. *Popul. Rep. J 38:* 00–00.

Cohen, J. (1960). A coefficient for agreement for nominal scales. *Educ. Psychol. Measure. 20:* 37–46.

Cohen, J. (1968). Weighted kappa: nominal scale agreement with provision for scaled disagreement or partial credit. *Psychol. Bull. 70:* 213–220.

Cohen, J. (1977). *Statistical Power Analysis for the Behavioral Sciences,* rev. ed. New York: Academic Press.

Cohen, J. and Cohen, P. (1983). *Applied Multiple Regression/Correlation Analysis for the Behavioral Sciences* (2nd ed.). Hillsdale, NJ: Lawrence Erlbaum Associates.

Coleman, J. S., Katz, E., and Menzel, H. (1966). *Medical Innovation: A Diffusion Study.* New York: Bobbs Merrill.

Converse, J. M., and Presser, S. (1986). *Survey Questions: Handcrafting the Standardized Questionnaire.* Newbury Park, CA: Sage.

Cook, T. D. and Campbell, D. T. (1979). *Quasi-experimentation: Design and Analysis Issues for Field Settings.* Boston: Houghton Mifflin.

Cordray, D. S. (1993). Strengthening causal interpretations of nonexperimental data: the role of meta-analysis. In L. Sechrest (ed.) *Program Evaluation: A Pluralistic Enterprise. New Directions for Program Evaluation, No. 60,* pp. 59–96. San Francisco: Josey Bass.

Crain, R. L. (1966). Flouridation: the diffusion of an innovation among cities. *Soc. Forces 44(4):* 467–476.

Cronbach, L. J., Ambron, S. R., Dornbusch, S. M., Hess, R. D., Hornik, R. C., Phillips, D. C., Walker, D. F., and Weiner, S. S. (1980). *Toward Reform of Program Evaluation.* San Francisco: Jossey-Bass.

Cronbach, L. J. and Furby, L. (1970). How we should measure "change"—or should we? *Psychol. Bull. 74(1):* 68–80.

Davis, D., Barrington, T., Phoenix, U., Gilliam, A., Collins, C., Cotton, D., and Chen, H. (2000). Evaluation and technical assistance for successful HIV program delivery. *AIDS Education and Prevention, 12, Supplement A,* 115–125.

Debus, M. (1990). *Methodological Review: A Handbook for Excellence in Focus Group Research.* Washington DC: Academy for Educational Development.

DeFleur, M. L. (1987). The growth and decline of research on the diffusion of news. *Commun. Res. 14(1):* 109–130.

Dehar, M. A., Casswell, S., and Duignan, P. (1993). Formative and process evaluation of health promotion and disease prevention programs. *Eval. Rev. 17:* 204–220.

Deutschmann, P. J. and Danielson, W. A. (1960). Diffusion of knowledge of the major news story. *Journalism Q. 37:* 345–355.

DHS (Demographic and Health Survey) (1989). Maternal and Child Health in Bolivia: Reports on the In-depth DHS Survey in Bolivia 1989. Columbia, MD: Macro Systems.

DHS (Demographic and Health Survey) (1994). Encuesta Nacional de Demografia y Salud 1994. Columbia, MD: Macro Systems.

Dignan, M. B. and Carr, P. A. (1992). *Program Planning for Health Education and Promotion,* 2nd ed. Philadelphia: Lea Febiger.

Dillman, D. A. (1978). *Mail and Telephone Surveys: The Total Design Method.* New York: John Wiley and Sons.

Durlak, J. A. and Lipsey, M. W. (1991). A practioner's guide to meta-analysis. *Am. J. Commun. Psychol. 19:* 291–332.

Ennett, S. T. and Bauman, K. E. (1993). Peer groups structure and adolescent cigarette smoking: a social network analysis. *J. Health Soc. Behav. 34:* 226–236.

Eulau, H. (1980). The Columbia studies of personal influence. *Soc. Sci. History 4:* 207–228.

Faden, R. R. and Beauchamp, T. L. (1986). *A History and Theory of Informed Consent.* New York: Oxford University Press.

Farquhar, J. W., Fortmann, S. P., Flora, J. A., Taylor, C. B., Haskess, W. L., Williams, P. T., Maccoby, N., and Wood, P. D (1990). Effects of communitywide education on cardiovascular disease risk factors: the Stanford five-city project. *JAMA 264(3):* 359–365.

Feingold, P. C. and Knapp, M. L. (1977). Anti-drug abuse commercials. *J. Commun. 27:* 20–28.

Finnegan, J. R., Viswanath, K., Hannan, P. J., Weisbrod, R., and Jacobs, D. R. (1989). Message discrimination: a study of its use in a campaign research project. *Commun. Res. 16(6):* 770–792.

Fishbein, M. and Ajzen, I. (1975). *Belief, Attitude, Intention and Behavior: An Introduction to Theory and Research.* Boston: Addison-Wesley.

Fishbein, M., Middlestadt, S. E., and Hitchcock, P. J. (1994). Using information to change disease-related behaviors: an analysis based on the theory of reasoned action. In R. J. DiClemente and J. L. Peterson (eds.) *Preventing AIDS: Theories and Methods of Behavioral Interventions,* pp. 61–78. New York: Plenum Press.

Fisher, A. A. and de Silva, V. (1986). Satisfied IUD acceptors as family planning motivators in Sri Lanka. *Stud. Fam. Plan. 17:* 235–242.

Fisher, A. A., Laing, J. E., Stoeckel, J. E., and Townsend, J. W. (1991). *Handbook for Family Planning Research Design,* 2nd ed. New York: The Population Council.

Flay, B. R. (1986). Efficacy and effectiveness trials (and other phases of research) in the development of health promotion programs. *Prev. Med. 15:* 451–474.

Flay, B. R. (1987a). Mass media and smoking cessation: a critical review. *Am. J. Public Health 77(2):* 153–159.

Flay, B. R. (1987b). *Selling the Smokeless Society.* Washington, DC: American Public Health Association.

Flay, B. R. and Cook, T. D. (1989). Three models for summative evluation of prevention campaigns with a mass media component. In R. E. Rice and C. K. Atkin (eds.) *Public Communication Campaigns,* pp. 175–200. Newbury Park, CA: Sage.

Flay, B. R., McFall, S., Burton, D., and Warnecke, R. B. (1993). Health behavior changes through television: the roles of de facto and motivated selection processes. *J. Health Soc. Behav. 34:* 322–335.

Fliegel, F. C. and Kivlin, J. E. (1966). Attributes of innovations as factors in diffusion. *Am. J. Sociol. 72:* 235–248.

Flora, J. A., Maccoby, N., and Farquhar, J. W. (1989). Communication campaigns to prevent cardiovascular disease: the Stanford community studies. In R. E. Rice and C. K. Atkin (eds.) *Public Communication Campaigns*, 2nd ed., pp. 233–252. Newbury Park, CA: Sage.

Fortmann, S. P., Flora, J. A., Winkleby, M. A., Schooler, C., Taylor, C. B., and Farquahar, J. W. (1995). Community intervention trials: reflections on the Stanford five-city project. *Am. J. Epidemiol. 142:* 576–586.

Fox, R. J., Crask, M. R., and Kim, J. (1988). Mail survey response rate: a meta-analysis of selected techniques for inducing response rate. *Public Opin. Q. 52:* 467–491.

Freedman, R. and Takeshita, J. Y. (1969). *Family Planning in Taiwan*. Princeton, NJ: Princeton University Press.

Freimuth, V. S. and Taylor, M. (1998). Are mass mediated health campaigns effective? A review of the empirical evidence. Paper prepared for the National Heart, Lung, and Blood Institute, National Institutes of Health, Bethesda, MD.

GAO/PEMD (General Accounting Office/Program Evaluation and Methodology Division) (1991a). *Designing Evaluations*. Washington, DC: U.S. General Accounting Office.

GAO/PEMD (General Accounting Office/Program Evaluation and Methodology Division) (1991b). *Using Structured Interview Techniques*. Washington, DC: U.S. General Accounting Office.

Gaziano, C. (1983). The knowledge gap: an analytical review of media effects. *Commun. Res. 10(4):* 447–486.

Gitlin, T. (1978). Media sociology: the dominant paradigm. *Theory and Society 6:* 205–253.

Gittelsohn, J., Harris, S., Burris, K., Kadegamic, L., Landman, L. T., Sharma, A., Wolever, T., Logan, A., Barie, A., and Zinman, B. (1996). Use of ethnographic method for applied research on diabetes among Ojibwa-Cree Indians in Northern Ontario. *Health Educ. Behav. 23:* 365–382.

Glanz, K., Lewis, F. M., Rimer, B. K. (Eds.) (1977). *Health Behavior and Health Education*. San Francisco, CA: Jossey-Bass.

Glass, G. V. (1976). Primary, secondary, and meta-analysis of research. *Educ. Res. 5:* 3–8.

Gordis, L. (1996). *Epidemiolgy*. Philadelphia: W. B. Saunders.

Gorsuch, R. L. (1974). *Factor Analysis*. London: W. B. Saunders.

Green, L. W. and Kreuter, M. W. (1991). *Health Promotion Planning: An Education and Environmental Approach*. Mountain View, CA: Mayfield.

Green, L. W., Richard, L., and Potvin, L. (1996). Ecological foundations of health promotion. *Am. J. Health Promotion 10:* 270–281.

Greer, A. L. (1977). Advances in the study of diffusion of innovation health care organizations. *Health Soc. 55(4):* 505–532.

Griliches, Z. (1957). Hybrid corn: an exploration in the economics of technical change. *Econometrica 25:* 501–522.

Guba, E. G. and Lincoln, Y. S. (1981). *Effective Evaluation: Improving the Usefulness of Evalaution Results Through Responsive and Naturalistic Approaches*. San Francisco: Jossey-Bass.

Hale, J. L. and Dillard, J. P. (1995). Fear appeals in health promotion: too much too little or just right? In E. Maibach and R. Parrott (eds.) *Designing Health Messages: Approaches from Communication Theory and Public Health Practice*, pp. 65–80. Newbury Park, CA: Sage.

Hamblin, R. L., Jacobsen, R. B., and Miller, J. L. L. (1973). *A Mathematical Theory of Social Change*. New York: John Wiley and Sons.

Hardy, M. A. (1993). *Regression with Dummy Variables*. Newbury Park, CA: Sage.

Harris, R. J. (1985). *A Primer of Multivariate Statistics*. New York: Academic Press.

Hawkins, R. P., Wiemann, J. M., and Pingree, S. (eds.) (1988). *Advancing Communication Science: Merging Mass and Interpersonal Processes*. Newbury Park, CA: Sage Annual Reviews.

Hayduk, L. A. (1987). *Structural Equation Modeling with LISREL*. Baltimore: Johns Hopkins University Press.

Healey, J. F. (2001). *Statistics: A Tool for Social Research* (6th Ed.). New York: Wadsworth.

Helitzer-Allen, D., Makhambera, M., and Wangel, A. M. (1994). The need for more than focus groups. *Reprod. Health Matters 3:* 75–82.

Henry, G. T. (1990). *Practical Sampling*. Newbury Park, CA: Sage.

Holtgrave, D. R., Tinsley, B. J., and Kay, L. S. (1995) Encouraging risk reduction: a decision-making approach to message design. In E. Maibach and R. Parrott (eds.) *Designing Health Messages: Approaches from Communication Theory and Public Health Practice*. Newbury Park, CA: Sage.

Homans, G. (1950). *The Human Group*. New York: Harcourt Brace.

Hornik, R. C. (1989). Channel effectiveness in development communication programs. In R. E. Rice and C. K. Atkin (eds.) *Public Communication Campaigns*, pp. 309–330. Newbury Park, CA: Sage.

Hornik, R., Contreras-Budge, E., McDivitt, J., McDowell, J., Yoder, P. S., Zimicki, S., and Rasmuson, M. (1992). *Communication for Child Survival: Evaluation of HEALTHCOM Projects in Ten Countries*. Philadelphia: Annenberg School for Communication, University of Pennsylvania.

Hosmer, D. W. and Lemeshow S. (1989). *Applied Logistic Regression*. New York: John Wiley and Sons.

Hovland, C. I., Janis, I. L., and Kelly, H. H. (1953). *Communication and Persuasion*. New Haven, CT: Yale University Press.

Hunter, J. E. and Schmidt, F. L. (1990). *Methods of Meta-analysis*. Newbury Park, CA: Sage.

Huntington, D. and Schuler, S. R. (1993). The simulated client method: evaluating client-provider interactions in family planning clinics. *Stud. Fam. Plan. 24:* 187–193.

Hyman, H. H. and Sheatsley, P..B. (1947). Some reasons why information campaigns fail. *Public Opin. Q. 11:* 412–423.

Jöreskog, K. G. and Sörbom, D. (1989). *LISREL: Analysis of Linear Structural Relationships by Maximum Likelihood, Instrumental Variables and Least Squares Methods*. Mooresville, IN: Scientific Software.

Katz, E. (1957). The two-step flow of communication: an up-to-date report on a hypothesis. *Public Opin. Q. 21:* 61–78.

Katz, E. (1987). Communication research since Lazarsfeld. *Public Opin. Q. S57:* S25–S45.

Katz, E. and Lazarsfeld, P. F. (1955). *Personal Influence: The Part Played by People in the Flow of Mass Communications*. New York: Free Press.

Katz, E., Levine, M. L., and Hamilton, H. (1963). Traditions of research on the diffusion of innovations. *Am. Sociol. Rev. 28:* 237–253.

Keller, A. (1991). Management information systems in maternal and child health/family planning programs: a multi-country analysis. *Stud. Fam. Plan. 22:* 19–30.

Kim, M. S. and Hunter, J. E. (1993). Relationships among attitudes, behavioral intentions, and behavior: a meta-analysis of past research, part 2. *Commun. Res. 20:* 331–264.

Kim, Y. M., Rimon, H. G., Winnard, K., Corso, C., Mako, V., II, Sebioniga, L., Bablola, S., and Huntington, D. (1992). Improving the quality of service delivery in Nigeria. *Stud. Fam. Plan. 23:* 117–126.

Kincaid, D. L. (2000). Social networks, ideation, and contraceptive behavior in Bangladesh: a longitudinal analysis. *Soc. Sci. Med. 50:* 215–231.

Kincaid, D. L., Merritt, A. P., Nickerson, L., Buffington, S. D., de Castro, M. P., and de Castro, B. M. (1996). Impact of a mass media vasectomy promotion campaign in Brazil. *International Family Planning Perspectives, 22,* 169–175.

King, J. A., Lyons Morris, L. L., and Fitz-Gibbon, C. T. (1987). *How to Assess Program Implementation.* Newbury Park, CA: Sage.

Kish, L. (1965). *Survey Sampling.* New York: John Wiley and Sons.

Kish, L. (1987). *Statistical Design for Research.* New York: John Wiley and Sons.

Klapper, J. (1960). *The Effects of Mass Communication.* New York: Free Press.

Kotler, R. and E. Roberto. (1989). *Social Marketing: Strategies for Changing Public Behavior.* New York: Free Press.

Kotler, P. and Zaltman, G. (1971). Social marketing: an approach to planned social change. *J. Marketing 35:* 3–12.

Kovar, M. G. (2000). Four million adolescents smoke: or do they? *Chance 13(2):* 10–14.

Kraemer, H. C. and Thieman, S. (1987). *How Many Subjects?: Statistical Power Analysis in Research.* Newbury Park, CA: Sage.

Krippendorff, K. (1980). *Content Analysis: An Introduction to Its Methodology.* Newbury Park, CA: Sage.

Krueger, R. A. (1994). *Focus Groups: A Practical Guide for Applied Research.* Newbury Park, CA: Sage.

Kuder, G. F. and Richardson, W. M. (1937). The theory of the estimation of test reliability. *Psychometrika 2:* 151–160.

Kuhn, T. S. (1970). *The Structure of Scientific Revolutions.* Chicago: University of Chicago Press.

Kvalem, I. L., Sundet, J. M., Riv , K. I., Eilertsen, D. E., and Bakketeig, L. S. (1996). The effect of sex education on adolescents' use of condoms: applying the Solomon four-group design. *Health Educ. Q. 23:* 34–47.

Kwait, J., Valente, T. W., & Celentano, D. D. (In press). Interorganizational Relationships Among HIV/AIDS Service Organizations in Baltimore: A Network Analysis. *Journal of Urban Health.*

Lachin, J. M. (1981). Introduction to sample size determination and power analysis for clinical trials. *Controlled Clin. Trials 2:* 93–113.

Lapham, R. J. and Mauldin, W. P. (1985). Contraceptive prevalence: the influence of organized family planning programs. *Stud. Fam. Plan. 16(3):* 117–137.

Lasater, T. M., DePue, J. D., Wells, B. L., Gans, K. M., Bellis, J., and Carleton, R. A. (1990). The effectiveness and feasibility of delivering nutrition education programs through religious organizations. *Health Promotion Int. 5(4):* 253–258.

Latkin, C. A., Mandell, W., Oziemkowska, M., Celenatano, D. D., Vlahov, D., and Ensminger, M. (1995). Using social network analysis to study patterns of drug use among urban drug users at high risk for HIV/AIDS. *Drug Alcohol Depend. 38:* 1–9.

Lazarsfeld, P. F., Berelson, B., and Gaudet, H. (1948). *The People's Choice,* 2nd ed. New York: Columbia University Press.

Lefebvre, R. C., Lasater, T. M., Carleton, R. A., and Peterson, G. (1987). Theory and delivery of health programming in the community: the Pawtucket heart health program. *Prev. Med. 16:* 80–95.

Levy, J. A. and Fox, S. E. (1998). The outreach-assisted model of partner notification with IDUs. *Public Health Rep. 113(S1):* 160–169.

Lipsey, M. W. (1990). *Design Sensitivity: Statistical Power for Experimental Research.* Newbury Park, CA: Sage.

Loether, H. J. and McTavish, D. G. (1980). *Descriptive and Inferential Statistics: An Introduction.* Boston: Allyn and Bacon.

Lomas, J., Enkin, M., Anderson, G. M., Hanna, W. J., Vayda, E., and Singer, J. (1991). Opinion leaders vs. audit feedback to implement practice guidelines: delivery after previous cesarean section. *JAMA 265:* 2202–2207.

Maccoby, N. (1988). The community as a focus for health promotion. In S. Spacapan and S. Oskamp (eds.) *The Social Psychology of Health,* pp. 175–206. Newbury Park, CA: Sage.

Maccoby, N. and Farquhar, J. W. (1975). Communication for health: unselling heart disease. *J. Commun. 25(3):* 114–126.

Maccoby, N., Farquhar, J. W., Wood, P. D., and Alexander, J. (1977). Reducing the risk of cardiovascular disease: effects of a community-based campaign on knowledge and behavior. *J. Commun. Health 3(2):* 100–114.

Maibach, E. and Cotton, D. (1995) Moving people to behavior change: a staged social cognitive approach to message design. In E. Maibach and R. Parrott (eds.) *Designing Health Messages: Approaches from Communication Theory and Public Health Practice,* pp. 41–64. Newbury Park, CA: Sage.

McElroy, L., Bibeau, D., Steckler, A., and Glanz, K. (1988). An ecological perspective on health promotion programs. *Health Educ. Q. 15:* 351–377.

McGraw, S. A., McKinlay, S. M., McClements, L., Lasater, T. M., Assaf, A., and Carleton, R. A. (1989). Methods in program evaluation: the process evaluation system of the Pawtucket Heart Health Program. *Eval. Rev. 13(5):* 459–483.

McGuire, W. J. (1989). Theoretical foundations of campaigns. In R. E. Rice and C. K. Atkin (eds.) *Public Communication Campaigns,* pp. 39–42. Newbury Park, CA: Sage.

Mcguire, W. J. (2001). Input and output variables currently promising for constructing persasive communications. In R. Rice and C. Atkin (Eds.). Public Communication Campaigns 3rd (ed.). Thousand Oaks: Sage.

McQuail, D. (1987). Processes of media effects. In D. McQuail (ed.) *Mass Communication Theory: An Introduction,* pp. 251–295. Newbury Park, CA: Sage.

Mendelsohn, H. (1973). Some reasons why information campaigns can succeed. *Public Opin. Q. 37:* 50–61.

Merton, R. K., Fiske, M., and Kendall, P. L. (1956). *The Focused Interview.* New York: Free Press.

Miles, M. B. and Huberman, A. M. (1994). *Qualitative Data Analysis: An Expanded Sourcebook.* Newbury Park, CA: Sage.

Mittelmark, M. B., Luepker, R. V., Jaocbs D. R., Bracht, N. F., Carlaw, R. W., Crow, R. S., Finnegan, J., Grimm, R. H., Jeffery, R. W., Kline, F. G., Mullis, R. M., Murray, D. M., Pechacek, T. F., Perry, C. L., Pirie, P. L., and Blackburn, H. (1986). Community-wide prevention of cardiovascular disease: Education strategies of the Minnesota heart health program. *Preventive Medicine, 15,* 1–17.

Mody, B. (1991). *Designing Messages for Development Communication: An Audience Participation-based Approach.* Newbury Park, CA: Sage.

Mohr, L. B. (1992). *Impact Analysis for Program Evaluation.* Newbury Park, CA: Sage.

Monahan, J. L. (1995) Thinking positively: using positive affect when designing health messages. In E. Maibach and R. Parrott (eds.) *Designing Health Messages: Approaches from Communication Theory and Public Health Practice,* pp. 81–98. Newbury Park, CA: Sage.

Monette, D. R., Sullivan, T. J., and DeJong, C. R. (1998). *Applied Social Research: Tool for the Human Services,* 4th ed. New York: Harcourt Brace.

Nas, T. F. (1996). *Cost–benefit Analysis: Theory and Application.* Newbury Park, CA: Sage.

Needle, R. H., Coyle, S. L., Genser, S. G., and Trotter, R. (1995). *Social Networks, Drug Abuse, and HIV Transmission,* NIDA Research Monograph #151. Rockville, MD: National Clearinghouse for Alcohol and Drug Information (NCAID).

Nunnally, J. C. (1978). *Psychometric Theory.* New York: McGraw-Hill.

Pedhazur, E. J. (1982). *Multiple Regression in Behavioral Research: Explanation and Prediction,* 2nd ed. New York: Holt, Rinehart, and Winston.

Pentz, M. A., Dwyer, J. H., Mackinnon, D. P., Flay, B. R., Hansen, W. B., Wang, E. Y., and Johnson, C. A. (1989). A multicommunity trial for primary prevention of adolescent drug abuse. *JAMA, 261(22):* 3259–3266.

Pentz, M. A., Trebow, E. A., Hansen, W. B., Mackinnon, D. P., Dwyer, J. H., Johnson, C. A., Flay, B. R., Daniels, S., and Cormack, C. (1990). Effects of program implementation on adolescent drug use behavior: the Midwestern Prevention Project (MPP). *Eval. Rev. 14(3):* 264–289.

Perry, C. L., Kelder, S. H., Murray, D. M., and Klepp, K. I. (1992). Community-wide smoking prevention: long-term outcomes of the Minnesota Heart Health Program and the Class of 1989 Study. *Am. J. Public Health 82(9):* 1210–1216.

Petty, R. E. and Cacioppo, J. T. (1981). *Attitudes and Persuasion: Classic and Contemporary Approaches.* Dubuque, IA: Brown.

Piotrow, P. T., Kincaid, D. L., Rimon, J., and Rinehart, W. (1997). *Health Communication: Lessons for Public Health.* New York: Praeger.

Prochaska, J. O., Diclemente, C. C., and Norcross, J. C. (1992). In search of how people change: applications to addictive behaviors. *Am. Psychol. 47:* 1102–1114.

Prochaska, J. O. and Velicer, W. (1997). The transtheoretical model of health behavior change. *Am. J. Health Promotion 12:* 38–48.

Puska, P., Koskela, K., McAlister, A., Mayranen, H., Smolander, A., Moisio, S., Viri, L., Korpelainen, V., and Rogers, E. M. (1986). Use of lay opinion leaders to promote diffusion of health innovations in a community programme: lessons learned from the North Karelia project. *Bull. World Health Organ. 64(3):* 437–446.

Puska, P., Nissinen, A., Tuomilehto, J., Salonen, J. T., Koskela, K., McAlister, A., Kottke, T. E., Maccoby, N., and Farquhar, J. W. (1985). The community-based strategy to prevent coronary heart disease: conclusions from the ten years of the North Karelia project. *Ann. Rev. Public Health 6:* 147–193.

Ratzan, S. (2001). Global population, health and nutrition communication: A review of the literature. Washington DC: USAID.

Ray, M. L. (1975). Marketing communication and the hierarchy-of-effects. In P. Clarke (ed.) *New Models for Mass Communication Research,* pp. 147–176. Newbury Park, CA: Sage.

Reger, B., Wootan, M. G., & Booth-Butterfield, S. (1999). Using mass media to promote health eating: A community-based demonstration project. *Preventive Medicine, 29,* 414–421.

Reiss, E. C., Duggan, A. K., Adger, H., and DeAngelis, C. (1994). The impact of anti-drug advertising: perceptions of middle and high school students. *Arch. Pediatr. Adolesc. Med. 148:* 1262–1268.

Rice, R. E., and J. E. Katz (Eds.). (2001). *The Internet and Health Communication.* Thousand Oaks, CA: Sage.

Rice, R. E. and Foote, D. (1989). A systems-based evaluation planning model for health communication campaigns in developing countries. In R. E. Rice and C. K. Atkin (eds.) *Public Communication Campaigns,* 2nd ed. Newbury Park, CA: Sage.

Roberts, D. F., Henriksen, L., and Christenson, P. G. (1999). *Substance Use in Popular Movies and Music. Office of National Drug Control Policy.* Rockville, MD: National Clearinghouse for Alcohol and Drug Information (NCADI).

Roethlisberger, F. and Dickson, W. (1939). *Management and the Worker.* Cambridge, MA: Harvard University Press.

Rogers, E. M. (1973). *Communication Strategies for Family Planning.* New York: Free Press.

Rogers, E. M. (1995). *Diffusion of Innovations,* 4th ed. New York: Free Press.

Rogers, E. M. and Storey, J. D. (1987). Communication campaigns. In C. R. Berger and S. H. Chaffee (eds.). *Handbook of Communication Science,* pp. 817–846. Newbury Park, CA: Sage.

Rogers, E. M., Vaughan, P. W., Swalehe, R. A., Rao, N., Svenkerud, P., and Sood, S. (1999). Effects of an entertainment–education radio soap opera on family planning in Tanzania. *Stud. Fam. Plan. 30:* 193–211.

Rosen, E. (2000). *The Anatomy of Buzz: How to Create Word-of-Mouth Marketing.* New York: Doubleday.

Rosenberg, M. (1964). *The Logic of Survey Analysis.* New York: Free Press.

Rosenstock, I. M. (1974). Historical origins of the health belief model. *Health Educ. Monogr. 2:* 328–335.

Rosenstock, I. M. (1990). The health belief model: explaining health behavior through expectancies. In K. Glanz, F. M. Lewis, and B. K. Rimer (eds.) *Health Behavior and Health Education,* pp. 00–00. San Francisco: Jossey-Bass.

Rosner, B. A. (2000). *Fundamentals of Biostatistics* (5th ed.). Pacific Grove, CA: Duxbury.

Rossi, P. H., & Freeman, H. E. (1993). *Evaluation: A systematic approach* (5th ed.). Newbury Park, CA: Sage.

Rossi, P. H., Freeman, H. E., and Lipsey (1999). *Evaluation: A Systematic Approach,* 6th ed. Newbury Park, CA: Sage.

Roter, D. L. and Hall, J. A. (1988). Patient–physician communication: a descriptive summary of the literature. *Patient Educ. Counsel. 12:* 99–119.

Ryan, R. and Gross, N. (1943). The diffusion of hybrid seed corn in two Iowa communities. *Rural Sociol. 8:* 15–24.

Saba, W., Valente, T. W., Merritt, A. P., Kincaid, D. L., Lujan, M., and Foreit, J. (1994). The mass media and health beliefs: using media campaigns to promote preventive behavior. Paper presented at the 121st Annual Meeting of the American Public Health Association, San Francisco, CA.

Salmon, W. C. (1998). *Causality and Explanation.* New York: Oxford University Press.

Scheaffer, R. L., Mendenhall, W., and Ott, L. (1990). *Elementary Survey Sampling.* Boston: PWS-Kent.

Schuler, S. R., Choque, M. E., and Rance, S. (1994). Misinformation, mistrust, and mistreatment: family planning among Bolivian market women. *Stud. Fam. Plan. 25(4):* 211–221.

Scott, J. (2000). *Network Analysis: A Handbook,* 2nd ed. Newbury Park, CA: Sage.

Scriven, M. (1967). The methodology of evaluation. In R. W. Tyler, R. M. Gagne, and M. Scriven (eds.) *Perspectives of Curriculum Evaluation,* pp. 39–83. Chicago: Rand McNally.

Scriven, M. (1972). The methodology of evalution. In C. H. Weiss (ed.) *Evaluating Action Programs: Readings in Social Action and Education,* pp. 123–136. Boston: Allyn and Bacon.

Sears, D. O. and Freedman, J. L. (1967). Selective exposure to information: a critical review. *Public Opin. Q. 31:* 194–213.

Sechrist, L., West, S. G., Phillips, M., Redner, R., and Yeaton, W. (1979). Some neglected problems in evaluation research: strength and integrity of treatments. *Eval. Stud. Rev. Annu. 4:* 15–35.

Shadish, W. R., Cook, T. D., and Leviton, L. C. (1991). *Foundations of Program Evaluation: Theories of Practice.* Newbury Park, CA: Sage.

Shannon, C. E. and Weaver, W. (1949). *The Mathematical Model Theory of Communication.* Urbana, IL: University of Illinois Press.

Shapiro, S. S. and Francia, R. S. (1972). An approximate analysis of variance test for normality. *J. Am. Stat. Assoc. 67:* 215–216.

Shapiro, S. S. and Wilk, M. B. (1965). An analysis of variance test for normality (complete samples). *Biometrika 52:* 591–611.

Shea, S. and Basch, C. E. (1990a). A review of five major community-based cardiovascular disease prevention programs. Part I: Rationale, design and theoretical framework. *Am. J. Health Promotion 4(3):* 203–213.

Shea, S. and Basch, C. E. (1990b). A review of five major community-based cardiovascular disease prevention programs. Part II: Intervention strategies, evaluation methods, and results. *Am. J. Health Promotion 4(4):* 279–287.

Siegel, M. and Biener, L. (2000). The impact of an antismoking media campaign on progression to established smoking: results of a longitudinal youth study. *Am. J. Public Health 90:* 380–386.

Siegel, M. and Doner, L. (1998). *Marketing Public Health: Strategies to Promote Social Change.* Gaithersburg, MD: Aspen.

Singhal, A. and Rogers, E. M. (1999). *Entertainment–Education: A Communication Strategy for Social Change.* Mahwah, NJ: Lawrence Erlbaum Associates.

Snyder, L. B. (1990). Channel effectiveness over time and knowledge and behavior gaps. *Journalism Q. 67:* 875–886.

Snyder, L. B. (2001). How effective are mediated health campaigns? In R. E. Rice and C. K. Atkin (eds.) *Public Communication Campaigns,* 3rd ed., pp. 181–190. Newbury Park, CA: Sage.

Snyder, L. B. and Hamilton, M. A. (In press). A meta-analysis of U.S. health campaign effects on behavior: emphasize emforcement, exposure, and new information and beware the secular trend. In R. Hornik (ed.) *Public Health Communication: Evidence for Behavior Change.* Hillsdale, NJ: Lawrence Erlbaum Associates.

Snyder, L. B., Hamilton, M. A., Mitchell, E. W., Kiwanuka-Tondo, J., Fleming-Milici, F., and Proctor, D. (In press). The effectiveness of mediated health communication campaigns: meta-analysis of commencement, prevention, and cessation behavior campaigns. In R. Carveth and J. Bryant (eds.) *Meta-analysis of Media Effects.* Mahwah, NJ: Lawrence Erlbaum Associates.

Solomon, R. L. (1949). An extension of control group design. *Psychol. Bull. 46:* 137–150.

Stake, R. E. (1980). Program evaluation, particularly responsive evaluation. In W. B. Dockrell and D. Hamilton (eds.) *Rethinking Educational Research*, pp. 72–87. London: Hodder and Stoughton.

Star, S. A. and Hughs, H. G. (1950). Report on an educational campaign: the Cincinnati plan for the United Nations. *Am. J. Sociol. 55:* 389–400.

Stephenson, M. T. and Witte, K. (2001). Creating fear in a risky world: generating effective health risk messages. In R. E. Rice and C. K. Atkin (eds.) *Public Communication Campaigns*, 3rd ed., pp. 88–102. Newbury Park, CA: Sage.

Stoebenau, K., & Valente, T. W. (1999). The Role of Network Analysis in Community-Based Program Evaluation: A Case Study from Highland Madagascar. Paper presented at the 19th annual meeting of the International Network for Social Network Analysis, Vancouver, Canada.

Stokols, D. (1996). Translating social ecological theory into guidelines for community health promotion. *Am. J. Health Promotion 10:* 282–297.

Strecher, V. J. and Rosenstock, I. M. (1997). The health belief model. In K. Glanz, F. M. Lewis, and B. K. Rimer (Eds.) *Health Behavior and Health Education*, pp. 41–59. San Francisco, CA: Jossey-Bass.

Suchman, E. A. (1967). *Evaluative Research: Principles and Practice in Public Service and Social Action Programs.* New York: Russell Sage Foundation.

Sudman, S. (1976). *Applied Sampling.* New York: Academic Press.

Thompson, M. S. (1980). *Benefit–Cost Analysis for Program Evaluation.* Newbury Park, CA: Sage.

Tye, J. B., Warner, K. E., and Glantz, S. A. (1987). Tobacco advertising and consumption: evidence of a causal relationship. *J. Public Health Policy 8:* 492–508.

Unger, J. B., Cruz, T. B., Schuster, D., Flora, J. A., and Johnson, C. A. (2001). Measuring exposure to pro- and anit-tobacco marketing among adolescents: intercorrelations among measures and associations with smoking status. *J. Health Commun. 6:* 11–29.

Valente, T. W. (1993). Diffusion of innovations and policy decision-making. *J. Commun. 43:* 30–45.

Valente, T. W. (1995). *Network Models of the Diffusion of Innovations.* Cresskill, NJ: Hampton Press.

Valente, T. W. (1996). Social network thresholds in the diffusion of innovations. *Soc. Networks 18:* 69–79.

Valente, T. W. (1997). On Evaluating Mass Media's Impact. *Studies in Family Planning, 28,* 170–171.

Valente, T. W. and Bharath, U. (1999). An evaluation of the use of drama to communicate HIV/AIDS information. *AIDS Educ. Prev. 11:* 203–211.

Valente, T. W. and Davis, R. L. (1999). Accelerating the diffusion of innovations using opinion leaders. *Ann. Am. Acad. Polit. Soc. Sci. 566:* 55–67.

Valente, T. W., Foreman, R. K., Junge, B., Valhov, D. (1998). Satellite exchange in the Baltimore needle exchange program. *Public Health Reports, 113(S1):* 91–96.

Valente, T. W., Kim, Y. M., Lettenmaier, C., Glass, W., and Dibba, Y. (1994). Radio and the promotion of family planning in The Gambia. *Int. Fam. Perspect. Plan. 20:* 96–100.

Valente, T. W., Paredes, P., and Poppe, P. R. (1998b). Matching the message to the process: behavior change models and the KAP gap. *Hum. Commun. Res. 24:* 366–385.

Valente, T. W., Poppe, P. R., Alva, M. E., de Briceno, V., and Cases, D. (1995) Street theater as a tool to reduce family planning misinformation. *Int. Q. Commun. Health Educ. 15:* 279–289.

Valente, T. W., Poppe, P. R., and Merritt, A. P. (1996). Mass media generated interpersonal communication as sources of information about family planning. *J. Health Commun. 1:* 259–273.

Valente, T. W. and Rogers, E. M. (1995). The origins and development of the diffusion of innovations paradigm as an example of scientific growth. *Sci. Commun. Interdisciplinary Soc. Sci. J. 16:* 238–269.

Valente, T. W. and Saba,W. P. (1998). Mass media and interpersonal influence in the Bolivia National Reproductive Health Campaign. *Commun. Res. 25:* 96–124.

Valente, T. W., Watkins, S., Jato, M. N., Van der Straten, A., & Tsitsol, L. M. (1997). Social network associations with contraceptive use among Cameroonian women in voluntary associations. *Social Science and Medicine, 45,* 677–687.

Walker, J. L. (1969). The diffusion of innovations among the American states. *Am. Polit. Sci. Rev. 63:* 880–899.

Wallack, L. (1981). Mass media campaigns: the odds against finding behavior change. *Health Educ. Q. 8:* 209–260.

Wallack, L., Dorfman, L., Jernigan, D., and Themba, M. (1993). *Media Advocacy and Public Health: Power for Prevention.* Newbury Park, CA: Sage.

Wasserman, S. and Faust, K. (1994). *Social Networks Analysis: Methods and Applications.* Cambridge, UK: Cambridge University Press.

Webb, E. J., Campbell, D. T., and Schwartz, R. D. (1966). *Unobtrusive Measures: Nonreactive Research in the Social Sciences.* Chicago: Rand McNally.

Weisbrod, R. R., Pirie, P. L., and Bracht, N. F. (1992). Impact of a community health promotion program on existing organizations: the Minnesota Heart Health program. *Soc. Sci. Med. 34(6):* 639–648.

Weiss, C. (1972). *Evaluation Research: Methods for Assessing Program Effectiveness.* Englewood Cliffs, NJ: Prentice-Hall.

Weiss, C. H. (1997). How can theory-based evaluation make greater headway? *Eval. Rev. 21:* 501–524.

Wells, B. L., DePue, J. D., Buehler, C. J., Lasater, T. M., and Carleton, R. A. (1990). Characteristics of volunteers who deliver health education and promotion: a comparison with organization members and program participants. *Health Educ. Q. 17(1):* 23–35.

Wholey, J. S. (1979). *Evaluation: Promise and Performance.* Washington, DC: Urban Institute.

Wickizer, T. M., Von Korff, M., Cheadle, A., Maeser, J., Wagner, E. H., Pearson, D., Beery, W., and Psaty, B. M. (1993). Activating communities for health promotion: a process evaluation method. *Am. J. Public Health 83:* 561–567.

Wiebe, G. D. (1951/52). Merchandising commodities and citizenship on television. *Public Opin. Q. 15:* 679–691.

Williams, F. (1986). *Reasoning with Statistics: How to Read Quantitative Research,* 3rd ed. San Francisco: Holt, Rinehart, and Winston.

Winkleby, M. A., Taylor, C. B., Jatulis, D., and Fortman, S. P. (1996). The long-term effects of a cardiovascular disease prevention trial: the Stanford five-city project. *Am. J. Public Health 86:* 1773–1779.

Witkin, B. R. and Altschuld, J. W. (1995). *Planning and Conducting Needs Assessments: A Practical Guide.* Newbury Park, CA: Sage.

Yin, R. K. (1989). *Case Study Research: Design and Methods.* Newbury Park, CA: Sage.

Zillman, D. and Bryant, J. (eds.) (1985). *Selective Exposure to Communication.* Hillsdale, NJ: Lawrence Erlbaum Associates.

Appendix A

POTENTIALLY HELPFUL WEBSITES

http://www.itrs.usu.edu/AEA/index.html

STUDY PLANNING SOFTWARE

http://www.gao.gov
www.statsol.ie/nquery.html (Nquery, for power analysis)
www.cdc.gov/epo/epi/epiinfo.htm (Epi Info, freeware)
members.aol.com/johnp71/javastat.html (Interactive Statistical Calculation
   Pages)
www2.chass.ncsu.edu/garson/pa765/index.shtml (statistical information)
www.stanford.edu/~davidf/webresources.html
www.utoronto.ca/chp/hcu (University of Toronto's Health Communication
   Unit)
www.socio.com (evaluation resources from Sociometrics)
hivinsite.ucsf.edu/prevention/evaluating_programs/ (Center for AIDS Prevention Studies)

EVALUATION SOFTWARE

http://www.kcenter.com/mer/

HEALTH EDUCATION/COMMUNICATION LISTSERVS

listserv@siu.edu (type: subscribe hedirs-l your-name)
listproc@unc.edu (type: subscribe heat your-name)
hltheduc@interactive-healthcare.com (type: subscribe on the subject line)
listserv@yorku.ca (type: subscribe click4hp your-name)

MEDIA RESEARCH FIRMS

www.arbitron.com
www.mediamark.com
www.nielsenmedia.com

QUALITATIVE ANALYSIS SOFTWARE

NUD*IST: www.qsr.com.au
ANTHROPAC: www.analytictech.com/APAC.htm
ATLAS.ti: www.atlasti.de/atlasneu.html

Appendix B

This questionnaire was created with assistance from the Information, Education, and Communication (IEC) subcommittee of the National Reproductive Health Program (NRHP) of Bolivia. The NRHP and its subcommittees were formed with financial and technical assistance from the U.S. Agency for International Development (USAID) and the Bolivian government. The Latin American division of the Johns Hopkins University Center for Communication Programs in Baltimore and La Paz, Bolivia was influential in providing assistance to the IEC subcommittee. It was pilot tested and modified by the Bolivian public opinion firm Encuestas y Estudios, S. A., located in La Paz, with offices in Santa Cruz and Cochabamba. The survey was originally fielded in Spanish and translated into Aymara and Quechua.

BOLIVIA NATIONAL REPRODUCTIVE HEALTH
PROGRAM EVALUATION

Date __/__/__

Good morning/afternoon. My name is _____. I am an interviewer
with the company Encuestas y Estudios. We are interested in knowing what you
think about health. The information you provide us will be valuable for the work
that we are doing. You assistance in helping by answering the following questions would be sincerely appreciated. (*Instructions for interviewer are in italic
type.*)

1. Age of respondent:_____   1a. Sex of respondent: male [1] female [2]

2. What is your marital status?
Married/cohabitating [1]   Single [2]   Widow/Widower [3]   Divorced [4]

3. Do you have or have you had children?
Yes [1]   No [2]   (*If the respondent does not have children and has never had
children, go to question 9.*)

4. Have any of them died?
Yes [1]   No [2]   (*If none have died, go to question 7.*) NA* [99]

5. *If any have died →* How many children have died?
1 [1]   2 [2]   3 [3]   More than 3 [4] DR [92]   NA [99]

6. *If any have died →* At what age did they die? (*Note the age at which each
child died.*)
BOYS   GIRLS (*There should be as many ages noted as there are children who have died.*)

_____   _____
_____   _____
_____   _____
_____   _____
_____   _____   NA [99]

7. How many living children do you have?:_____
☐ Number of boys:_____
☐ Number of girls:_____   NA [99]

8. Age of each child: (*There should be as many ages indicated as there are children.*)
BOYS   GIRLS

_____   _____
_____   _____
_____   _____   NA [99]
_____   _____

*DK, don't know; NA, not applicable; DR, didn't respond; NR, non response.

9. How many siblings do you have:_____
    ☐ Number of brothers:_____
    ☐ Number of sisters:_____

10. What is the monthly income of your family? *(You should include the contributions of all members of the family. Verify the accuracy of the response with the possessions of the interviewee.)*
No income [1]   80–140 Bs. [2]   141–500 Bs.[3]   501–800 Bs. [4]
801–1100 Bs. [5]   More than 1100 Bs. [6] DK/NA [92]

11. What is your level of education?
None [1]   Basic [2]   Middle school [3]   High school [4]   Technical [5]
University [6]   NA [92]

12. *Only for those who answered 1 or 2 on question 11* → Can you read a magazine or newspaper without difficulty?
Without difficulty [1]   With difficulty [2]   Don't know how to read [3]
NR [92]   NA [99]

13. What is your occupation?
Professional [1]   Office worker [2]   Business owner [3]   Laborer [4]
Farmer [5]   Unemployed [6]   Do housework [7]   Student [7]   Retired [8]
Artist [9]   Other [10]

14. *Only for women* → Are you currently pregnant? *For men* → Is your partner currently pregnant?
Yes [1]   No [2]   Don't know [3]   NA [92]

15. Do you want to have another child?
Yes [1]   No [2]   Don't know [3]   NA [92]

16. I am going to read you a statement. Please tell me to what extent you agree or disagree with each of the statements. (3 = Agree; 2 = Undecided; 1 = Disagree)

	AGREE	NEUTRAL	DISAGREE
a. People who use methods to avoid having children are in a better economic situation.	3	2	1
b. People who use methods to avoid having children can give their children a better education.	3	2	1
c. The use of contraceptive methods assures marital stability.	3	2	1
d. Family planning permits the mother to be more healthy.	3	2	1

	AGREEE	NEUTRAL	DISAGREE
e. Couples that practice family planning have time to give more care and love to their children.	3	2	1
f. Family planning allows you to take better care of your children.	3	2	1
g. Couples that plan their families have more time to participate in other activities.	3	2	1
h. When a woman gets pregnant without wanting to, she can have many problems.	3	2	1
i. I can become pregnant if I am not careful.	3	2	1
j. One partner should use a method so that the woman does not get pregnant.	3	2	1
k. Abortion is a form of family planning.	3	2	1

17. In a couple, is it the woman or the man that should talk about family planning methods?
Man [1]   Woman [2]   Either one [3]   [4] Neither [5] DK [91] NR [92]

18. *Only for women* → If your partner was opposed to your using a method, would you use it anyway, think about using it or not using it, or definitely not use it.
Would use it [1]   Would think about using it [2]   Would not use it [3]
DK [91]   DR [92] NA [99]

19. Are there different methods that a couple can use so that the woman doesn't become pregnant? Which of these methods have you heard of ? (*Allow the interviewee to respond spontaneously, note the responses in column 19, mark 1 if the respondent knows the method and 0 if the method is not known.*)

20. *For all the methods that the respondents cannot spontaneously recall, ask* → Have you heard of _____? *Next to the name and explanation of the method that appears in the first column, note the responses in column 20 , mark 1 if the respondent recognizes the method and 0 if the respondent doesn't recognize the method. If the method was recalled spontaneously, leave the column blank.*)

21. *For all the methods that were recalled, whether spontaneously or with assistance* → Have you used it before? (*Ask until you obtain responses for all of the methods known and note the response in column 21. Mark 1 if the method was ever used or 2 if it was never used; leave blank spaces next to methods that are not known.*)

22. *If the respondent has used a method before* → At what age did you use the method for the first time? *(Note responses in column 22.)*

23. *If the respondent has used a method before* → Are you currently using the method? *(Mark the results in column 23. If the respondent has used a method, place the age at first use and mark if the respondent is currently using that method.)*

METHOD	METHODS KNOWN						USED FOR FIRST TIME (COLUMN 22)	CURRENTLY USING? (COLUMN 23)	
	SPONTANEOUSLY (COLUMN 19)		WITH ASSISTANCE (COLUMN 20)		USED BEFORE (COLUMN 21)				
	YES	NO	YES	NO	YES	NO		YES	NO
a. Abstinence: Abstaining from sex to avoid pregnancy	1	0	1	0	1	0		1	0
b. Withdrawal: Ejaculate outside the vagina	1	0	1	0	1	0		1	0
c. Calendar/rhythm: Avoid sex on the "dangerous days"	1	0	1	0	1	0		1	0
d. Condom: rubber sheath used by the man during sex	1	0	1	0	1	0		1	0
e. Spermicide: foam or tablets placed into the vagina during sex	1	0	1	0	1	0		1	0
f. The Pill: pills that are taken each day	1	0	1	0	1	0		1	0
g. Injectibles, Depro-provera: Injection taken by the woman every 3 months	1	0	1	0	1	0		1	0
h. IUD: Device placed in the uterus by the doctor	1	0	1	0	1	0		1	0
i. Vasectomy: an operation on the man to prevent having any more children	1	0	1	0	1	0		1	0
j. Hysterectomy: an operation on the woman to prevent having any more children	1	0	1	0	1	0		1	0
h. Traditional methods: herbs, etc.	1	0	1	0	1	0		1	0

24. *For everyone except those who said they had a vasectomy or hysterectomy* → Do you plan to use or continue using a method in the future?
Definitely not [1]   Probably not [2]   Probably yes [3]   Definitely yes [4]
DK [91]   NR [92]   NA [99]

25. *For those who responded that they were currently using a method (question 23)* → How long have you been using he method? → *(If in question 23 the response was more than one method, ask the respondent which was used the most.)*
_____(months)   DK [91]   NR [92] NA [99]

26. *For those who responded that they were currently using a method* → Where did you get information about the method you are currently using? → *If in question 23 the response was more than one method, ask the respondent which was used the most.*

Pharmacy [1]   Clinic/hospital [2]   Doctor [3]   Another place [4]
Other people [5]   Other_____   DK [91]   NR [92]   NA [99]

27. *For those who responded that they were currently using a method (question 23)* → Before using this method, did you discuss with your partner the convenience of using or not using the method?

→ *If in question 23 the response was more than one method, ask the respondent which was used the most.*

Yes [1]   No [2]   DK [91]   NR [92]   NA [99]

28. *For those who responded that they had used a method before (question 21) and also said they were not currently using a method (question 23)* → Did you or your partner stop using contraceptive methods because there were problems with the method or because it was very expensive?

Had problems [1]   Expensive [2]   Other_____   DK [91]   NR [92]
NA [99]

29. *For all* → I am going to read you a phrase. Please tell me if the phrase is true or false:

	FALSE	TRUE	DON'T KNOW
a. Hysterectomy is a permanent method of family planning.	1	2	3
b. The IUD can perforate the uterus.	1	2	3
c. When the women uses injectibles to avoid pregnancy, she can never have more children.	1	2	3
d. Pregnancy can occur as soon as a woman starts taking the pill.	1	2	3
e. The condom can prevent venereal diseases.	1	2	3
f. After the birth of a child, it is necessary that the mother visits the health center to obtain care within 2 weeks.	1	2	3
g. If the woman forgets to take the pill for more than 2 days, she shouldn't use another contraceptive method until the next month.	1	2	3
h. The dangerous days for pregnancy are the first days after the period.	1	2	3
i. A woman should have a cervical exam each year.	1	2	3
j. After the doctor places an IUD inside the woman, it is not necessary that she visit again for follow-up care.	1	2	3

	FALSE	TRUE	DON'T KNOW
k. When a woman uses pills, they accumulate in her uterus.	1	2	3
l. The insertion of the IUD takes only a few minutes.	1	2	3
m. A person with a venereal disease can infect a health person if they have sex.	1	2	3
n. Foam and tablets are used after the sex act.	1	2	3

30. If a mother has several children, is in a difficult economic situation, and has recently become pregnant, would this justify an abortion or not?
Yes [1]   No [2]   DK [91]   NA [92]

31. Do you know what reproductive health is?
Limit the number of children [1]   Receive prenatal care [2]
Have the number of children you want to have [3]   Reproduce health [4]
Have healthy sex organs [5]   Live better [6]   Medical examination [7]
Breast-feeding [8]   Postnatal counseling [9]   Other [10]   DK [91]   NA [92]

Ask questions 32–37 as if you don't know what reproductive health is.
32. On a scale of 1 to 7, how important is reproductive health to you? 7 means very import and 1 means not important at all.
1   2   3   4   5   6   7   NA [92]

33. *For whatever the previous response was* → Why?
For the well-being of the family, couple, mother and child [1]   Other_____
                                                              DK [91]   NA [92]

34. Who do you talk to about reproductive health? *(Note who is talked to most)*
Husband/wife/partner [1]   Parents [2]   Children [3]   Other relatives [4]
Friends [5]   Doctor/health professional [6]   Other [7]
Don't talk to anyone [8]   NA [92]

35. Through what medium did you learn about reproductive health? *(Note the medium the was most seen, heard, etc.)*
TV [1]   Radio [2]   Newspaper [3]   Posters [4]   Friends [5]   Other [6]
Did not understand [90]   DK [91]   DR [92]

36. Have you heard any program on reproductive health on the micros (minibuses)?
Yes [1]   No [2]   NA [92]

37. Do you know where to find reproductive health services?
Health centers/clinics/hospital [1]   Pharmacy [2]   Doctor [3]   Other [4]
                                                              DK [91]   NR [92]

38. In the last 6 months have you visited any location to obtain information about family planning?
Yes [1]   No [2]   NR [92]

39. In the last 6 months have you visited any location to obtain information about reproductive health?
Yes [1]   No [2]   DR [92]

40. *If the response is yes* → Where or at what location did you get that information?
Health center/clinic/hospital [1]   Pharmacy [2]   Doctor [3]
Other_____   DK [91]   NR [92]

41. *If in the response was yes in question 39* → When you went to this location (clinic, hospital, etc.) what services did you receive?
Only information [1]   Family planning methods [2]   Prenatal care [3]
Postnatal care [4]   Other_____   DK [91]   NR [92]   NA [99]

42. *If in the response was yes in question 39* → What motivated you to go to this place?
Radio [1]   TV [2]   Friend/acquaintance [3]   Relative [4]
Him- or herself [5]   Doctor [6]   Other health professional [7]
Other_____   DK [91]   NR [92]   NA [99]

43. Have you or your partner ever gone to obtain prenatal care?
Yes [1]   No [2]   NR [92]

44. If you or your partner were pregnant would you go to get prenatal care?
Yes [1]   No [2]   NR [92]

45. Do you know the precautions a woman should take after she gives birth?
Go to the doctor [1]   Don't lift weights [2]   Eat well [3]   Rest [4]
Don't get wet [5]   Don't drink alcohol [6]   Other_____   None [90]
                                                                          DK [91]   NR [92]

46. *For those that have children* → Who attended to the birth of your child?
(Note the most important)
Doctor [1]   Nurse [2]   Midwife [3]   Friend [4]   Husband [5]
Mother-in-law [6]   Mother [7]   Other [8]   NR [92]   NA [99]

47. In order of importance could you tell me which people are most capable of assisting in a birth? *(Note 1 for the most important, etc. 3 maximum)*

	ORDER OF IMPORTANCE
Mother-in-law	
Midwife	
Doctor	
Nurse	
Mother	
Husband	
Friend	
Others (specify)	

48. In your opinion, should you breast-feed immediately after birth, or wait a few hours?

Immediately after birth [1]   After a few hours [2]   DK [91]   NR [92]

49. Until what age should you continue breast-feeding your baby?

Less than 6 months [1]   6 months [2]   6 months to 1 year [3]

1 to 2 years [4]   More than 2 years [5]   DK [91]   NR[92]

50. *If respondent has children* → Until what age did you breast-feed your last child?

Less than 6 months [1] 6 months [2]   6 months to 1 year [3]

1 to 2 years [4]   More than 2 years [5]   Still breast-feeding [90]

                                           DK [91]   DR [92]   NA [99]

51. During the first 6 months of life, do you think the child should be only breast-fed or should be given other liquids in addition to breast milk?

Breast-feed only [1]   Breastfeed + other liquids [2]   DK [91]   NR [92]

52. During the first 6 months of life, do you think the child should be only breast-fed or should be given foods in addition to breast milk?

Breast-feed only [1]   Breastfeed + other foods [2]   DK [91]   NR [92]

53. In the last 6 months have you talked with your partner about ways to prevent pregnancy?

Yes [1]   No [2]   NR [92]

54. In the last 6 months have you talked with your partner about the number of children you would like to have?

Yes [1]   No [2]   NR [92]

55. Does your partner want more chilren than you want, fewer children than you want, or the same number of children that you want?

More children [1]   Fewer children [2]   The same number of children [3]

                                           DK [91]   NR [92]

56. During which hours do you normally listen to the radio Monday–Friday? Saturday? and Sunday? *(Circle the hours during which respondent most often listens to the radio)*

DAYS	12 TO 5 AM	5 TO 7 AM	7 TO 9 AM	9 TO 12 AM	12 TO 2 PM	2 TO 6 PM	6 TO 9 HRS	AFTER 9 PM	DON'T LISTEN
Monday–Friday	1	2	3	4	5	6	7	8	25
Saturday	9	10	11	12	13	14	15	16	26
Sunday	17	18	19	20	21	22	23	24	27

Don't have a radio nor listen to radio [28]   DK [91]   DR[92]

59. *If respondent listens to the radio* → What radio station do you listen to most often? *(In addition to the name of the station, mark whether the station is AM or FM)*

_____AM [ ] FM [ ]   DK [91]   NR [92]   NA [99]

60. In the last 6 months, have you heard any commercials on reproductive health, family planning, or maternal health?
Yes [1]   No [2]

If the response is no, move to question 64 and mark NA in 61, 62, and 63.

61. *If the response was yes for question 60* → Could you please tell me what you heard on the radio in those commercials?
Commercial 1_____   DK [91]   NR [92]   NA [99]
Commercial 2_____
Commercial 3_____

62. *If the response was yes for question 60* → Thinking about the radio commercials you heard about reproductive health, can you tell me one of the messages in these commericals.

_____   DK [91]   NR [92]

NA [99]

63. *If the response was yes for question 60* → Did you like the reproductive health commercials a lot, a little, or not at all?
A lot [1]   A little [2]   Not at all [3]   NR [92]   NA [99]

64. During which hours do you normally watch TV from Monday to Friday? Saturday? and Sunday?

DAYS	BEFORE 7 AM	7 TO 9 AM	9 TO 12 AM	12 TO 2 PM	2 TO 6 PM	6 TO 8 PM	8 TO 0 PM	AFTER 10 PM	DON'T WATCH
Monday–Friday	1	2	3	4	5	6	7	8	25
Saturday	9	10	11	12	13	14	15	16	26
Sunday	18	19	20	21	22	23	24	27	

No time to watch television [28]   DK [91]   NR [92]

67. *If respondent watches TV* → Which channel to you watch most often?
2   4   5   6   7   8   9   10   11   13   Other [90]   DK [91] NR [92] NA [99]

68. In the last 6 months, have you seen any commercials on reproductive health, family planning, or maternal health?
Yes [1]   No [2]

69. *If the response was yes, go to question 68* → Please tell me what you saw on TV in those commercials.
Commercial 1_____   _____ .   DK [91] NR [92] NA [99]
Commercial 2_____
Commercial 3_____

70. *If the response was yes for question 68* → Thinking about the TV commercials you saw about reproductive health, can you tell me one of the messages in these commericals?

_____   DK [91] NR [92] NA [99]

71. *If the response was yes to question 68* → Did you like the commercials a lot, a little, or not at all?

A lot [1]   A little [2]   Not at all [3]   NR [92]   NA [99]

72. I am going to show you several images of commericals from TV. One by one, please tell me which you do and do not remember.

COMMERCIALS	RECALL	DO NOT RECALL
Spot A Secretary	1	0
Spot B Testimony	1	0
Spot C Prenatal care	1	0
Spot D Postnatal care	1	0
Spot E Ringer 1	1	0
Spot F Clinic 1	1	0
Spot G Breast-feeding	1	0
Spot H Family planning	1	0
Spot I Ringer 2	1	0
Spot J Abortion	1	0
Spot K Birth	1	0
Spot L Clinic 2	1	0

73. I will now read you several messages from radio and TV. One by one, please tell me if you remember them or not. If you do remember them I will also ask if you remember them from radio or TV. Finally, I will ask if you agree or disagree with each of the messages. *(If a respondent answers radio and TV, note that which is listened to or watched most.)*

MESSAGE	REMEMBER YES	REMEMBER NO	ON RADIO OR TV RADIO	ON RADIO OR TV TV	DON'T KNOW	AGREE YES	AGREE NO
a. The government is trying to reduce maternal mortality from childbirth and abortion.	1	0	1	2	91	1	0
b. Reproductive health means the well-being of the mother, the child, and the couple.	1	0	1	2	91	1	0
c. Information on reproductive health can be obtained at clinics and health centers.	1	0	1	2	91	1	0
d. In order to avoid problems during birth, it is important to obtain prenatal care.	1	0	1	2	91	1	0

| | REMEMBER | | ON RADIO OR TV | | | AGREE | |
MESSAGE	YES	NO	RADIO	TV	DON'T KNOW	YES	NO
e. Women should give birth only under the attention of a health professional.	1	0	1	2	91	1	0
f. It is important to breast-feed only until a child is 6 months old.	1	0	1	2	91	1	0
g. Couples should decide together which method of family planning they will use.	1	0	1	2	91	1	0
h. Family planning means having the number of children you want, when you want them.	1	0	1	2	91	1	0
i. There are various methods of family planning. Two of these are the rhythm (or calendar) method and the IUD.	1	0	1	2	91	1	0
j. Reproductive health has many benefits.	1	0	1	2	91	1	0
k. Family planning is a way to prevent abortion.	1	0	1	2	91	1	0
l. Reproductive health depends on the couple.	1	0	1	2	91	1	0

74. I am going to show you four logos. For each of them, please tell me whether or not you have seen the logo and where you saw the logo.

	LOGO 1	LOGO 2	LOGO 3	LOGO 4
Television				
Posters				
Magazines				
Newspapers				
Press releases				
Emblems				
Health centers				
Others (specify)				
Didn't see logo				

75. *For those who saw logo 3* → You told me you have seen logo 3; please tell me if you like the logo a lot, a little, or not at all.
A lot [1]   A little [2]   Not at all [3]   DK [91]   NR [92]   NA [99]

76. Please tell the the names of the people with whom you discuss personal issues. You may give me only the first name if you prefer.

You

1 2 3 4 5	Name 1: _____			
1 2 3 4 5	1 2 DK	Name 2: _____		
1 2 3 4 5	1 2 DK	1 2 DK	Name 3: _____	
1 2 3 4 5	1 2 DK	1 2 DK	1 2 DK	Name 4: _____
1 2 3 4 5	1 2 DK	1 2 DK	1 2 DK	1 2 DK	Name 5: _____

With no one[0]

If only one name was given, note it and move to question 79.

77. On a scale of 1 to 5, order the names of the persons according to your level of affinity or closeness with that person.
(with 1 the closest and 5 the least close).   NA [99]

78. Please tell me which of these people knows one another and which are total strangers.

NA [99]

79. Is [Name 1] a man or woman?

NA [99]

NAME 1		NAME 2		NAME 3		NAME 4		NAME 5	
MAN	WOMAN	MAN	WOMAN	MAN	WOMAN	MAN	WOMAN	MAN	WOMAN
1	2	1	2	1	2	1	2	1	2

80. What is the native language of [Name 1]? *(Repeat for each name.)* And your native language?

NA [99]

	NAME 1	NAME 2	NAME 3	NAME 4	NAME 5	YOU
Spanish	1	1	1	1	1	1
Aimara	2	2	2	2	2	2
Quichua	3	3	3	3	3	3
Other	4	4	4	4	4	4
Don't know	9	9	9	9	9	9

81. For each of the persons you have named, could you tell me their level of education?

	NAME 1	NAME 2	NAME 3	NAME 4	NAME 5
None	1	1	1	1	1
Basic	2	2	2	2	2
Intermediate	3	3	3	3	3
Middle	4	4	4	4	4
Technical	5	5	5	5	5
University	6	6	6	6	6
Don't know	9	9	9	9	9

82. How often do you talk to [Name 1]?

NA [99]

	NAME 1	NAME 2	NAME 3	NAME 4	NAME 5
Daily	4	4	4	4	4
Weekly	3	3	3	3	3
Monthly	2	2	2	2	2
Occasionally	1	1	1	1	1
Don't know	9	9	9	9	9

83. How long have you known [Name 1]? *(Repeat for all of the names.)*

NA [99]

	NAME 1	NAME 2	NAME 3	NAME 4	NAME 5
Years					
Don't know					

84. I am going to show you a list *(show Table 2)* of some possible relations that you can have with people. Most people have more than one relation with a person. Each time I give the name of one of the people you have named, please tell me the type of relation you have with this person. *(circle all the relationships named)*

NA [99]

	NAME 1	NAME 2	NAME 3	NAME 4	NAME 5
Spouse/partner	1	1	1	1	1
Parents	2	2	2	2	2
Siblings	3	3	3	3	3
Children	4	4	4	4	4
Other family	5	5	5	5	5
Co-worker	6	6	6	6	6
Neighbor	7	7	7	7	7
Friend	8	8	8	8	8
Advisor	9	9	9	9	9
Other	10	10	10	10	10

85. I am going to show you a list of several themes that people discuss *(show Table 3)*. Please tell me the three most important themes that you talk about with [Name 1].

NA [99]

	NAME 1	NAME 2	NAME 3	NAME 4	NAME 5
Work	1	1	1	1	1
Cost of living	2	2	2	2	2
Food	3	3	3	3	3
Parents or relatives	4	4	4	4	4
Children	5	5	5	5	5
Religion	6	6	6	6	6
Health	7	7	7	7	7
Sex	8	8	8	8	8
Books, art, or cultura	9	9	9	9	9
Television	10	10	10	10	10
Crime, violence	11	11	11	11	11
Politics	12	12	12	12	12
Economy	13	13	13	13	13
Socal aquaintances, friends	14	14	14	14	15

	NAME 1	NAME 2	NAME 3	NAME 4	NAME 5
Clothing, fashion	15	15	15	15	15
Climate	16	16	16	16	16
Others	90	90	90	90	90

86. Please tell me the age of [Name 1]? *(Repeat for each name.)*

NA [99]

	NAME 1	NAME 2	NAME 3	NAME 4	NAME 5
Age					
Don't know	91	91	91	91	91

87. What religion does [Name 1] practice? What religion do you practice?

	NAME 1	NAME 2	NAME 3	NAME 4	NAME 5	YOU
Catholic	1	1	1	1	1	1
Evangelist	2	2	2	2	2	2
Other	3	3	3	3	3	3
None	4	4	4	4	4	4
Don't know	91	91	91	91	91	91

88. The following table contains a list of the goods that people can possess. Which of these does [Name 1] have? *(Repeat for each name, continue until you get all the goods possesed by each person.)* And can you tell me which of these you have?

	NAME 1	NAME 2	NAME 3	NAME 4	NAME 5	YOU
TV	1	1	1	1	1	1
Radio	2	2	2	2	2	2
VCR	3	3	3	3	3	3
Refrigerator	4	4	4	4	4	4
Car	5	5	5	5	5	5
Telephone	6	6	6	6	6	6
Own house	7	7	7	7	7	7
Drinking water	8	8	8	8	8	8
Don't know	91	91	91	91	91	91

89. Do you know if [Name 1] approves (1) or disapproves (2) of family planning? *(Repeat for each name.)*

NA [99]

NAME 1			NAME 2			NAME 3			NAME 4			NAME 5		
YES	NO	DK	YES	NO	DK	YES	NO	DK	YES	NO	DK	YES	NO	DK
1	2	91	1	2	91	1	2	91	1	2	91	1	2	91

90. Do you know if [Name 1] uses or does not use any method of family planning? *(Repeat for each name.)*

NAME 1			NAME 2			NAME 3			NAME 4			NAME 5		
YES	NO	DK	YES	NO	DK	YES	NO	DK	YES	NO	DK	YES	NO	DK
1	2	91	1	2	91	1	2	91	1	2	91	1	2	91

91. Of the people you mentioned, which do you think are in favor of family planning?

1   2   3   4   5   DK [91]   NR [92]   NA [99]

92. Of the people you mentioned, who do you think practice family planning?

1   2   3   4   5   DK [91]   NR [92]   NA [99]

Appendix C

INFORMED CONSENT

Good morning/afternoon. My name is _____, and I am a researcher from _____. We are doing a survey in this area to learn about various health issues that may affect you and your family. We are also interested in programs you may have seen or heard on the mass media. All of your answers will be kept strictly confidential and only reported in aggregate form. Would you be willing to answer these questions, which will take approximately 20 minutes? [If the respondent says "no" then say, "thank you for your time," and end the interview.] [If the respondent says "yes," then say the following: "Thank you for agreeing to participate. If there are any questions you don't want to answer, please let me know and I will skip them. Again, thank you for agreeing to talk with me."]

Appendix D

SAMPLE BUDGET ITEMS FOR HEALTH
PROMOTION PROGRAM EVALUATION PROJECT

The budget assumes a 6-month $1,000,000 media campaign with pre- and post-cross-sectional surveys. The sample size is 800/wave, respondents are selected via random-digit dialing, assuming a 50% response rate, and interviews are conducted via telephone.

	RATE/DAY	NO. DAYS	COST ($U.S.)
Planning and design			
Principal investigator	$600	5	3000
Research assistant	$200	20	4000
Administrative assistant	$100	10	1000
Formative research (8 FGDs)			
Principal investigator	$600	6	3600
Research assistant	$200	40	8000
Administrative assistant	$100	20	2000
Facility rental, incentives, and refreshments			2000

	RATE/DAY	NO. DAYS	COST ($U.S.)
Instrument development and testing			
Principal investigator	$600	7	4200
Research assistant	$200	50	10,000
Administrative assistant	$100	10	1000

	RATE	NUMBER	COST
Survey administration costs			
Printing	$0.50	2000	1000
Phone numbers	$0.10	4000	400
Phone charges (completed, 20 minutes)	$0.07/minute	1600	2240
Phone charges (not completed, 4 minutes)	$0.07/minute	1600	448
Data entry	$10/question	1600	16,000
Data analysis and interpretation			
Principal investigator	$600	10	6000
Research assistants	$200	80	16,000
Administrative assistants	$100	5	500
Study coordination travel and meeting expenses			
Meetings with programmer	$250	6 meetings	1500
Conference presentation	$2000	3 people	6000
Dissemination			
Principal investigator	$600	5	3000
Research assistants	$200	30	6000
Administrative assistants	$100	10	1000
Printing of evaluation report	$5000		5000
Supplies			
Office supplies (paper, disks, etc.)			3500
Computer software licences			3000
Computer hardware upgrades			5000
Totals			
PI total no. days	33		
RA total no. days	220		
AA total no. days	55		
Subtotal			115,388
Indirect costs (overhead) @ 30%			34,616.40
Total			150,004.40

AA, administrative assistant; FGDs, focus discussion groups; PI, principal investigator; RA, research assistant.

Index

299

Lightning Source UK Ltd.
Milton Keynes UK
08 December 2010

164076UK00001B/6/P